LANGUAGE DELAYS AND DISORDERS

From Research to Practice

LANGUAGE DELAYS AND DISORDERS

From Research to Practice

LYDIA R. SMILEY, PH.D.

Florida Atlantic University
Boca Raton Campus
Boca Raton, Florida

PEGGY A. GOLDSTEIN, ED.D

Florida Atlantic University
Davie Campus
Davie, Florida

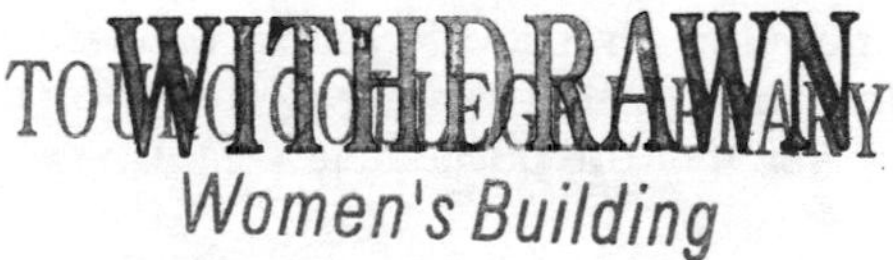

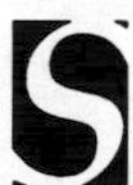

SINGULAR PUBLISHING GROUP, INC.
SAN DIEGO · LONDON

Singular Publishing Group, Inc.
401 West "A" Street, Suite 325
San Diego, California 92101-7904

Singular Publishing Group Ltd.
19 Compton Terrace
London, N1 2UN, UK

e-mail: singpub@mail.cerfnet.com
Website: http://www.singpub.com

Second Printing May 1998

Typeset in 11/14 Bookman by So Cal Graphics
Printed in the United States of America by Bang Printing

Library of Congress Cataloging-in-Publication Data

Smiley, Lydia Ruffner, 1946–
Language delays and disorders : from research to practice / Lydia R. Smiley, Peggy A. Goldstein
p. cm.
Includes bibliographical references and index.
ISBN 1-56593-694-9
1. Language disorders. I. Goldstein, Peggy, A. II. Title.
RC423.S56 1997
616.85'5—dc21

97-28437
CIP

CONTENTS

CONTRIBUTOR

DEENA LOUISE WENER, PH.D., CCC-SLP
Assistant Professor
Department of Health Sciences
Florida Atlantic University
Boca Campus
Boca Raton, Florida

PREFACE

Language issues can act like a spider web in the world of students with disabilities. Reaching into the crevices of every aspect of every interaction of every day, this labyrinth strengthens or weakens communication effectiveness in world knowledge, academic understanding, skills development, relationship building, and self-concept. Unfortunately, many professionals working with students who have disabilities feel uncomfortable about knowing what language is, how to recognize language difficulties, understanding their effects on other areas of learning, and most importantly knowing how to improve language skills in order to improve social and academic outcomes.

This text is designed to provide professionals with basic competencies in language development and disorders so that they can feel more confident dealing with language issues. Language and its various component areas (i.e., phonology, morphology, syntax, semantics, and pragmatics) are defined. The text is organized so that typical or normal development is presented first followed by problems related to each component area, including, when appropriate, their relationship to academic and social performance. Finally, some current best practices in intervention are presented.

This text was written for practicing and future professionals working with students with disabilities in an academic environment—primarily special education teachers, speech-language pathologists, and general education teachers. However, inclusion has generated a fresh batch of specialty practitioners who could also benefit from such a text, for example, behavior specialists, special education facilitators, transition specialists, and support specialists.

It is our contention that professionals who really *know* language and continuously evaluate students' language performance are the most likely to design programs that will produce positive outcomes. They will recognize the student's language abilities and their overlap with academics. They will anticipate problems and encourage programming that promotes language learning. For example, if 8-year-old Brandon consistently omits the past tense form of verbs, it may mean that he does not possess earlier grammatical forms in the developmental sequence or it may mean he doesn't understand the concept of time. And if he doesn't understand these aspects of time, it may be reflected in concepts such as "before," "after," "yesterday," which may be evidenced in math, history, and the organization of his life (e.g., "When will mom return from work?").

What is unique about this text is the bridge that we build between the research on typical and atypical language development and the research on language intervention. It is this bridge from research to practice that we hope will help build knowledgeable and effective professionals, who in turn will help build effective academic and social learners.

Several individuals deserve special thanks for their contributions to this book: Deena Wener for her contribution of Chapter 2, Ron Taylor (POP) for his insightful feedback, and David Lee, who probably provided us the freshest perspective and, therefore, the most useful suggestions. And finally, a special thanks goes to all our students, both graduate and undergraduate, who each year shared our excitement about language by providing a wealth of examples of language behavior and who consistently told us that we needed a better book. We hope we have provided an adequate response.

CHAPTER

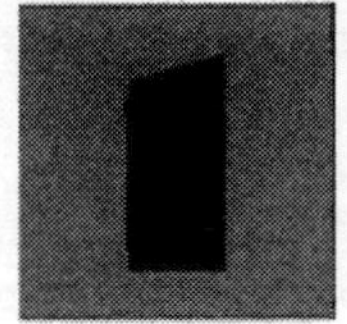

AN OVERVIEW OF LANGUAGE

Language is one of the most mysterious products of the human mind. It is a means of communication and socialization as well as a vehicle for thought. It is highly complex and is learned incredibly rapidly. Language development is intriguing in and of itself, but for professionals serving students with disabilities, an understanding of language development and intervention is paramount for three basic reasons: (a) language ability is related to academic success, (b) there is a strong relationship between students with disabilities and language deficiencies, and (c) language deficits may be the earliest indicator of other problems (Goldstein, 1994). In other words, early identification of language abilities may grant us the opportunity to provide early intervention and possibly alleviate or minimize later problems for the many children who will eventually have other classifications such as learning disabilities (Haring et al., 1992).

A majority of students with a variety of disabilities have language delays and disorders; therefore, as practitioners we must address those needs. The relationship between poor language skills and learning disabilities (Cantwell & Baker, 1987; Wallach & Butler, 1994; Wiig & Semel, 1984) or mental retardation (Schiefelbusch, 1993) has been well documented. More recently, the relationship between communication problems and behavior disorders (Prizant & Wetherby, 1990) or attention-deficit hyperactivity disorder (ADHD) (Westby & Cutler, 1994) has been recognized. Most important, because language problems are highly correlated with academic and social outcomes, language intervention for students with disabilities may not only improve language functioning but also enhance development in a host of related areas.

It is not surprising that children who have difficulty learning language will likely have difficulty with reading and language arts skills (Felton, 1992; Kamhi & Catts, 1989; Olswang & Bain, 1991). However, a language delay may also result in poor problem solving abilities (Haring et al., 1992) and poor information storage and retrieval (Nippold, 1992). In addition, a child's language abilities may affect social outcomes such as peer relations, family relations, and later employment (Bursuck, 1989; Gerber, 1991; Hummel & Prizant, 1993; Lapadat, 1991; Mellard & Hazel, 1992). It is our contention that, if teachers and clinicians know language and its manifestations in social and academic tasks, they will implement programs that integrate language and evaluate student performance on a continuous basis.

This chapter attempts to define language and all its intricate components. Based on this information, a definition of language disorders is discussed. The focus of the text is language; language and speech are not synonymous. As we shall see, *language* is a code in which symbols stand for meaning and the rules that govern that code; *speech* is the physical production of that code.

A DEFINITION OF LANGUAGE

There are many definitions of language in existence today just as there are many disciplines involved in language. Owens (1992) defined language as a socially shared code or conventional system for representing concepts through the use of arbitrary symbols and rule-governed combinations of these symbols. Reed (1994) simply stated that language is a code in which we make specific symbols stand for something else. Bloom (1988) defined language as a code by which ideas about the world are represented through a conventional system of arbitrary signals for communication. Wardhaugh (1977), a linguist, suggested that **language** is a system of arbitrary vocal symbols used for human communication.

To better understand the definition of language, and the concepts within it, major terms in these definitions will be discussed individually. To maximize this understanding, however, it is important to first examine the components of spoken language.

The Major Components of Language

Spoken languages are generally considered to be made up of five components. There are rules to be mastered in each component, and they are mastered simultaneously, not separately. The components of language overlap and in some cases the determination of the component is somewhat arbitrary. However, it is possible to have a language disorder in only one or two components of language and be quite competent in the others. For purposes of discussion, we will discuss each component separately while reminding the reader to keep in mind the overlapping and simultaneous development that exists. These components are phonology, morphology, syntax, semantics, and pragmatics; each component is briefly defined here and then discussed in depth later in the text.

Phonology

This component of language, **phonology**, deals with the system of speech sounds and the rules governing their use. These are the rules that indicate what sounds occur, what sound combinations are acceptable, and where those sounds and combinations of sounds may occur for a specific language. The unit of sound on which this text focuses is the **phoneme,** which is the minimally significant unit of sound. The phoneme is significant in that, if it were to be replaced with another phoneme, a meaning change would result. For example, the following words are the same except for the beginning phoneme in each: *bat, cat, hat, sat.* The following words vary only in the final phoneme: *bat, back, bad, bag*; and the following differ only in the medial position: *sit, sat, set, seat.* All of the previous words are made up of three phonemes; each set has only one differing phoneme; and yet each word in each set has a different meaning, thus the unit of sound that changed was significant.

Morphology

This component, **morphology**, involves the rules governing the use of the minimally significant unit of meaning, the **morpheme**. Morphemes may be free or bound. Free morphemes have meaning on their own and may not be broken into any smaller units and still maintain that meaning, for example, *happy*. A bound morpheme has meaning only when attached to another morpheme. For example, *un* alone has no meaning, but when attached to *happy*, as in *unhappy*, it acquires the meaning of *not*, that is, not happy. When attached to *tie*, *wrap*, or *lock*, as in *untie*, *unwrap*, or *unlock*, it means to reverse the action. Or consider *er*, which has a different meaning when attached to *teach* (*teacher*) than when attached to *big* (*bigger*). The meaning of a bound morpheme can only be determined when it is attached to another morpheme.

Syntax

Syntax refers to the rules of word function and word order; it encompasses the rules for forming phrases, clauses, and sentences. For example, it governs how we change the declarative, *You are going to the movies*, to the interrogative, *Are you going to the movies*? Syntax allows us to combine *The truck is red* and *The truck is mine* to create *The truck which is red is mine.*

Semantics

Semantics is a system of rules governing the meaning of words and word combinations. Included in this component would be multiple meanings of words such as *run* and the figurative meanings of words such as *blue*. Other figurative language usage, such as idioms (*kick the bucket*), metaphors (*the eye of a needle*), similes (*eats like a pig*), and proverbs (*don't put the cart before the horse*), would also be semantic aspects of language.

Pragmatics

Whereas phonology, morphology, syntax, and semantics generally relate to the structure of language, **pragmatics** is the use of language. The illocutionary forces of language, that is, our intents, are governed by rules of pragmatics. Socialization skills such as conversation are governed by rules of pragmatics as well. For example, the rules of conversation require that the speaker wait for his or her turn and then speak about something that is related to the previous speaker's comments.

Some nonlinguistic cues may also be included in our knowledge of the use of language. Requesting a favor has nonlinguistic (e.g., smiling nicely) as well as linguistic components. These components include both **kinesics** (e.g., gestures, body posture and movement, eye contact, and facial expressions) and **proxemics** (physical distance). These nonlinguistic components will be further discussed later in this chapter.

In order to function successfully in communication, the rules of all of these components must be mastered to some degree. There are, of course, age-appropriate aspects to this mastery, and there are cultural and subcultural differences in the rules. If a speaker has not mastered the rules, he or she may be experiencing a language delay or disorder and may need assistance in replacing some of his or her language behaviors with more age-appropriate usage. If a speaker has mastered a different set of rules, that is, the rules of another culture or subculture, he or she may need assistance in acquiring an additional set of rules to be used in appropriate contexts.

Human Communication

With knowledge of the five major components of language—phonology, morphology, syntax, semantics, and pragmatics—in mind, we may now return to the task of defining language by discussing the most common terms found in our definitions. As previously mentioned, Wardhaugh (1977) defined **language** as a system of arbitrary vocal symbols used for human communication. This definition contains most of the concepts of agreement among definitions of language. First and foremost, language is a **system**; if it were not systematic, language could not be used and understood consistently. It is both a system of sounds and a system of meaning. The rules of phonology within a specific language determine that only certain sounds and combinations of those sounds are acceptable. Within the English language, a proficient speaker will recognize that the word *lamb* is acceptable in *Mary had a little lamb*, but *Mary had a little bmal* is not acceptable nor is *Mary had a little lbam.* The proficient speaker of English has learned which combinations of sounds are acceptable and which are not. The American geneticist who creates a new animal would certainly not call it an *mbal*, for although that may be a very acceptable combination of sounds in other languages, it is not in English.

Just as a language is a system of sounds in which certain sounds and certain combinations of those sounds can be used over and over to form units of meaning, it is also a system of meaning in which those units can be used over and over in an infinite number of ways to express both simple and complicated ideas. Once again, however, the proficient speaker of a language will recognize that these units of meaning can be combined in an infinite number of ways, but with limits. *Mary had a little lamb* is certainly an acceptable combination of units of meaning, and *A little lamb had Mary* might also be acceptable in a different context; however, *Mary a little had lamb* or *A had little lamb Mary* would certainly result in some strange looks from proficient speakers of English. Although a language is a system that offers its speakers unlimited possibilities of expression, it is also a system of rules to which a speaker must adhere if he or she hopes to be understood.

Although a language is necessarily systematic, it is also **arbitrary** in many aspects. Once a particular language is mastered, its systematic rules allow some predictability, but there is no way of knowing in advance what a particular word means from hearing it or what morphemes will be used to mark regular plural nouns. The fact that a *table* is called a *table* in English has nothing to do with how it looks or feels. Tables certainly exist in other languages, but they are not usually called *tables*. What these particular pieces of furniture are called in one language versus another is arbitrary.

Standard American English has specific rules for what morpheme to use to indicate the plural of a word; these rules are based on the ending sounds of a noun. Knowing that those morphemes include the three regular plural markers, as found in *dogs*, *cats*, and *horses*, allows us to predict the plurals of other nouns or even of such nonsense words as those used by Berko Gleason (1958, 1971) in her Experimental Test of Morphology: *wug*, *bik*, and *gutch*. However, is there any predictable or logical reason for the selection of these three particular sounds, or phonemes, as indicators of plural? No. Do other languages also use these same sounds to indicate plurals or do they use another indicator or set of indicators for plural markers? Although the plural concept exists in all languages, how each language marks it is arbitrary.

Let's observe an even more complicated, but still systematic, syntactic rule in English, that of the optional deletion process. For the statement *Mary could have gone, and the lamb could have gone, too,* the speaker could choose to say *Mary could have gone and the lamb could have, too,* or *Mary could have gone and the lamb, too,* but what about *Mary could have gone and the lamb have, too?* There are options in the deletion rule of syntax, but they obviously are limited. Once learned, the options can be predicted, but the particular options are arbitrary.

The specifics of a language are arbitrary. The determination of what objects are called in Spanish, how plurals are formed in French, what word order is acceptable in Russian, how the possessive is marked in German, and what sound combinations are allowed in Swahili are all arbitrary.

Symbol in the definitions of language refers to the fact that there is no connection, or minimal connection, between the sounds speakers use and the objects, actions, or ideas to which they refer. In only a few cases might there be a direct representational connection. Most obvious would be onomatopoeic words such as *buzz, hiss, bang, crash,* and *roar*, although even these words would not be obvious to speakers of Chinese or Greek. Actually, little evidence exists to refute the claim that languages are systems of arbitrary symbols (Wardhaugh, 1977). Vocabulary must be learned almost word-by-word.

A term in many definitions is **communication**, which is the major goal of language. The need for communication is strong and language allows speakers to talk about anything within the realm of their knowledge—and many things outside that realm of knowledge, too (Wardhaugh, 1977). Actually, there are two major purposes of communication: intraindividual and the more obvious interindividual communication. **Intraindividual communication**, that is, communication with oneself, includes one's inner thoughts, ideas, feelings, attitudes, and other cognitive activities. Research on verbal mediation, rehearsal, self-instruction, and other cognitive and metacognitive activities increasingly supports the importance of language in all aspects of learning.

Interindividual communication takes at least two participants and in order to be successful requires not only a well-produced speech or **locutionary act**, but also the appropriate **illocutionary force** to express one's intention and a **perlocutionary force** to ensure that the listener's interpretation is correct (Austin, 1962). Some predictable clues exist in language and mastery of these clues is a part of successful communication. Learning to use and interpret correctly the simple sentence *He will be here* as opposed to a complementary clause such as *He said that he will be here* will allow for better communication. The first sentence leaves little doubt, whereas the second statement may be doubted. A true mastery of all aspects of interindividual communication allows a Perry Mason or Ben Matlock to skillfully extract confessions from witnesses on the stand (What if I were to tell you that we found a contact lens beside the pool . . . ?).

The term **vocal** in Wardhaugh's definition may seem to be controversial, but it is in no way meant to suggest that language exists only in a vocal form, nor that there are not components of spoken language that are not vocal. In fact, Owens (1992) reported it has been estimated that up to 60% of the information in face-to-face conversation may be transmitted through nonvocal means. Knapp (1972) suggested that less than 35% of social meaning is actually transmitted by words, whereas 65% of social meaning is conveyed through nonverbal communication. As pointed out in other sections of this chapter, these components enhance the meaning of the vocal message. Wardhaugh's use of the term vocal in his definition refers to the fact that the primary medium of language is sound. Writing exists as a secondary medium and is based on spoken language; its major purpose is to lend some permanence to spoken language. And sign languages that are separate but equal systems and not based on spoken language are typically used as alternatives to spoken language. Indeed, if we removed the term **vocal** from this definition of language, it would include sign languages as well. A language such as American Sign Language (ASL) is a system of arbitrary symbols used for human communication. It has its own systematic rules for movement and meaning which are predictable and often complex, but arbitrary. Although hearing individuals who attempt to learn ASL tend to associate its manual symbols with a visual or verbal icon (e.g., the bill of a cap as the symbol for boy or the string of a bonnet as the symbol for girl), the native ASL speaker learns these as symbols that are just as arbitrary as the spoken symbols of boy and girl are for the hearing child learning spoken English. However, because the purpose of this text is to mainly examine delays and disorders in spoken language, the term vocal will be assumed, unless otherwise indicated.

The term **human** in Wardhaugh's definition refers to the fact that the kind of system we are interested in is possessed only by humans and is very different from other systems. No system of animal communication makes use of a dual system of sound and meaning. It has been asserted that no other system allows its users to do all that human language allows. The criteria for making human language unique often include (a) reminiscing over the past, (b) speculating about the future, (c) telling lies at will, and (d) devising theories (Wardhaugh, 1977). Although this remains to be the case with most other species' communication systems, even the very sophisticated system of bees and dolphins, for example, the first three criteria may not be as unique as once thought. Primate language studies increasingly show that gorillas do reminisce about the past, as in the famous sign language user Koko's mourning over her lost cat (Patterson, 1978), and do tell lies, as in Koko's apparently blaming her actions on a research assistant (Linden, 1993). And the abstract-symbol user pygmy chimpanzee, Kanzi, certainly was speculating about the future when she devised a tool to retrieve a favorite treat from a locked box (Linden, 1993). Even in the wild, chimps plan future courses of action, manufacture and use tools, hold grudges, nurse resentments, experience prolonged grief at the loss of a loved one, form friendships, keep secrets, and lie (e.g., Sagan & Druyan, 1992). As yet, humans alone are known to theorize and even talk about talking, so with that in mind we will move on in our metalanguage discussion.

Language is a system of arbitrary vocal symbols used for human communication. As already observed, language is exceedingly complex, and yet it is learned incredibly rapidly by the normally developing child at a very young age. To further complicate the task of learning language, there are additional nonlinguistic aspects of communication to be mastered as well. An overview of some of these additional aspects follows.

FoxTrot
by Bill Amend
IT'S UNBELIEVABLE HOW MUCH HOMEWORK I HAVE TO DO TONIGHT!
I CAN'T REMEMBER THE LAST TIME I HAD THIS MANY THINGS DUE!
I DON'T KNOW WHAT ALL MY TEACHERS WERE THINKING!
IN THAT CASE, SWEETIE, WHY DON'T I DO THE DISHES?
© 1995 Bill Amend/Dist. by Universal Press Syndicate
I THOUGHT YOU HAD NO HOMEWORK...
IT'S ALL IN HOW YOU SAY IT.
AMEND

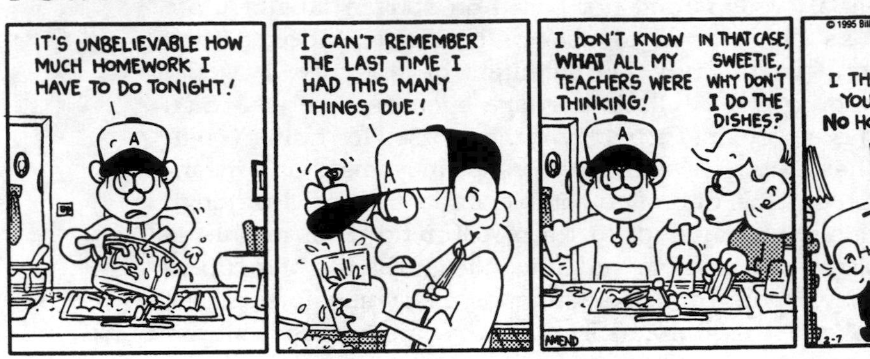

NONLINGUISTIC HUMAN COMMUNICATION

Language appears to be used most effectively when words, gestures, and behavior support one another and are appropriate for the speaker and listener and to the content and context of the message (Wardhaugh, 1977). "It wasn't what he said, it was how he said it." Tone and gestures can actually contradict what is said. Impressions may be formed based on how someone speaks, and in the case of different cultures and subcultures, misinterpretations may easily occur as signs are misread, not read at all, or given a significance they do not have. Certain behaviors may be judged as effeminate in a male, lethargic in a young person ("She acts just like a little old lady"), or arrogant in a speaker ("Did you hear the way he gave that report? He is so arrogant!"). A young woman who was putting herself through school by working in a bar recently reported an incredible scenario relating to judgments based on nonlinguistic systems of communication. This incident occurred at the bar during Monday night football. Monday after Monday, groups of men gathered in front of TV sets expressing their joys and frustrations through belly laughs, cheers, jumps, arm-waving, and jeers; no words required; all behavior understood and accepted. These men were having a good time. One Monday night, a group of women gathered in front of one set to watch football and began to exhibit exactly the same behavior at approximately the same noise level. By the end of the first quarter, this particular group of sports spectators had been asked twice to quiet down, and by halftime, they had been asked to leave the bar for being disruptive. It appears that judgments of acceptable behavior differed on the basis of group membership. The signs were misread or given an interpretation that did not exist. The manager and some of the customers were apparently applying a 1950's rule of acceptability to 1990's behavior. Both linguistic and nonlinguistic rules change with time as well as place.

In communication, it is important to avoid misjudgments and misinterpretations; therefore, it is necessary to be aware not only of the systems that exist in one's own language and culture, but also of the fact that there are differences in nonlinguistic signs, just as there are differences in linguistic symbols, in other languages and cultures, and within cultures. Wardhaugh (1977) delineated three systems that are superimposed on the already defined linguistic system to add extra dimensions of meaning. These three superimposed systems are referred to as paralanguage, kinesics, and proxemics.

Paralanguage

The paralinguistic system relates to modulation and is superimposed on the linguistic system to indicate attitude, emotion, or some other meaning. Paralanguage may be viewed as being composed of various scales; in normal communication, utterances typically fall in the center of the scale (Wardhaugh, 1977). For special circumstances, speakers move up or down a particular scale or scales. It is also possible to use these scales inappropriately, if the paralinguistic rules have not been mastered along with the linguistic rules of the language. The scales presented here are specific to American English. Appropriateness may vary among cultures and even within subcultures.

Loudness-to-Softness

The first scale is a scale of loudness-to-softness. In specific circumstances, there may be a call for overloudness or oversoftness. Certainly the street vendor trying to sell his or her wares will use a very loud voice to attract customers, and someone must be reinforcing the local commercial-makers for their very noisy productions for selling used cars or car insurance; this level of volume would never be used to advertise intimate moments together at an exquisite restaurant or to sell a seductive cologne or aftershave. These commercials would more likely be presented in a very soft volume. Another use for the soft end of the scale would be to invoke the feeling of suspense in storytelling, as in, *and then the wolf licked his lips and started quietly moving toward the little girl*, but what about, *It's a bird, it's a plane, it's Superman!?* And as Wardhaugh pointed out, lovers do not generally yell at each other while sitting and holding hands.

Pitch

A second scale is a pitch scale, that is, how high or how low the voice is pitched in speaking. This, too, varies with the situation and is another set of rules to learn. An extra high pitch may be used to indicate excitement or pleasure (*I'm so excited!*), whereas a low pitch is used to indicate displeasure, fatigue, or disappointment (*I'm so tired of telling you over and over again*). Or listen to the dog owner's *Good girl!* versus *Bad girl.* Some dogs might be quite confused if the wrong pitch were superimposed on these linguistic messages, as might some humans as well.

Rasping-to-Openness

A third scale is that of rasping-to-openness. The rasping end of the scale contains a great deal of friction as in *Ugh! More work!*—another notation of displeasure. At the other end of the scale is a very open resounding characteristic often used by religious or political orators, as in the now famous *I have a dream* speech by Martin Luther King, Jr.

Drawling-to-Clipping

A fourth scale is that of drawling-to-clipping. Drawling can indicate insolence or reservation, and clipping may be taken as sharpness or irritation. Which teacher do you think will be asked again, "May I skip this page and go out with the other kids?" Will it be the teacher who clips, *No!* or the one who drawls, *Noooo.* Children who are learning language in normal stages learn early who meant no and who might reconsider. They have learned to interpret the meanings attached to the drawling-to-clipping scale. For the student who has not learned the difference, the cost may be high.

Tempo

And finally, the tempo of an utterance can be varied, too. In general a well-rehearsed story will be told much faster than one being composed on the spot.

If a speaker is to be understood correctly and to correctly understand what is being said, all of these paralinguistic aspects of language must be mastered. If a speaker is often inappropriately loud or usually speaks too fast, this interferes with communication and may lead to isolation. Illocutionary and perlocutionary acts are much affected by the paralinguistic system. The same word or words may take on very different meanings depending on the use of this system.

Kinesics

Along with the paralinguistic system exists a system of gestures called kinesics. Kinesics includes signals such as eyebrow movements, facial twitches, changes in positioning of feet, use of hands, and shoulder shrugs. The appropriate use of gestures must be learned and there are variations among and within cultures. Americans move their heads up and down to agree and sideways to disagree; other cultures reverse the process or use different devices altogether (Wardhaugh, 1977). The Semang people from the Malay peninsula thrust the head forward to express agreement; the Ovimbundu people from Angola shake a hand in front of the face with the forefinger extended to express negation. There are differences in greetings among cultures, from nodding and hand-shaking to embracing and back-rubbing. Each of these routines is arbitrary, but perfectly natural for the group. Some uses may be gender-, age-, or situation-specific. Different parts of the body are used

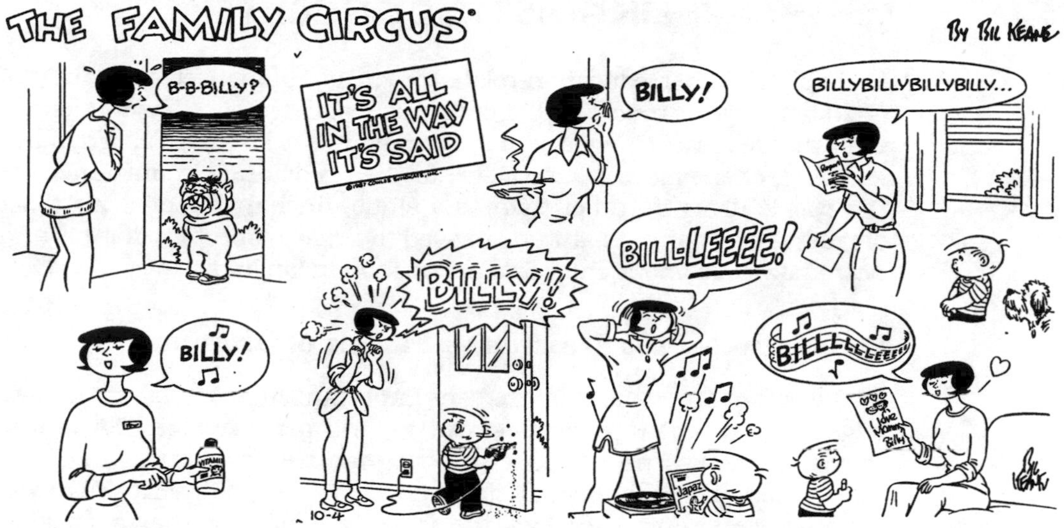

© Bil Keane. Reprinted with special permission of King Features Syndicate.

differently to communicate particular meanings with or without words. Use and interpretation of this system must be learned for efficient and successful communication.

Proxemics

Still another system of nonlinguistic communication is the system of proxemics, or how people use space between listeners and speakers. Appropriate distances depend on whether the speaker is speaking to an intimate friend, an acquaintance, or a superior, and what is acceptable and appropriate varies among and within cultures. North Americans typically require much more space to feel comfortable than do, for example, Hispanic populations. Invasion of this "comfortable zone" can result in many negative reactions and may lead to rejection and avoidance of the speaker. The listener is often so distracted by the discomfort that he or she feels that the message of the speaker is totally lost. Misinterpretation of social cues indicated by the stance of a group may lead to social problems for individuals who go barreling into an obviously closed and serious group to share a joke. This is one more system of rules that must be mastered if communication is to be successful.

Nonlinguistic systems may not be as complicated as the linguistic system, but they must be acquired. And even further, the two systems must be appropriately matched.

LINGUISTIC CONCEPTS

Probably no other education-related area has influenced the study of child language as much as that of linguistics. Linguistics has influenced our attitude toward language in the acceptance of language as a dynamic, living, changing tool, responsive to the needs and circumstances of the people using it, rather than as a static, unchanging prescribed set of rules. This change in attitude has led to a new respect for dialects and new knowledge about children's acquisition of language.

Descriptive Versus Prescriptive Models of Grammar

Two views of language that are very important in terms of our knowledge of child language are **descriptive** and **prescriptive grammars**. In the linguistic sense of the term **grammar**, we are referring to all the rules of language that one must learn to master it. A descriptive model of language simply describes the rules of language that a speaker uses; a prescriptive model of language prescribes which rules are correct and should be learned. The prescriptive model of language is the one most of us experienced in school when we were taught traditional "grammar." Specific rules were presented as the correct (or *proper*) way to speak.

Applying these models to studying child grammar, or language development, will illustrate the importance of thinking descriptively. In establishing norms for a child's development of the present progressive tense, for example, the use of a prescriptive model would require that we note when the correct (i.e., adult) form appears. Using a descriptive model would require that we note all formations of children's present progressive, and when they occur. By describing these formations, it has been found that children progress through stages as they master rules such as present progressive (i.e., the syntactic rule requiring the addition of an auxiliary verb and the grammatical morpheme *-ing*). Before the adult form of *Daddy is going* occurs, it is noted that a child expresses this structure first with no markers at all, as in *Daddy go*. The next occurrence of this structure includes the *-ing* marker for present progressive, thus, *Daddy going*. Next, the inclusion of the auxiliary verb *to be* occurs, *Daddy is going*. By describing what children actually say, rather than just noting whether or not the adult form occurs at specific ages, it has been determined that children learn the adult form of this structure in predictable sequential stages. At a particular stage of development, it is normal child grammar to say *Daddy going*. This is very important information in establishing stages of normal development, and thus in determining if there is a problem in language acquisition. In other words, using a descriptive model, we find that *Daddy going* may be correct, even though it is not the prescribed adult form.

The application of a descriptive model has also led to new respect for nonstandard dialects as different, rule-governed systems, as opposed to deficient productions of standard dialects. The rules of Standard American English have for a long time been considered by prescriptive grammarians as the correct and only acceptable way of speaking. For example, the prescriptive rule for forming the possessive in Standard English is to (a) place the object after the possessor and (b) add a marker to the possessor to indicate possession as in, *Give me John's hat.* A prescriptive model would require the investigator to simply note whether or not a speaker uses this formation as prescribed. The descriptive model would note how a speaker actually forms the possessive. By applying this model to a nonstandard dialect, Black English, it has been found that the rules differ depending on the context. In Black English, placing the object after the possessor is enough to indicate the possessive, as in *Give me John hat.* Possession is indicated by word order. The descriptive grammarian, in noting how the speaker of Black English forms the possessive, hears this same speaker, in response to "Whose hat do you want?" reply *I want John's!* The same possessive marker occurs in Black English as in Standard English, but the rules governing its use are different. In Black English, the possession is marked by word order, but when word order is not present, the extra possessive marker becomes necessary. The rule for marking possession is simply different. By using a descriptive model, it can now be determined which set of rules, if any, a speaker has mastered.

Linguistic Performance Versus Linguistic Competence

To fully understand language development and language disorders, the distinction between **linguistic performance** and **competence** must be considered. Linguistic performance refers to the expressive and receptive use of language and can be directly observed. Competence refers to a speaker's total knowledge of language which allows him or her to perform. This total knowledge of language includes the rules of language that are predictable and that allow us to judge the acceptability of different structures of a language.

Lindfors (1987, p. 25) provided the following examples to illustrate that competence. Place a check beside the sentences that you judge to be unacceptable. Given that you are a competent speaker of English, your checks should match those of other speakers who are competent in English. You may not be able to verbalize what made some of these acceptable and others not; it is a part of your total knowledge of language.

1. Mary married a drunken sailor.
2. It was a drunken sailor that Mary married.
3. It was Mary that married a drunken sailor.
4. That was it Mary married a drunken sailor.
5. It was drunken that Mary married a sailor.
6. It was nice that Mary married a sailor.
7. It was sailor that Mary married a drunk.
8. It was strange that Mary married a drunk.
9. It was a drunk that Mary married strange.
10. It was drunk that strange Mary married.
11. It was a drunk that strange Mary married.
12. That Mary married a drunken sailor was strange.
13. That Mary married a strange sailor was drunk.

14. That Mary married a drunk was sailor.
15. That Mary married a drunk was inevitable.
16. Mary's marrying a drunken sailor came as a surprise to us.
17. Mary's drunken sailor came to surprise us.
18. Sailor Mary's drunken to surprise us came.
19. What shall Mary do with a drunken sailor?
20. What with a drunken sailor Mary shall do?
21. Shall Mary do drunk with what a sailor?
22. Shall Mary have fun with such a sailor?
23. With what a sailor shall Mary do drunk?

Lindfors checked 4, 5, 7, 9, 10, 13, 14, 18, 20, 21, and 23. More than likely, your judgments are the same or similar, even though the sentences may be novel, that is, never heard before. This judgment may be made by a person who is competent in English even though he or she may not be able to verbalize the reasons for these choices. This intuitive knowledge is an indication of competence in English.

Unlike performance, competence is not affected by factors such as fatigue and anxiety; however, competence must be inferred from observation of performance. As a language disorder is present when there is a problem with competence, it becomes clear that a thorough analysis of linguistic performance must occur. Almost everyone has experienced difficulty in performance at some time. When you practiced your presentation last night in front of the mirror, it was perfect, but now that all those faces are staring at you, you have forgotten simple words, just can't pull them, and you seem to be speaking in simple sentences only. Or perhaps you just stayed up too late preparing at the last minute and now you're so tired that you can't seem to find the words you worked so hard on. You are having difficulty with your linguistic performance in this situation at this time, but don't worry, it's not a suddenly developed language disorder. Your linguistic competence is still there; however, if we were to evaluate your language only in this situation, a disorder might be suspected. A true evaluation of language must include more than one setting and must thoroughly describe language so that competence can be inferred. This description should include all the components of language that were defined earlier in the chapter.

DEFINITION OF A LANGUAGE DISORDER

The American Speech-Language-Hearing Association (1982) defined a language disorder in the following way: A **language disorder** is the impairment or deviant development of comprehension and/or use of a spoken, written, and/or other symbol system. The disorder may involve (1) the **form** of language (phonologic, morphologic, and syntactic systems), (2) the **content** of language (semantic system), and/or (3) the **function** of language in communication (pragmatic system) in any combination (p. 949). ASHA (1982) further differentiates a disorder from a **Communicative Variation:**

> Communicative difference/dialect is a variation of a symbol system used by a group of individuals which reflects and is determined by shared regional, social, or cultural/ethnic factors. Variations or alterations in the use of a symbol system may be indicative of primary language interferences. A regional, social, or cultural/ethnic variation of a symbol system should not be considered a disorder of speech or language. (p. 950)

Examples of language disorders in each of the areas of form, content, and function are illustrated in Table 1–1. The importance of analyzing the language of children and adolescents in order to prevent or minimize other problems has been well established. The need to integrate this knowledge into classroom intervention and evaluation has also been well established.

Language Analysis

It has become more and more apparent that without naturalistic context and spontaneity, a true sample of a student's language cannot be obtained. Most formal language tests are devoid of naturalistic context and often rely on elicited imitation of a model (Lund & Duchan, 1993). Children may fail to imitate, without context, that which they may produce spontaneously. In fact, Bloom and Lahey (1978) found that Peter, identified as an imitator in natural speech, could not fully imitate his own spontaneously produced sentences when presented to him the next day. For example, on Day 1, Peter, trying to get a colt's feet to fit into a barrel said, *I'm trying to get this cow in here.* When asked to imitate this same sentence the next day in a game of "Simple Simon says," Peter repeated, *Cow in here.* Missing from this situation were both contextual support and intention to speak. On the other hand, short sentences may be imitated correctly by a child who has no understanding or ability to produce them in spontaneous language. Some time ago, Fraser, Bellugi, and Brown (1963, 1970) found elicited imitation to be superior to spontaneous production and concluded that the equivalence of production and elicited information is not a totally sound assumption. Slobin and Welsh (1973) found similar results, but also demonstrated how imitation of long sentences may provide useful information. For example when asked to repeat *The pussy eats bread, and the pussy runs fast,* Echo responded with *Pussy eat bread, and he run fast.* There is evidence of the use of pronouns in Echo's response. However, the previous example of Peter indicates that caution should be used with further interpretation of the response.

Limitations of standardized assessment procedures are significant (Bain, Olswang, & Johnson, 1992). A valid assessment of language is needed for determining intervention programming goals and for obtaining frequent, repeated measurements regarding the effects of intervention. This needs to be an assessment of language in a naturalistic context and must involve the assessment of all components of language. Appendix A discusses how to obtain a representative sample of language and prepare it for analysis.

TABLE 1–1. Examples of language disorders.

PHONOLOGY
Nicholas is a 6½ -year-old who exhibits a phonological disorder characterized by many processes of phonology that occur earlier in normal development. In this example, Nicholas is manifesting final consonant deletion in his speech as he describes a picture.
Nicholas: da ca caw da mou (The cat caught the mouse).
MORPHOLOGY
Mikey is a 7-year-old student with learning disabilities. He exhibits many problems in the areas of both morphology and syntax. In this example, Mikey demonstrates a problem with overgeneralizing the rule for forming the regular third person singular present tense of an irregular verb.
Mikey: He dos (do + s) it all the time like that!
SYNTAX
In this example, Mikey illustrates a problem with a rule of syntax which requires that a verb particle (e.g., the *up* in *pick up*) be moved when used with a pronoun.
Mikey: My mom is picking up me today.
SEMANTICS
Melissa, a 10-year-old student receiving services for both learning disabilities and language disorders, exhibits problems in many of the components of language. The following example is taken from a discussion with her teacher about an upcoming trip to Indoor Sports with her mom. This excerpt illustrates her problems with word retrieval.
Teacher: What kinds of things do they have there?
Melissa: They have, let's see, they have a game like it's a big table and air blows up and you have like a little circle thing and you can move it across. (Melissa shows the shape of a circle with her hands.)
Teacher: Oh, OK. And can you tell me the name of the game?
Melissa: And if they get it across the other person wins.
Teacher: Do you know what the name for that game is?
Melissa: Uh, uh . . . I think it's called . . . Ping Pong!
PRAGMATICS
Leo, a 7-year-old, is in an ESOL program for speakers of English as a second language and a speech and language program and also is receiving medication for hyperactivity. This excerpt from a discussion with his teacher takes place while Leo is medicated. Leo exhibits problems with syntax, semantics, and pragmatics. This example illustrates Leo's difficulty with maintaining a topic in conversation.
Teacher: I want you to tell me all about your little brother.
Leo: He's really good, but um he's 5 months. And I got this new jacket from Brazil from my Dad.
Teacher: Did you get it for Christmas?
Leo: No, it's not from Christmas. It's because um I think it was because my birthday, because he's he's going to Brazil. He's already in Brazil with his father and his um brother. And . . . you saw my Dad once didn't you?

The following chapters will aid the reader in determining the existence of a language disorder in any of the previously delineated areas in order to design and implement plans for students who may have language disorders.

✓ SUMMARY CHECKLIST

☐ **Definition**
Language is a system of arbitrary vocal symbols used for human communication.

☐ **Major Components of Language**
Phonology
Morphology
Syntax
Semantics
Pragmatics

☐ **Human Communication**
Systematic
Arbitrary
Symbolic
Vocal
Intraindividual
Interindividual
Locutionary Act
Illocutionary Force
Perlocutionary Force

☐ **Nonlinguistic Human Communication**
Paralanguage
Kinesics
Proxemics

☐ **Important Linguistic Concepts**
Descriptive Model of Grammar
Prescriptive Model of Grammar
Linguistic Performance
Linguistic Competence

☐ **Definition of Language Disorder**
A language disorder is the impairment or deviant development of comprehension and/or use of a spoken, written, and/or other symbol system. The disorder may involve (1) the **form** of language (phonologic, morpholog-

ic, and syntactic systems), (2) the **content** of language (semantic system), and/or (3) the **function** of language in communication (pragmatic system) in any combination.

Communicative Variation

Language Analysis

Appendix A

CHAPTER

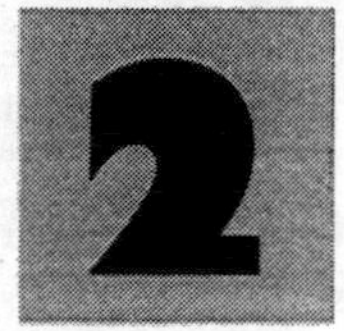

THEORIES OF LANGUAGE DEVELOPMENT

Contributed by Deena Louise Wener, Ph.D., CCC-SLP

An understanding of normal language development is critical to the understanding of language deficits, delays, and differences. Normal language development is frequently used as a guideline or referent by which language delays and disorders are assessed. In fact, a knowledge of normal language development is essential, not only in the evaluative process, but in the intervention process as well. Comparisons to normal development allow the teacher or therapist to establish current levels of function and starting points for intervention. Further, one's beliefs about how language is learned will shape how he or she works with children needing language intervention.

Children acquire language over a relatively brief span of time. It is, in fact, quite remarkable that children do develop language given that no real direct instruction in that language occurs. How and why they develop this skill is debated widely. Some theorists argue that our ability to learn language is innate or biologically predetermined, some that it is learned, and others that it is dependent on our social interactions and need to communicate. Regardless of the approach to which one ultimately subscribes, it cannot be argued that it would be impossible to identify deficits or disorders without an understanding of what "typical" language development is. Information on the developmental sequence that language follows allows the teacher or therapist to predict the language behaviors expected based on the age and cognitive development of the child.

Knowing how children acquire language may help educators to provide an environment that promotes and enhances language development. Establishing classroom environments that encourage the acquisition of language in natural settings is essential in assisting children with language delays or disorders. If language learning could occur in the classroom akin to how it is learned in the home prior to school, the child with a language delay or disorder might have increased opportunities for success. This would involve the teaching of language in context. For instance, items referred to would be present, situations and contexts for the introduction of vocabulary would be functional, and vocabulary selected would allow for the natural redundancy that occurs in the caregiver-child interaction. Further, it is important to remember that language learners progress from the concrete to the abstract. All too often, classroom environments for children with limited language abilities rely on pictorial or print examples, rather than initial presentation of the actual item or illustration of the action.

Five broad theoretical positions on how language develops are presented. These include (a) **Biological Maturation/Nativist**, (b) **Behavioral**, (c) **Psycholinguistic**, (d) **Semantic/Cognitive**, and (e) **Sociolinguistic/Social Interactionism**.

THEORIES OF LANGUAGE LEARNING

Through the study of typical language development, hypotheses have been developed as to how children acquire their language. One important universal is that all children, regardless of the language being learned, acquire that language in essentially the same developmental sequence. Theorists attempted to organize the information they observed and recorded it in reasonable outlines that explained language acquisition. There are differing theories on language development, just as there are differing theories on how children develop and learn in other areas. Most certainly, the best theory of how language develops is one that incorporates elements of all of the theories to be discussed. Although each theory has individual merit, each also has failings or elements that do not adequately explain all the behaviors one sees in the child developing language. Perhaps no single theory is capable of explaining all of the elements of language development. For this reason, there is no comprehensive, single theory or model for how language is acquired. It should also be noted that language development cannot be isolated completely from the acquisition of other behaviors and skills such as cognitive, physical, and social and emotional development.

It is important to point out the possibility that individual children will learn language differently. Language learning is affected, most likely, by variables such as learning styles, cultural/ethnic backgrounds, parenting styles, and home environments. Language learning may also be constrained by sensory, intellectual, or physical impairment. Human beings are not homogenous. The fact that individual experience plays such a large role in what we are exposed to and subsequently learn cannot be discounted. All of these factors, as well as developmental variability, make it extremely difficult to formulate a comprehensive all-encompassing theory as to how language develops.

The five theoretical areas discussed in this chapter encompass the main theories of language development. The final section takes a look at some of the directions in which language development theory may be heading. An overview of each theory and its strengths and weaknesses is presented.

Biological Maturation/Nativist

This theory of language development links the acquisition of language to **biological maturation**. Proponents of biological maturation theory see biological development as the only reasonable explanation for how language develops. They argue that this is the only explanation that makes sense given the universality of language. Children from all cultural and ethnic groups and from all socioeconomic levels develop language. What else, given this variability, might explain this development?

Nativist theory subscribes to the belief that the human brain is designed to learn language and that there are innate mechanisms that make language possible. In fact, language is considered to be a part of our genetic make-up as human beings. There are, however, some structures of the brain that have been identified as more critical to language learning and production. The left hemisphere of the brain, which is larger than the right hemisphere, appears to be more specialized for the processing and production of language. Although primarily focused on these biological factors, nativists do acknowledge that both genetics and the environment have some influence on the developing brain.

Factors such as cerebral asymmetry, brain weight and growth, and neuronal growth patterns all support the idea that language development may be a function of biological maturation. Left-right hemisphere asymmetries are present at birth and are known to be necessary for normal language functioning. Additionally, the degree of asymmetry appears to increase as we grow and develop. N.W. Nelson (1993) suggested that cerebral dominance is innate and not developed. Infants as young as 3 months of age exhibit the ability to discriminate speech. In the majority of cases, the processing of that speech is lateralized to the left hemisphere. The brain increases in size and weight most dramatically during the first 2 years of life by more than tripling its weight during that time. By 5 years of age, when children have clearly developed most of the rules and conventions of their language, the brain is 90% of its adult weight.

Strengths

The strength of this approach lies in its identification of cerebral structures associated with the production of speech and language. Cerebral asymmetries and areas in the brain associated with language processing and production have been identified clearly. There are recognizable and universal similarities that have been identified in the general development and configuration of the brain. Because most human beings will develop and use some form of language, the argument that there are innate mechanisms that facilitate this development appears to be a strong one.

Weaknesses

This theory does not recognize the contributions of cognition or social environment to language development. Nor does it adequately explain the generative nature of language, the fact that children produce novel sentences that they have never heard before and use linguistic structures that they have not been taught. Further, although it acknowledges the influence of environment on cerebral growth, this theory does not adequately address the phonetic, semantic, syntactic, morphemic, or pragmatic aspects of language. In essence, viewing language as innate leaves too many areas either ignored or not fully explained. How do we learn to use language in context? What active role does the child take as a language learner? How does the child's exposure to language affect his or her ability to learn language? These are just a few of the questions that biological maturation theory fails to address.

Behavioral

The behavioral theory of language development focuses on the processes of acquisition and not on the linguistic or biological system. The two areas of thought that have contributed most significantly to this theory are **information theory** and **learning theory**. Information theory suggests that the linguistic and nonlinguistic aspects of the speech situation determine the probability that a particular response will be produced. The occurrence of a particular word is thereby determined by the word or phrase preceding it. What jumps out immediately as a flaw in this thinking is that, in fact, there is no strict intrinsic model for the ordering of words. A word can be followed by numerous words or phrases. Word order is most likely determined by the message that the speaker wishes to convey and by the linguistic conventions of the speaker's language.

Learning theory, on the other hand, views language as a subset of other learned behaviors. Language, then, is a learned or conditioned response to stimuli. The primary proponent of learning theory was B.F. Skinner. Skinner (1957) explained that the processes of conditioning accounted for the establishment of the associations between arbitrary verbal stimuli and their internal representation. Skinner viewed language as a verbal behavior and, as a behavior, subject to all the rules of operant conditioning (stimulus-response-reinforcement). Skinner used the processes of operant conditioning to explain how selective reinforcement shaped verbal behavior by reinforcing a series of successive approximations. Imitation played a key role in language learning. Children imitated the language they heard and were reinforced for using that language. Language, then, was no different from any other human behavior. It was a behavior performed in response to specific stimuli that required specific responses. Consequently, it was believed that children were born with a general learning potential as part of their genetic make-up. Learning occurred through the shaping of responses and the environments in which these responses occurred. Language was shaped by the reinforcement of responses to specific stimuli (Lindfors, 1987). Lindfors further explained that "in the shaping of a very complex behavior such as language, there is a progressive selection or narrowing of responses which are positively reinforced" (1987, p. 97). Behavior was learned through modification and all behavior was operant (learned), according to Skinner. A stimulus would engender a response which was either reinforced, increasing the probability that it would occur again, or punished, decreasing the probability of its reoccurrence. The resulting change in behavior was *learning*. More complex behaviors were learned through chaining or shaping. **Chaining** is a process by which each step or stage serves as a stimulus for the next step or stage. **Shaping** occurs when a behavior is modified by the reinforcement of successive approximations of the target or intended response. In other words, parents or caregivers were the providers of the modeling and reinforcement necessary for the development of language. This reinforcement was provided following an infant's random vocalization. If that random vocalization approximated an actual word form, for example, *ma-ma* or *da-da*, the child received reinforcement from the caregiver, thereby increasing the likelihood of that vocalization being produced again.

The acquisition of phonology was explained by the processes of modeling and imitation. Skinner maintained that caregivers provided important models for the acquisition of the phonological aspects of language by reinforcing those sounds that come closest to those occurring in the language and ignoring sounds that did not occur in the language. Ignoring sounds that did not naturally occur in the language decreased the probability of their reoccurring or extinguished them completely. Infants produced many sounds that did not occur in their languages and through operant conditioning these sounds decreased in frequency of occurrence. The acquisition of words, as mentioned previously, occurred when a vocalization approximating an actual word was reinforced. Subsequent productions were modified through modeling and shaping and reinforced when the production approximated, more closely, the actual word. Words then became associated with the entities they represented. It was this process of conditioning that established the link between the word and its referent. Hence, the parent eventually became the stimulus for the production of the utterance *ma-ma* or *da-da*.

Sentences were acquired through the process of successive associative learning. Applying the principles of learning theory, children learned to associate one word with another in a left-to-right order. Children learned larger and larger functional units and how to combine them. Adult speakers continued to model and reinforce standard language productions. As the child became more adept at producing language, closer approximations were demanded by the caregiver and reinforcement was withheld until an acceptable utterance was produced.

Strengths

The strengths of this theory lie more in its application to remediation than in its explanation of language learning. Behavioral theory forms the foundation for a large portion of sociolinguistic theory. It places a heavy emphasis on the environment and input from the environment and the critical role they play in the development of language. Principles of operant and classical conditioning are readily apparent in many language remediation programs.

Weaknesses

There are, however, several important limitations to this explanation of language development. In reality, parents or caregivers reinforce a relatively small percentage of a child's total utterances. Additionally, early on, parents have a tendency to ignore grammatical errors and reinforce for content or speaking truth value. In other words, the parent reinforces or responds to the child based on the content of the child's utterance not the structure of it. Therefore, imitation alone may not be an adequate explanation for language development. Imitation does not account for common early language constructions such as *wented* or *camed*. Further, adult speech is fraught with idiomatic usage and loose grammatical construction and is a rather poor model. If a child truly learned language through imitation, then the logical extension would be that a child would have to hear every future sentence uttered. This is not only absurd, it is impossible. Behavioral theory ignores the generative nature of language and the fact that children and adults produce utterances that they have never heard or uttered previously. Behavioral theory also minimizes the contributions of comprehension and cognition to the acquisition of language. If we were to adhere to a strict behavioral interpretation of how language is acquired, then we would be suggesting that language is far more constrained and limited than it is in reality.

Lindfors (1987) pointed out other inadequacies in behavioral theory. She referred to the uniformity with which children acquired language as being *species uniform*. She further stated, "There is the other side of this *species uniform* coin, the *species specific* argument. The behaviorist position would predict that intelligent beings other than humans could acquire language too" (1987, p. 98). Although numerous studies have been conducted with primates learning sign language, no irrefutable evidence exists that primates learn and use language as humans do.

Psycholinguistic

Psycholinguistic theory, also referred to as linguistic rule induction (LRI) theory, came into prominence in the late 1950s and early 1960s. This theory of language development stressed language form and the foundation of mental processes on which those forms were built. The leading researcher in psycholinguistic theory was Noam Chomsky.

Chomsky (1965) attempted to describe not just the form of language, but the way in which we created that language and made judgments about it. Owens (1992, p. 35) observed that Chomsky concentrated "on the linguistic process *NOT* grammatical products." He adopted a scientific perspective on language.

Chomsky believed that all languages contained commonalities or *universal rules*. He reasoned that this had to be the case because some form of language is common to all people. Chomsky stated that all human beings acquired some form of language, even at the most basic levels, and that the difference that did occur in acquisition occurred in the degrees of acquisition. Complex language use and conversation were limited to humans. Like the nativist theorists, the proponents of psycholinguistic theory believed that language was biologically based and that as humans we had an innate capacity for language. This, however, was where the similarity ended. Biological maturation theory did not focus any attention on the structure of language.

Chomsky explained that linguistic processing took place at two levels: **phrase structure rules**, which were universal and common to all languages, and **transformational rules**, which were not universal and were related to the specific language. Phrase structure rules described the basic relationships that were the foundation for the organization of sentences independent of the language being described. Transformational rules defined how phrase structure components were rearranged and organized based on the specific language being used.

Each sentence uttered contained elements or individual units referred to as *constituents*. These constituents served specific functions within a sentence and were arranged hierarchically. Constituents in a sentence might be words or phrases acting as nouns, verbs, adverbs, or adjectives. Further, one word might serve several different functions.

Phrase structure rules began with the sentence as the basic unit.

$$S = NP + VP$$

The preceding formula states that a sentence may be written as a noun phrase (NP) plus a verb phrase (VP). In essence then, a sentence is composed of both a noun phrase and a verb phrase.

Chomsky's goal was to develop and present a finite set of rules governing sentence construction from which an infinite number of sentences might be generated. The only constraint on the variety of sentences that might be generated would be the limits of the speaker's vocabulary or words available for use as constituents in a sentence.

Transformational rules were sentence construction rules that were language specific and delineated how the constituents in the basic phrase structure sentence were rearranged. By allowing for the rearrangement, deletion, and addition of sentence elements, numerous sentence types could be created. Transformational rules explained how questions, negatives, passives, imperatives, and complex sentences with embedded subordinate clauses may be produced from basic phrase structure rules. Chomsky (1965) suggested that there was a two-tier mental model for the acquisition of linguistic rules: **deep structure,** which was the underlying meaning, and **surface structure,** which was the sentence actually produced. Transformational rules spelled out the relationship between the deep structure and the surface structure that was produced. A complete grammar, Chomsky explained, had three components: syntax, phonology, and semantics. Syntax was viewed as the most important part of grammar, the part that allowed the speaker to generate sentences. Phonology and semantics were ancillary and for interpretive purposes only.

Chomsky viewed the child as a sort of *mini-recorder*. In order to acquire language, the child had to make assumptions about the rule systems underlying language and then test those assumptions in actual use. All children progressed from single-word to multiword utterances and eventually to sentences. Chomsky further noted that developmental milestones were similar across children and occurred independently of cognition. Because Chomsky believed that there (a) was a biological basis for language, (b) were universal rules that governed all languages, and (c) were similarities in language development across children, he postulated that there was an inborn mechanism in humans for the acquisition of language. He named this mechanism the LAD, or **language acquisition device**. Universal phrase structure rules were contained within the LAD. So, in essence, the newborn is preprogrammed or *prewired* for language. However, the LAD, although innate, requires linguistic input to be activated. The child hears language, analyzes it, and then deduces the rules underlying that language. The LAD requires a jump-start, if you will, from the environment in order for language to develop. Because most language learning occurred prior to a child's becoming competent at using inductive reasoning, some aspects of grammar had to be preprogrammed, Chomsky argued. The child learning language has an innate system of "constraints and biases that lead a child to treat linguistic evidence in specific ways" (N.W. Nelson, 1993, p. 61). Lindfors (1987) referred to the child as *a little linguist*, a metaphor that she felt was useful because it identified the child as an active participant in the language learning process. The end product is an internalized system of finite rules that allow the generation of an infinite number of sentences. Unlike the behaviorists who promoted the idea that language was *taught*, Chomsky observed that very little, if any, direct teaching actually takes place during the language development process. In fact, there is very little relationship between the language produced initially by the child (single-word and two-word utterances) and the language the child hears from the adults in the environment. It is then the environmental activation of the LAD that allows children to develop and use the rules underlying language.

Strengths

Psycholinguistic theory does a good job of describing and explaining linguistic processing. The primary emphasis is on **linguistic competence** (what one knows about language) and not **linguistic perfor-**

mance (what one says). Language is not externally imposed, as suggested in behaviorist theories, but develops as a result of internal processing. Psycholinguistic theory provides us with a logical and well-defined rule system governing how words are combined into various sentence types.

Weaknesses

There are some rather important flaws in Chomsky's linguistic processing theory. It virtually ignores the phonetic, semantic, and pragmatic aspects of language. If language form is not linked to semantic content, there is no way to explain the recognition of syntactically correct sentences that do not make sense. As mentioned before, psycholinguistic theory does not explain the single- and two-word utterances that children produce while acquiring language. Following with this line of thinking, it is important to recognize that Chomsky's grammar was based on adult grammar and not on the early grammar produced by children. Psycholinguistic theory places little emphasis on the environment and social and cognitive growth. Consequently, it does not explain why children use language to describe and accompany their experiences. Finally, Chomsky's contention that children who fail to develop language normally have defective LADs seems far too easy an explanation with little substance to support it. It is important to note, however, that Chomsky did not intend to describe the processes involved in language acquisition. Chomsky's goal was to describe and explain linguistic processing (Owens, 1992). In this regard, Chomsky's theory is a strong one.

Semantic/Cognitive

The only challenge, in the early 1960s, to syntactic theory were the **semantic** and **cognitive theories** of language acquisition. Semantic theorists contended that a full description of language required the inclusion of semantics. It is semantics that allows us to distinguish between utterances that make sense and those that do not.

C. Fillmore (1968) proposed **case grammar**, a generative system that sought to explain the influence of semantics on syntax. Case grammar was not innate. It involved a set of universal concepts that specified the relationships that existed between nouns and verbs. A case was the semantic role or function of a specific noun phrase. Thus, sentence structure was dependent on the "semantic function of nouns in relation to verbs" (Owens, 1992, p. 48). Fillmore identified seven universal cases for nouns: agentive, dative, experiencer, factitive, instrumental, locative, and objective. Nouns could serve many functions. They could serve as the initiator of an action or *agentive* (The *boy* cooked his dinner), as a person affected by the action of the verb or *dative* (The ball hit the *girl*), or as the person who is experiencing something or *experiencer* (The *man* was feeling sad).

Additionally, nouns might represent the person or object resulting from the action of the verb or *factitive* (John baked a *cake*), or an inanimate object or force that causes an action but is not the initiator of that action or *instrumental* (The *key* opened the door). *Locative* cases describe the location or spatial orientation of the acrion. *Objective* cases are "the most neutral" (Owens, 1992, p. 49) and describe nouns whose feelings or actions are dependent on the meaning of the verb. A noun may be used in all cases for which it meets the criteria. "Much like Chomsky's transformational grammar, case grammar is an attempt to describe a generative system based on usage rules. These universal semantic cases form a structure that underlies and provides a basis for syntax" (Owens, 1992, p. 50).

The most notable proponents of semantic theory in the 1970s were Bloom and Lahey (1978). They described language as a code produced through the interactions of form (phonology, morphology, syntax), content (semantics), and use (pragmatics). Nicolosi, Harryman, and Kreschek (1996) defined phonology as the study of the sound system of a language including pauses and stress (p. 212); morphology as the study of how morphemes are put together to form words (p. 173); syntax as the rules that dictate the acceptable sequence, combination, and function of words in a sentence (p. 269); semantics as the study of the meaning of language including the relationship between language, thought, and behavior (p. 243); and pragmatics as the set of rules governing the use of language in context (p. 216).

Language form encompasses the area of phonology which includes both segmental (phonemes, syllables) and suprasegmental (intonation, pauses, stress) features. It also includes morphology, which encompasses substantive words which are content words such as verbs, nouns, adjectives, and adverbs, and relational words which may be content words or function words such as prepositions, conjunctions, articles, and auxiliary verbs. Morphology further includes the *inflections* added to words. Inflections are noun, verb, and adjective suffixes that alter words to express grammatical meanings. Examples of inflections are the plural *–s* added to nouns and the present progressive *–ing* added to verbs. The last component of spoken form is syntax, which describes word order, which is both linear and hierarchical.

Language content or semantics involves object knowledge, object relations, and event relations. Object knowledge refers to particular objects and to classes of objects. Object relations involve the reflexive relations of existence and disappearance, the intraclass relations of attribution and quantity, and the interclass relations of action, state, and possession. The last component of content is event relations, which deal with the temporal, causal, and epistemic (the act or ways of knowing) relations.

Language use or pragmatics encompasses the functions of language, personal (intrapersonal or intraindividual), and social (interpersonal or interindividual), as well as the linguistic and nonlinguistic contexts in which language is used. It is this element of language that governs how we initiate language, the type of language we use, and the conventions we use with various conversational partners. It is the integration of form, content, and use that leads to the knowledge of development of language. Figure 2–1 illustrates the interactions of form, content, and use according to Bloom & Lahey's theory (1978).

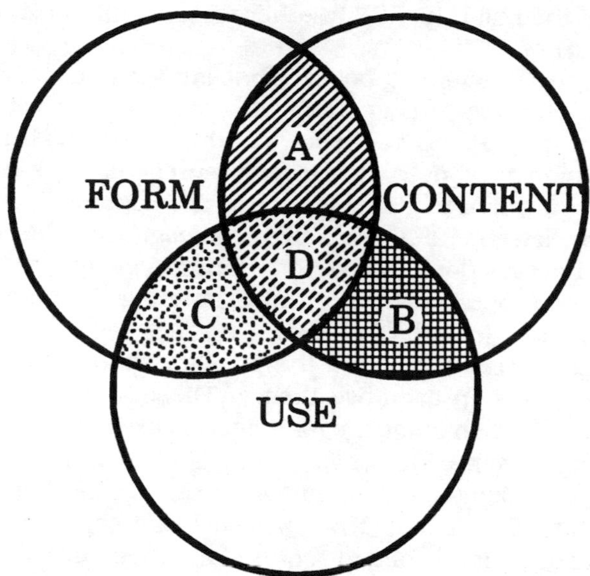

Figure 2–1. The interaction of content/form/use in language. (From *Language Development and Language Disorders* (p. 291), by L. Bloom and M. Lahey, 1978. New York: John Wiley. Copyright 1978 by John Wiley & Sons. Reprinted by permission of Allyn & Bacon.)

The intersection or overlap of these three areas (shaded area in Figure 2–1) represents our knowledge of language (Lahey, 1988). Bloom and Lahey described eight phases of language development. The boundaries of the first five phases were determined by the mean length of the child's utterance. The **mean length of utterance (MLU)** is the "average length of oral expressions as measured by a representative sampling of oral language; usually obtained by counting the number of morphemes per utterance and dividing by the number of utterances" (Nicolosi et al., 1996, p. 168). Each of Bloom and Lahey's phases represents the appearance of new language skills across a series of content categories which might express, for example, existence, nonexistence, recurrence, rejection, denial, attribution, possession, action, or time concepts. According to Bloom and Lahey, children's single-word, two-word, multiword utterances, and eventually sentences are produced to express content or meaning. Form and use are determined by the meaning the child wishes to convey. Bloom (1970) found syntactic rules inadequate for describing the different meanings that could be expressed by the same surface structure. Structure was directly related to the intended meaning and not to syntax, as postulated by Chomsky. Bloom (1970), Chafe (1970), Lakoff (1971), and Leech (1970) all believed that the underlying semantic bases of language developed prior to the development of syntax. According to Owens (1992), "Children learn basic relationships between entities within the environment, and these relationships are reflected in the semantic structures produced by the child" (p. 52). In other words, children talk about the things they know.

Cognitive theorists also believe that language develops based on experiences. Jean Piaget is credited with the classic work on cognitive theory. According to Piaget's theory, children progress through stages that allow them to construct internal representations of the world. "There is no Piagetian model of language development" (Owens, 1988, p. 135). N.W. Nelson (1993) explained that cognitive "development can be explained across domains by postulating a general set of cognitive structures and processes, among which language holds no particularly special position" (p. 67).

N.W. Nelson (1993) outlined the primary assumptions about language development in cognitive theory. These assumptions included the fact that, although language may not be viewed as innate, the nonlinguistic, cognitive precursors for language are. Language is only one of several symbolizing abilities that occur during the process of cognitive maturation. Bowerman (1974) believed that cognitive factors must be present in order for a child to acquire language. Among these factors were the ability to represent objects and events not perceptually present (object permanence) and the development of cognitive abilities related to the concepts of space and time. Additionally, the child must be able to derive linguistic processing strategies from the general cognitive processes and to formulate strategies to serve as the structural components for linguistic rules.

Even though single-word utterances presumably are free of structure, they do demonstrate the existence of underlying cognitive processes. Early two-word utterances are far from random. Meaning is signaled by word order and specific words fulfill specific roles. Syntactic markers are mapped over basic word order rules to form sentences and deal with semantic functions that do not agree with the word-order rules. McLean and Snyder-McLean (1978) hypothesized that the perceptual relationships that children make and their subsequent understanding of their worlds are the by-products of the cognitive domain.

Strengths

Semantic/Cognitive theorists and their views on language acquisition appear to conform more closely to actual child utterances and how a child represents the world verbally. In fact, case grammar is readily adaptable to the simple structures found in a child's early multiword utterances. Further, these theorists present language acquisition against the general backdrop of child development. It seems only logical to link a child's development of language with development in other areas as well.

Weaknesses

Although cognitive development may be important to the development of language, cognition alone does not provide a satisfactory explanation for language acquisition. There are children who appear intact cognitively, but who do not develop language. The greatest gap is in the explanations of how cognitive abilities are actually linked to language acquisition. There is no description as to how cognitive concepts are coded linguistically. Last, the semantic relationships of Bloom and Lahey are still drawn from the adult perspective of how the child is representing reality.

Sociolinguistic/Social Interactionism

Theories of learning, syntax, and semantics really only focus on fragments of language. The **sociolinguistic** view of language centers on the communication *unit* used to impart information. In this theory, language is not removed from the communicative context. It is the context that is viewed as the primary determinant of how and what language will be used. Language is used for communication and does not occur in a vacuum. The underlying reason for the use of language is social and communicative. Social and communicative contexts are essential to the conveyance of meaning. **Social Interactionism** suggests that the primary motivation for language acquisition is the individual's desire to communicate. This desire and need to communicate dictate the form and content that will best express the speaker's intended meanings. Also influencing the form and content of an utterance are the speaker's assumptions about the listeners and their knowledge.

Bates and MacWhinney (1987) proposed an information processing model called the **Parallel Distributed Processing Model** (PDP). It was based on the computer model of **information processing**. Information processing focuses on how language is learned. It stresses that the communicative function is what creates the language structure. Bates and MacWhinney dubbed their PDP model the *competition model*. The PDP mechanism, they believed, was innate. Initially all phonetic patterns, words, and syntactic forms *compete* equally to represent meaning. With ongoing experience, certain activation patterns are strengthened and others are weakened. During the course of language development, patterns that match with accumulated evidence win the competition and are selected for use in communication. Development is gradual and occurs in stages. N.W. Nelson (1993) stated that "information processing views hold a functionalist focus in common with the social interaction views. They hold a generalist focus in common with cognitivist views" (p. 66). Bates and MacWhinney (1987) argued against a structure of language divided into linguistic categories (phonology, morphology, syntax, semantics, and pragmatics), feeling instead that children learning language divided it across traditional linguistic boundaries. Human beings are processors of information. That information is then used to build internal models of the external reality.

More traditional sociolinguistic theorists ground their observations in **speech act** theory. Speech act theory views language as having two broad pragmatic functions: intrapersonal or intraindividual, which is used for memory, problem solving, and concept development, and interpersonal or interindividual, which is used for communication. A speech act is "a unit of linguistic communication, which is expressed according to grammatical and pragmatic rules and which functions to convey a speaker's conceptual representations and intentions" (Dore, 1974, p. 344).

Speech acts have propositional force, which relates to the meaning of the utterance, and illocutionary force, which relates to the speaker's intention. In speech act theory, a single utterance with a fixed form and semantic context can fulfill several intentions. A single speech act can be altered by gestures, intonation, and facial expression. Conversely, several different forms can fulfill a single intention.

The concept of speech acts was first introduced by John Austin (1962), who analyzed speech acts in three parts: locutions (propositions), illocutions (intentions), and perlocutions (the listener's interpretations). Searle (1965) strengthened Austin's theory by proposing five speech act categories: representatives (an assertion conveying belief or disbelief), directives (demands or commands), commissives (vows or promises), expressives (expression of psychological state), and declaratives (statements of fact). Austin and Searle, however, were explaining adult speech and not the speech of a child.

Dore (1974) identified the *primitive speech act* (PSA). He defined a PSA as an "utterance, consisting formally of a single act or a single prosodic sound-intonation pattern which functions to convey the child's intention before he acquires sentences" (p. 345). PSAs are different from adult speech act forms. Dore identified nine categories of PSAs: labeling, repeating, answering, requesting action, requesting answer, calling, greeting, protesting, and practicing. Primitive speech acts eventually develop into adultlike speech acts.

In sociolinguistic theory, the primary communication context in the acquisition of language is the child-caregiver interaction. These are the interactions that set the stage for language learning. Research has shown that infants are able to discriminate phonemes, intonation patterns, voices, and speech from nonspeech within the first few months of life. Infants, in fact, show a distinct preference for the human face and speech. Parents or caregivers respond to specific infant behaviors as meaningful social communication. Early child-caregiver interactions are regulated by eye-gaze. It is the consistency of maternal or caregiver behaviors that enable the infant to predict and anticipate. There are two general sets of behaviors or routines that are common in the **caregiver-child interaction**. The first is **joint action** routines or dialogues such as *peek-a-boo, so big*, and *pat-a-cake*. The second is **joint reference**. Joint reference refers to the concentration or focusing of attention by both participants on a common object, person, or activity. The establishment of joint reference and the accompanying caregiver verbalizations are critical to the development of meaning.

It is well known that caregivers modify their speech, in most cases unconsciously, so that it will be comprehensible to the child. A prime example of this modification is a type of speech known as *motherese*. Reed (1994) explained that the term motherese was used because "most investigations of adults' language to children have focused on the mothers' speech rather than the fathers' speech" (p. 54). The role of motherese in language development may be referred to as the **motherese hypothesis** (Bernstein & Tiegerman, 1993). This refers to the way a mother or caregiver regulates her or his speech according to the infant's needs or level of language learning. It is, in essence, child-oriented language. Caregivers employ variations in articulation, pitch, and loudness to convey messages to the infant. The length and complexity of a caregiver's utterances will vary depending on the child's age and language ability. (Reed, 1994). Adults also modify the way they respond to a child's utterances, often using *expansions* and *recasts* (Reed, 1994) to elaborate on or clarify meaning.

The child is able to convey a range of intentions prior to ever uttering a first word. Gestures, vocalizations, and facial expressions are used to initiate joint action and joint reference. Earliest one-word utterances are generally names or words for familiar people, animals, or objects and are used to gain attention or request. Caregivers then expand the forms and meanings of early utterances by offering a reply, comment, modification, or model of an expanded production. Language acquisition is therefore entrenched in and dependent upon the social, communicative context.

N.W. Nelson (1993) drew the following assumptions about language acquisition from social interaction theory:

1. Language develops because humans are motivated to communicate socially;
2. Development is characterized by the production of intentional and symbolic speech acts;
3. Acquisition of language requires dynamic, dyadic interactions;
4. Parents and caregivers adjust their linguistic output to accommodate the child.

Strengths

The true strength of sociolinguistic theory is its emphasis on the function and use of language and the social aspects of language. The act of communication itself is the reinforcement for continued interaction. It stresses the roles of the caregiver in providing modeling and feedback to assist in the acquisition of language. It takes into account the very profound effect exerted by both the environment and the context in which the communication occurs.

Weaknesses

Sociolinguistic theory is the newest of the language acquisition theories and as yet has no uniform or agreed-on classification system. And, alone, the social interactionist view of language development does little to illuminate how a symbol is associated with a referent. Further, it offers no clear explanation for the acquisition of the structure of language.

CONCLUSION

This chapter has attempted to provide an overview of the main theories concerning the acquisition of language. Although each theory has strong points, no one theory is fully capable of explaining the phenomenon of language acquisition, and each has gaps and failings. However, each of these theoretical points of view has made an important contribution to our thinking about and understanding of language and how it is acquired. It continues to amaze students of language development that a child, by age 3, has learned most of the basic rules governing the use and production of language.

Investigators have begun looking at the possibility of a gene that may carry language ability. This innateness of language is unique to humans and investigators and theorists continue to search for a quantifiable or scientific explanation of this ability. Another promising area of investigation is the study of the disruption in language that occurs following a neurological lesion and how that might be used to explain what is *normal*. It is felt that studying how language breaks down will provide clues to how language is formed. The development of sophisticated radiological imaging techniques has also allowed theorists to study such components as blood flow and sites of neural excitation during the production of language and other language-based activities. Certainly there is much yet to be discovered about language and how it develops. As was mentioned at the start of this chapter, most likely the best explanation for how children acquire their language will be found by combining elements found in a number of the theoretical positions.

✓ SUMMARY CHECKLIST

☐ **Theories of Language Learning**

Biological Maturation/Nativist

Strengths

Weaknesses

Behavioral

Information Theory

Learning Theory

Strengths

Weaknesses

Psycholinguistic

Phrase Structure Rules

Transformational Rules

Deep Structure

Surface Structure

Language Acquisiton Device (LAD)

Strengths

Weaknesses

Semantic/Cognitive

Case Grammar

Language Form

Language Content

Language Use

Strengths

Weaknesses

Sociolinguistic/Social Interactionism

Parallel Distributed Processing Model (PDP)

Information Processing

Speech Act

Joint Action

Joint Reference

Motherese Hypothesis

Strengths

Weaknesses

CHAPTER

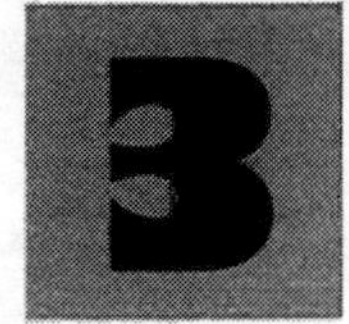

THE DEVELOPMENT OF PHONOLOGY

DEFINING PHONOLOGY

Phonology is the study of the sound system of a language, including what those sounds are and the system of rules underlying the pronunciations of words, that is, the rules of combining and sequencing these sounds. The smallest significant unit of sound is the **phoneme**; it is significant in that it signals a change in meaning, as in the words *cat* and *mat*, in which the first speech sound, or phoneme, has changed. There are between 40 and 46 phonemes in American English, depending on one's dialect. Phonemes are actually made up of a group of **phones** (allophones) which are not significant to the perception of speech. For example, the beginning sound in *top* in slightly different from the second sound in *stop*. If the reader of this text places a hand in front of his/or her mouth while speaking these two words, it should be noticed that a puff of air (aspiration) occurs in the beginning sound of *top*, but not in the second sound of *stop*. This difference, however, does not indicate a separate speech sound and would not signal a change in meaning if the two phones were interchanged.

Phones are variants of sounds that speakers and listeners of a language tend to ignore. The level of representation with which this text will be concerned is the level of the phoneme, the significant unit of sound. The phoneme is the segment that speakers have learned from listening to speech in infancy to discern as being significant to meaning. This occurs even though speakers are not speaking in discrete segments, but rather in continuous waves of sound, as can be seen in the spectrogram of *The springtime is warm and clear* shown in Figure 3–1. It is from this stream of sound that an infant must distinguish the significant segments of sound in the language he or she is learning. Adults rather easily distinguish these segments in a language they have mas-

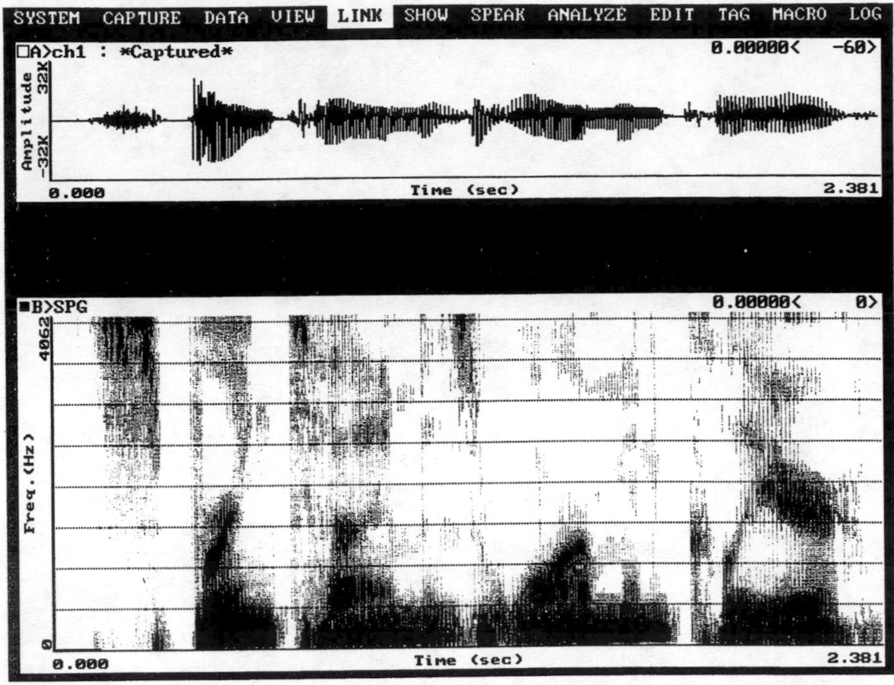

Figure 3–1. Sound spectrogram of adult speech: The springtime is warm and clear.

tered, but even an adult would find it a difficult, if not impossible, task to segment the sounds in an unknown language just from listening to a speaker of that language.

PHONEMIC NOTATION

Traditional letters of the alphabet may have more than one pronunciation (e.g., the *c* in *city* and *cut*), and the same pronunciation may have more than one orthographic representation, or spelling (e.g., the vowel sound in *bait*, *bale*, *beige*, and *bay*). Furthermore, these pronunciations and spellings may be different in other languages with the same alphabet (e.g., French and Spanish). For these reasons and others, linguists have developed a phonemic alphabet in which one symbol corresponds to one sound. Phonemic symbols are written between slashes to distinguish them from other symbols; the beginning sound of *code* is written as /k/, the whole word is /kod/. A number of phonemic alphabets for English are currently in use. For example, the initial phoneme in *yet* may be /y/ or /j/, depending on the system used. The important aspect of phonemic notation is that one symbol represents one sound, or phoneme; it is quite easy to convert from one transcrip-

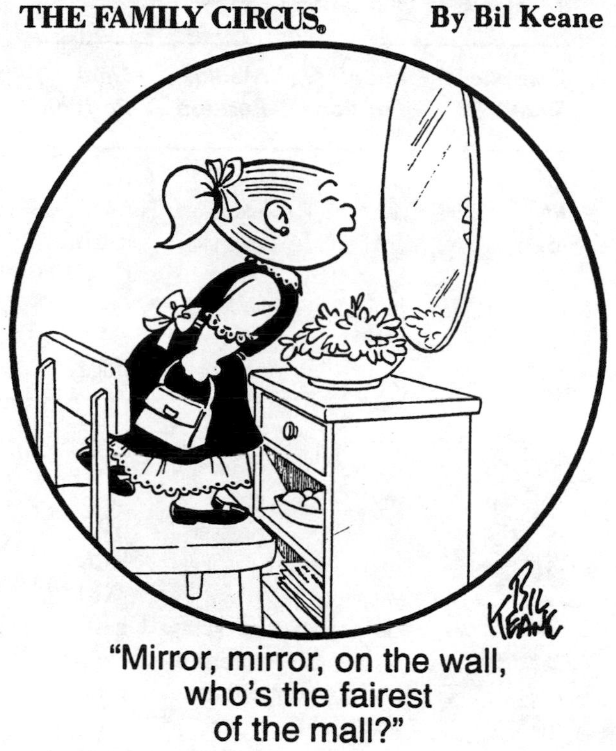

"Mirror, mirror, on the wall, who's the fairest of the mall?"

tion system to another. We have found that the use of a phonemic notation system helps adults return to being aware of sounds of the language, as opposed to thinking of graphemic symbols (letters). The use of a phonemic system ensures that we are all using the same pronunciation as we discuss specific words and sounds. Each spoken language employs certain phonemes. In English, these sounds are classified as consonants and vowels. The distinction is based mainly on sound production characteristics that are discussed later in this text.

Consonants of English

The phonemic alphabet used in this text for consonant sounds is presented in Table 3–1. At the bottom of the table the most common alternate forms used in education and speech-language pathology are noted. Beside each symbol is an example of a word, in regular orthography, in which that phoneme occurs in the initial position, the medial position, and the final position.

In some positions, a blank will be noted. This occurs in places where our rules of phonology do not allow the occurrence of a specific sound in a specific position in a word. For example, the phoneme rep-

TABLE 3–1. Consonants of English.

Consonant Sound	Initial Position	Medial Position	Final Position
/p/	pin	apple	rap
/t/	tin	jester	rat
/č/*	chin	catcher	catch
/k/	kin	backer	rack
/b/	bin	fibber	rib
/d/	din	grinder	rid
/ǰ/**	gin	ranger	ridge
/g/	goat	beggar	rig
/f/	fin	differ	laugh
/θ/	thigh	ether	bath
/ð/	thy	either	bathe
/s/	sin	dresser	bass
/š/***	shin	washer	bash
/v/	vat	liver	give
/z/	zip	razor	has
/ž/****		measure	mirage
/m/	mat	simmer	ham
/n/	gnat	sinner	sin
/ŋ/		ringer	sing
/r/	rat	stirring	stir
/l/	life	taller	tall
/y/	yet	layer	
/h/	hat	ahead	
/w/	win	lower	
/hw/	whew		

Alternate forms: */tʃ/ **/dʒ/ ***/ʃ/ ****/ʒ/

resented by /ŋ/ occurs only at the end of a syllable or word, and /ž/ occurs only in the medial or final position in English, although other languages such as French often use it in the initial position (e.g., *Jean*). Speakers of Swahili use words that begin with /ŋ/ as in *ngoma* for *drum*. The final phonemes on the chart in Table 3–1, sometimes referred to as semivowels, occur only in the initial position of a syllable (see examples for medial in Table 3–1) or word. It should also be noted that the /t/ and /d/ become a **flap** when they occur between two vowels, the first of which is stressed and the second of which is unstressed, as in *matter* and *madder*.

Other restrictions on the use of phonemes exist as well. For example, some combinations of phonemes, or consonant clusters, can occur only in specific positions, and there are restrictions on the number of consonants that may be clustered (Wardhaugh, 1977). The maximum initial consonant cluster in English is three, the first of which must be /s/. These clusters are illustrated in *scream* /skr-/, *sclerosis* /skl-/, *skewer* /sky-/, and *squelch* /skw-/. Generally, no other consonant can occur after the initial consonants /n/, /z/, /r/, or /l/, although some dialects have /ny-/ in the beginning of *new*. Initial consonants such as /f/, /p/, or /k/ may only be followed with /r/, /l/, /y/, or /w/. In final positions, there are similar restrictions on possible sequences, or clusters, and these are different than the rules for initial clusters. For example, the /-ks/ at the end of *six* and the /-ksθs/ at the end of *four-sixths* may not occur in the initial position. The cluster /gs/ may not occur in either position, whereas /-gz/ may occur in the final position (as in *dogs*), but not in the initial position. The combination /gz/ illustrates another phonological rule in English, the rule of **assimilation,** in which the plural morpheme becomes voiced, voiceless, or syllabic depending on the features of the last sound of the word to which it is attached. Thus, *dog* ending in a voiceless consonant is *dog/z/*, *cat* ending in a voiceless consonant is *cat/s/*, and *bus* with a fricative at the end is *bus/əz/*.

One might argue that some consonant clusters or sounds are simply too hard to pronounce and that is why they don't occur. However, these constraints may apply only to English, just as these particular phonemes may occur only in English. Other languages use some of the same phonemes as English, plus additional sounds, and even some other articulation possibilities. Furthermore, the rules for combinations and placements of these phonemes also differ. Although English does not allow /tl/ in the intitial position, some languages may have words that begin with this consonant cluster. English does allow the /tl/ to occur in words such as *greatly* (but note the different syllables). Spanish makes no distinction between /s/ and /z/, but has two *trill* /r/ phonemes, that is, /r/ phonemes that are tapped against the upper ridge of the mouth. These are difficult for English speakers to distinguish. In Zulu, there are different varieties of /t/, /k/, and /p/ that are distinguished by the amount of aspiration or breathiness (Owens, 1992). All information about the consonants of a language is part of the phonological knowledge, or competence, of the proficient speaker of that language. The proficient speaker is also aware of how context and meaning affect the pronunciation of a word, such as *have*, as in *I have (hav) some work to do tonight* as opposed to *I have (haff) to go now*.

Vowels of English

The phonemic alphabet used in this text for vowel sounds is presented in Table 3–2. Beside each symbol is an example of a word, in regular orthography, in which that phoneme occurs. The use of these symbols allows us to indicate that we perceive that the words *seat*, *fleet*, *key*, *piece*, and *Pete* all contain a common vowel sound (long E /i/), although our standard orthography does not indicate this commonality. We can also indicate the difference in pronunciation that may occur for words such as *lead* (/lid/ and /lɛd/) and it allows for a logical representation of illogical spellings of words such as *canoe* (/kənu/). Furthermore, we can indicate the different pronunciations that speakers of different dialects may use for the same word. For example, the word *caught* may be /kɔt/ for some speakers of English and /kat/ for oth-

TABLE 3–2. Vowels of English.

Vowel Sound	*Example*
/i/	beat
/ɪ/	bit
/e/	bait
/ɛ/	bet
/æ/	bat
/ʌ/	but
/ə/	above, comma
/a/	body
/u/	boot
/ʊ/	put
/o/	boat
/ɔ/	bought
Diphthongs	
/aɪ/	bite
/aʊ/	bout
/ɔɪ/	boy

ers. Some of us eat *eggs* /egz/ for breakfast, whereas others have *eggs* /ɛgz/; some of us *catch* /kɛč/ and others *catch* /kæč/ fish.

Most of the symbols in Table 3–2 indicate that vowel sounds are single phonemes; however, note that the last three vowels are represented by more than one symbol. These vowel sounds are called **diphthongs**. A diphthong is the blend of two vowels within the same syllable (Owens, 1996). The sound begins with one vowel and glides toward another position. When the word *my* is said slowly, the speaker can hear and feel the shift from one vowel to another. A diphthong dips! Figure 3–2 illustrates this effect with a spectrogram showing the vowel sounds /a/, /ɪ/, and /aɪ/ consecutively.

Another important characteristic of vowels is that they can lose their distinctiveness before certain consonants. The most significant of these is the /r/ as in fair /fɛr/, far /far/, and fear /fɪr/. A teacher who is attempting to teach students to listen to vowel sounds should keep this in mind.

Suprasegmental Units

Other phenomena that may be important in analyzing the sound system of a language are suprasegmental units (Wardhaugh, 1977). Paralinguistic features such as stress and pitch can affect language syntactically and semantically. The words *perfect* and *permit* may vary in stress depending on the context. For example, when the teachers *per-*

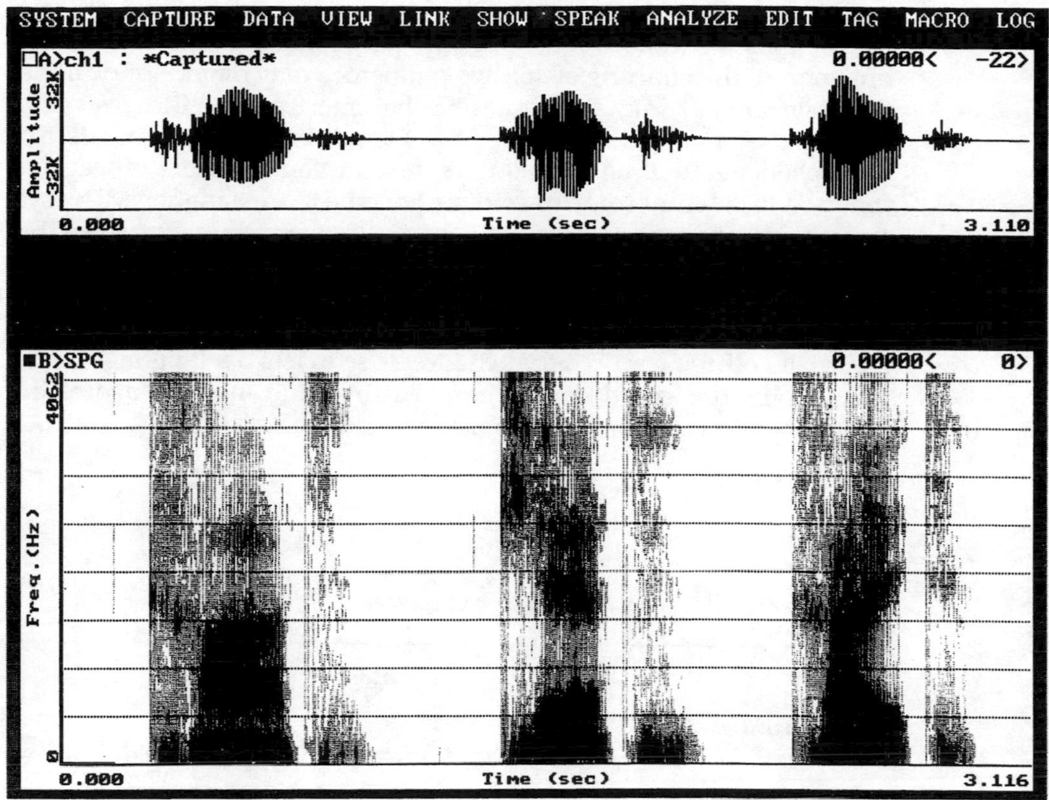

Figure 3–2. Sound spectrogram of adult speech: cat /kat/, kit /kɪt/, kite /kaɪt/.

fect the lesson, they may have a *perfect* day. Or they may issue a *permit* to *permit* the students to play. Another stress pattern may involve pauses between words, referred to as **juncture**. The difference in a compound word and a phrase may be a matter of juncture, as in *a brief case*, not a *briefcase*, or *the green house*, not the *greenhouse*. How does the word *alienation* differ from the TV show *Alien Nation*? Although there are symbols to indicate the differences in stress, pitch, and juncture, these will not be presented in this text. The important factor is that readers keep these paralinguistic features in mind. It is also clear at this point that syntactic and semantic information need to be taken into account when analyzing phonemes.

PHONEMIC CLASSIFICATION

Segmental phonemes differ from one another along particular dimensions. Traditional classification of English phonemes is based on articulation information. Each sound has a unique set of articulatory features. Consonants can be described by the place and manner of articulation, and by the presence or absence of voicing. Although vowels are all voiced, they may be described in terms of tongue height and positioning. As with phonemic alphabets, there are several different feature systems in use today. Not only may some of the features differ, but some of the charting of specific phonemes may differ. For example, the phoneme /h/ may sometimes be characterized as a fricative, or, as it is here, sometimes classified as a glide. What is important is that each phoneme is given a unique representation in terms of features, that is, it is different from any other phoneme in the language. The system for consonants presented in Table 3–3 is somewhat simplified, but is most useful for our purposes. The system for vowels presented in Table 3–4 is fairly standard in terms of the features that are included. These systems closely resemble those presented by Parker and Riley (1994). It is these features that children use to learn a language, and it may also be the knowledge of these features that makes learning our illogical written system of language more difficult.

TABLE 3–3. Place, manner, and voicing of consonant phonemes in English.

Place (From Front to Back)	*Manner*					
	Stop	***Fricative***	***Affricate***	***Glide***	***Liquid***	***Nasal***
Bilabial						
Voiceless	p			hw		
Voiced	b			w		m
Labiodental						
Voiceless		f				
Voiced		v				
Interdental						
Voiceless		θ				
Voiced		ð				
Alveolar						
Voiceless	t	s				
Voiced	d	z			l	n
Palatal						
Voiceless		š	č			
Voiced		ž	ǰ	y	r	
Velar						
Voiceless	k					
Voiced	g					ŋ
Glottal						
Voiceless						
Voiced				h		

TABLE 3–4. Most common vowel sounds of English.

Height of Tongue	***Frontness of Tongue***			
	Front			***Back***
High				
Tense		i		u
Lax	ɪ			ʊ
Mid				
Tense	e			o
Lax	ɛ		ʌ	
			ə	
Low				
Tense				ɔ
Lax	æ		a	
Lip Rounding		Spread		Round

Consonant Sounds of American English

A **consonant** is a speech sound produced when the speaker either stops or severely constricts the airflow in the vocal tract (Akmajian, Demers, Farmer, & Harnish, 1990). The **vocal tract** is the space within which speech sounds are made and includes the oral pharynx, the oral cavity, and the nasal cavity (Akmajian et al, 1990). Consonant phonemes are described in terms of three physical dimensions of articulation: place, manner, and voicing.

Place of Articulation

For each consonant phoneme, the vocal tract is constricted at one of several places. The location is described in terms of the articulator and the point of contact. In other words, place is the *what and where* of the phoneme articulation. Each consonant phoneme is described in terms of the following places.

Bilabial. Bilabial is derived from the morphemes for two (*bi*) + lips (*labial*), because the primary point of constriction in making these sounds is at the lips (/p,b,m,w,hw/). Consider the initial sounds of *man* /mæn/ and *ban* /bæn/.

Labiodental. Labiodental is derived from the morphemes for lip (*labio*) + teeth (*dental*). The primary constriction is between the lower lip and upper teeth (/f,v/). Consider the initial sounds of *fat* /fæt/and *vat* /væt/.

Interdental. Interdental is from the morphemes for between (*inter*) + teeth (*dental*). The primary constriction is between the tongue and the upper teeth (/ð,θ/. Consider *thy* /ðaɪ/ and *thigh* /θaɪ/.

Alveolar. Alveolar comes from the alveolar ridge, which is the bony ridge of the mouth right behind the upper teeth. The primary constriction is between the tongue and the alveolar ridge (/t,d,s,z,n,l/). Consider *team* /tim/ and *seam* /sim/.

Palatal. The palate is the bony roof of the mouth. The primary constriction is between the tongue and the palate (/č,ž,š,ǰ,r,y/). Consider *chin* /čɪn/ and *shin* /šɪn/.

Velar. Velar is from the velum, the soft tissue immediately behind the palate. The primary constriction is between the back of the tongue and the velum (/k,g,ŋ/). Consider *came* /kem/ and *game* /gem/.

Glottal. Glottal refers to the glottis, the space between the vocal cords. The primary constriction is at the glottis (/h/). Consider *hope* /hop/.

The beginning sounds of *man* and *ban* are both bilabials and yet the speaker of English recognizes these as two distinct phonemes. This tells us that some other descriptive dimension is needed to make this distinction. For *man* and *ban*, that dimension is the manner of articulation.

Manner of Articulation

For each consonant phoneme, the vocal tract is constricted in a specific way. This dimension of articulation describes *how* the sound is made. Each consonant phoneme is described in ways of constricting the vocal tract. The first four manners are related to the flow of the airstream; the last two are related to curvature of the tongue.

Stop. Two articulators (teeth, tongue, lips, etc.) are used to completely block, that is, stop, the flow of air through the vocal tract (/p,b,t,d,k,g/). Consider the initial sounds of *pit* /pɪt/ and *bit* /bɪt/.

Fricative. Two articulators are brought together to interfere with the flow of air, but not block it completely. In other words, friction results, thus the term fricative (/f,v,θ,ð,s,z,š,č/). Consider the beginning sounds in *fat* /fæt/ and *vat* /væt/.

Affricate. Affricates begin like stops by completely closing the vocal tract and then end like fricatives with a narrow opening (/č, ǰ/). Consider the words *chin* /čɪn/ and *gin* /ǰɪn/.

Nasal. The airflow through the mouth is blocked and forced through the nasal passage (/m,n,ŋ/). In other words, we close for a stop and then release the air through the nose. Consider the beginning (and ending) sounds in the words *man* /mæn/ and *Nan* /næn/.

Liquid. Liquids share the properties of consonants and vowels; the tongue is raised and sometimes curved as the air flows smoothly through the oral cavity (/l,r/). Consider the words *lake* /lek/ and *rake* /rek/.

Glide. The vocal tract is constricted but not enough to interfere with the airflow (/w,y,h,hw/). These phonemes also share the properties of both consonants and vowels and are sometimes referred to as semivowels. Consider the words *wet* /wɛt/ and *yet* /yɛt/.

Flap. The tongue is tapped to the alveolar ridge. As the reader will recall, this occurs when a /t/ or /d/ is between a stressed and an unstressed vowel, as in *matter* and *madder*, or *butter*. Notation systems require the use of a symbol at the phonetic level to represent this sound, for example, [D], to distinguish between the /t/ and /d/ and the flap. As this distinction may be important in the application of written language, we will use it in phonemic transcriptions; thus, *matter* is /mæDər/.

The distinction between the beginning sounds of the words *man* and *ban* is now clear; although they are both bilabial in place of articulation, the manner differs. *Man* begins with a nasal, whereas *ban* begins with a stop. However, *pan* and *ban* both begin with bilabial stops. One more dimension needs to be included to distinguish between the beginning sounds of these words. This dimension is voicing.

Voicing

For any phoneme that is articulated, the vocal cords are either vibrating (/b,d,g,v,ð,z,ž,ǰ,m,n,ŋ,l,r,w,y/) or not vibrating (/p,t,k,hw,θ,č,s,š,h/). Compare *zoo* /zu/ (voiced) and *Sue* /su/ (voiceless). Note from Table 3–3 that many consonant phonemes come in pairs. The voicing feature is sometimes referred to as voice onset time (VOT) because the distinction in a word is when the voicing begins, at the beginning of the phoneme (voiced) or at the end of the phoneme (voiceless) as the next phoneme begins. Consider *thy* /ð/ and *thigh* /θ/.

Using all three of these dimensions of articulation, we see that the beginning sounds in *fat* and *vat* are both labiodental fricatives, but /f/ is voiceless and /v/ is voiced. The beginning sounds of *bet* and *get* are both voiced stops, but /b/ is a bilabial and /g/ is a velar, thus the distinction between these two sounds is place of articulation. If we examine the beginning sounds of *man* and *ban*, we find that the /m/ and /b/ are both voiced and both are bilabials. To determine the distinction between these sounds, manner of articulation is necessary. With these dimensions, all consonant sounds of English can be described uniquely. However, vowel sounds require a different set of physical dimensions. These dimensions are described next.

Vowel Sounds of American English

Whereas consonants are formed by obstructions, either partial or total, **vowels** are phonemes that are produced with an open vocal tract operating as a resonating chamber (Akmajian et al., 1990). Vowels are described in terms of the following dimensions as noted in Table 3–4. Included are most of the vowels of American English used by most speakers. Others may exist for different dialects.

Tongue Height

For the articulation of each vowel phoneme, the tongue is either relatively **high** in the mouth (/i,ɪ,u,ʊ/), **mid** (/e,ɛ,ʌ,ə,o/), or **low** (/æ,a,ɔ/). Compare the vowel sounds in *beat* /bit/ (high) and *bat* /bæt/ (low).

Frontness

For each vowel phoneme, the tongue is either relatively **front** (/i,ɪ,e,ɛ,æ/) or **back** (/ʌ,ə,a,u,ʊ,o,ɔ/). Compare *beet* /bit/ (front) and *boot* /but/ (back).

Lip Rounding

For each vowel phoneme, the lips are either relatively **round** (/u,ʊ,o,ɔ/) or **spread** (/i,ɪ,e,ɛ,æ,ʌ,ə,a/). Compare *boat* /bot/ (round) and *bait* /bet/ (spread).

Tenseness

For each vowel phoneme, the vocal musculature is either relatively **tense** (/i,e,u,o,ɔ/), or **lax** (/ɪ,ɛ,æ,ʌ,ə,a,ʊ/). Compare *bait* /bet/ (tense) and *bet* /bɛt/ (lax). Note that tense and lax are roughly equivalent to what most of us know as long and short vowel sounds.

With these physical dimensions, the vowel sounds of American English may be distinguished. When vowels and consonants are grouped together with consideration for the required constraints in English, we can find that meaning often evolves. When just one of the phonemes in a unit of meaning (or word) is changed, the meaning changes. Two words that differ in only one phoneme but have a different meaning are known as **minimal pairs** of words, as in:

map (/mæp/)	map (/mæp/)	map (/mæp/)	mope (/mop/)
nap (/næp/)	mat (/mæt/)	mope (/mop/)	dope (/dop/)

Children can distinguish between minimal pairs of words that contain most English contrasts by age 35 months (Menyuk & Menn, 1979).

To understand the full significance of this accomplishment, recall that language is spoken as a continuous stream of sounds, not in segments. Listening to the language of a speaker of an unfamiliar language makes it easier for us to realize that language is indeed a continuous stream, not segmented phonemes. One of the authors observed herself, in response to her cats' begging to be fed, saying, "/ardifɛdyə/." Somehow they, as masters of the English language, understood that she had said "I already fed you." And somehow infants move from what must seem to be a stream of noise to a full-fledged, highly complex, abstract adult system of sounds and meaning in at least one language (Lindfors, 1987). And as will be seen, it is the articulatory features that children will use in learning to discriminate significant sounds.

ACQUISITION OF PHONOLOGY

Children acquire phonology in stages that occur as a part of the development of meaning in language. In fact, as we have seen, phonemes are often dependent on meaning (as in *permit* the noun vs. *permit* the verb). However, before any meaningful linguistic distinctions are made, infants are able to make some fine perceptual discriminations in speech sounds. It would seem that children must be born with the ability to distinguish complex speech sounds.

Perceptual Discriminations

Within days after birth, infants are highly responsive to speech or sounds of similar pitch. In fact, speech seems highly rewarding for infants as they are shown to be much more responsive to human speech than to other sounds (Reich, 1986).

Through monitoring of changes in heart rate and pacifier-sucking rate, researchers have demonstrated that not only are infants responsive to speech at a very early age, but also that they can make fine discriminations between a number of speech sounds as early as age 1 month. For example, Morse (1972) reported that infants' sucking rate changed when a repetitive stimulus of /pa/ changed in place-feature to /da/, or in voicing-feature to /ba/. However, it will be much later before distinctions in units of meaning, as in words, can be made as the child must learn which of the many differences in speech sounds actually mark differences in linguistic meaning. It is during the first few months that infants discriminate between angry and friendly verbal expression, and between male and female voices (Clark & Clark, 1977).

Interestingly, children typically acquire phonemic segments that are common among world languages before they acquire those that are relatively rare. For example, the universal /a/ sound and the nearly universal /i,u/ are early acquired vowels (Vs). Front consonants tend to develop before back consonants (Cs); stops and nasals are generally acquired before liquids and fricatives; this coincides with the most common elements of world languages. Earliest syllable occurrences in development are of the form CV. The simplest syllable found among world languages is that of CV and all languages have a CV syllable. In fact, almost all syllables in Japanese words are made up of CV, as in *Fujiyama* (Parker & Riley, 1994). Although English has a very complex syllable structure, children's early occurring syllables will be of the CV form.

Prelinguistic Vocalization

Early vocalizations of infants may be considered acoustic signals, or noises, produced by the babies' moving articulators around as they progress to the more controlled production of speech sounds used in the language or languages they hear around them. Even profoundly deaf infants move through the early stages of production.

Crying and Cooing

Babies' first sounds from birth up to about 2 months may be described as vegetative sounds (e.g., burping, coughing) and reflexive crying (inhalation and exhalation). After the first month, differentiated crying (for wetness, hunger, illness) is noted and cooing appears. **Cooing** can be described as the production of clear vowels, often in isolation, and is referred to by Reich (1986) as happy sounds. The earliest **cooing** is made up of /a,i,u/ sounds. Between 2 and 3 months, consonant-vowel (CV) patterns begin to appear and back sounds that resemble velar consonants (e.g., /k/ and /g/) are combined with vowels (Lund & Duchan, 1993). During this time children appear to be vocalizing in a random way, using a wide range of sounds with no pattern or control (Lindfors, 1987). From 4 to 7 months, vocal play begins with longer syllable sequences (Lund & Duchan, 1993). Additional consonants (e.g., /p,b,d/ and nasals) are added.

Babbling

During the second 6 months, the vocalizations are different. Repetition of syllables and intonational patterns begin as do self-monitoring and self-imitation. Early CV repetitions result in such forms as /mama/ and /papa/, that is, nasals and stops with vowels. These represent extreme contrasts between consonants and vowels and account for the constituents common to the majority of *mama-papa* terms across languages (Jakobson, 1962). Jakobson reported that consonant clusters appear in no more than 1.1% of the 1,072 parental terms counted by Murdock in his 1957 anthropological *world ethnographic samples* of child language. One could assume that a great deal of reinforcement occurs after these early repetitive syllable sound productions.

Repetitive chaining of syllables increases during the second 6 months, and consonants resemble those of adults in some ways. From 9–12 months, different sounds are used across the syllable sequence, and imitation of others occurs. This has been referred to as both *echolalia* and *jargon* as the child seems to be simulating adults. Nonnative sounds decrease in number (Owens, 1992). The suprasegmental features of language (intonation, stress, rhythm) are more evident, and some of the prebabbling vocalizations are gone (Lindfors, 1987). In other words, children begin to sound as if they are talking, albeit with meaningless forms.

Also appearing are **vocables**, or short segments that are consistent and context specific. These include ritualized games (*peek-a-boo*), emotional states (*uh-oh*), or frequently occurring communicative acts (*da* + point, *bye-bye*) (Lund & Duchan, 1993). These are not yet considered *words* as they do not occur outside of specific contexts.

Linguistic Production

Phonology of First Words

At about 10 months, children produce their first words through planned, controlled speech. From this time until about 18 months, children gradually acquire meaningful words. These words may not be adult forms, although children may produce more advanced forms of words first and then "progress" to less adult forms (Moskowitz, 1970). First words tend to be words whose referents are familiar objects or events (e.g., /ba/ for *bottle*) and tend to have a simple CV syllable structure which may or may not be duplicated (e.g., /baba/). The consonants are typically front stops or nasals, although children vary in their choice of favorite sounds or syllables (Lund & Duchan, 1993). The early word stage may thus be different for different children. The key elements of this stage are a shift to greater control of articulation and applying meaning to sounds. Children may reach a vocabulary of about 50 meaningful words, but their phonological ability is highly restricted and they produce great phonological variation. This stage, however is followed by another in which there is rapid phonological progression (Ingram, 1976).

Phonological Processes

From about 18 months to 4 years of age, the production of consonants in all syllable positions improves and consonant clusters appear. The use of a number of **phonological processes** (Stampe, 1972), or procedures to simplify speech, occurs. Ingram (1976) used these to characterize error patterns in phonological acquisition. These may be divided into processes related to syllable structure, assimilation, and phoneme substitution. The processes that are listed as characteristic of normal Standard English-speaking children follow.

Syllabic Structure Processes. The number of syllables or the consonant-vowel patterns of syllables are systematically changed.

Final consonant deletion: CVC becomes CV (/ke/ for *cake*)

Consonant cluster reduction: CC becomes C (/gin/ for *green*)

Unstressed syllable deletion: (/nænə/ for *banana*)

Reduplication of syllable: (/wawa/ for *water*)

Assimilation Processes. Adjacent phonemes or features become more alike. This may occur in either direction.

Prevocalic voicing of consonant: before a V (/di/ for *tea*)

Devoicing of final consonant: (/bɛt/ for *bed*)

Velar assimilation: (/gək/ for *duck*)

THE FAMILY CIRCUS. By Bil Keane
BIL KEANE
"But how can 'tato chips start with a P?"

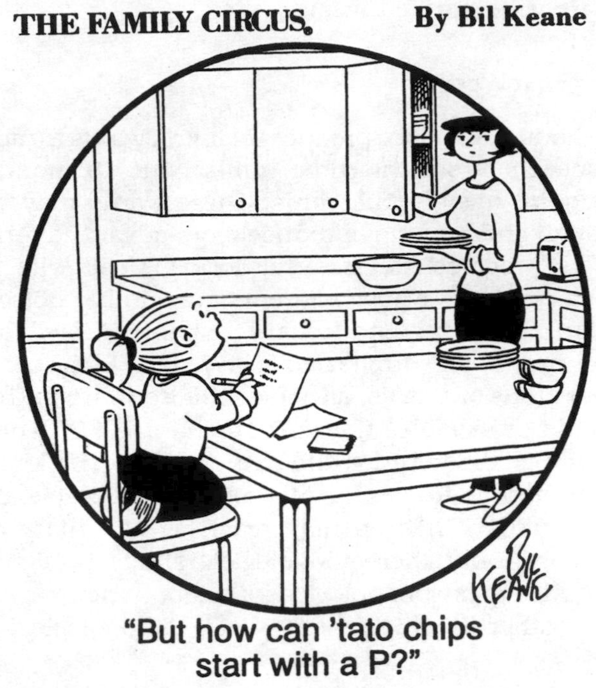

Consonant harmony: (/gagi/ or /dadi/ for *doggie*)

Nasalization of vowels: (/mæ̃/ for *man*)

Substitution Processes. Segments are modified, often depending on their position in a word.

Stopping: stops for fricatives (/dup/ for *soup*)

Fronting: alveolars for velars and palatals (/tot/ for *coat*)

Denasalization: vocal consonants for nasals (/do/ for *no*)

Gliding: glides for liquids (/wak/ for *rock*)

Vocalization: Vs for syllabic Cs (/æpo/ for *apple*)

A February, 1990, newsletter from Mead Hall, a parish day school of St. Thaddeus Episcopal Church in Aiken, SC, reported on a classic example of gliding overheard at the kindergarten Christmas program practice: "The teacher says to stand with your hands on your *yegs*," declared one young man. Another tapped him on the shoulder and corrected him with great assuredness, "It's not *yegs*, it's *wegs*."

Unfortunately, phonological processes are not always as simple as those illustrated here, because multiple processes may be occurring in one word. For example, a combination of gliding and reduplication could result in /wæwæ/ for *rabbit*. Stampe (1972) has described seven processes that may account for /bap/ for *lamb*!

The processes described before are common for both normal and abnormal language learners and for children learning different languages (Lund & Duchan, 1993). In describing developmental trends, Hodson and Paden (1991) reported that by age 4, normally developing English-speaking children have eliminated most of these processes that lead to errors, with the exception of liquid (/l,r/) deviations. Owens (1995) reported that cluster reduction, which usually disappears after age 4, is followed by a stage in which another sound is substituted for the omitted sound. Mastery of consonant clusters is not expected until about age 7.

Completion of the Phonemic Inventory

From about ages 4 to 7, children do continue development from the previous stage. Sander (1972) has proposed that it is more appropriate to determine age ranges, not ages, within which specific sounds are mastered by normally developing children. Included on Figure 3–3 are ages at which 50% of children use the sound correctly in all positions and the age at which 90% of an age group are using it. This is identified as the range of normal acquisition. When a child is not producing a sound above the age range presented, it can then be assumed that he or she is in the slowest 10% in development. This is more appropriate than a single age for each phoneme for, as can be seen, variability in development is the rule rather than the exception (Lund & Duchan, 1993).

By the end of this stage, children can pronounce most of their words in correct adult form. However, as more complex words are acquired, inaccurate productions can still be expected (e.g., *vegetables* and *spaghetti*). Ingram (1976) reported three different children's productions of vegetables as /vɛstaboz/, /vɛjəblz/, and /vɛnčtəblz/.

Morphophonemic Development

Morphophonemic knowledge is awareness of phonemic changes that occur based on morphemic information and develops in the period from 7 to 12 years of age. This includes complex rules such as the **vowel shift** rule which accounts for changes in pronunciation of morphemes when the part of speech changes. This is illustrated by shift in the vowels that occurs in *photograph-photography* and *explain-explanation.*

Another example includes knowledge of the suprasegmental stress system necessary to differentiate some compound words from phrases as in *greenhouse* and *green house, redhead* and *red head,* or *highchair* and *high chair.* Speakers must learn that phrases take stress at the end of a word and compound words at the beginning. Atkinson-King (1973) found that 5-year-olds did not know this rule; the closer children were to age 12, the more likely they were to have learned it.

Metalinguistic Knowledge

Metalinguistic knowledge is the ability to think about the components of language. It is not until children begin to learn to read that

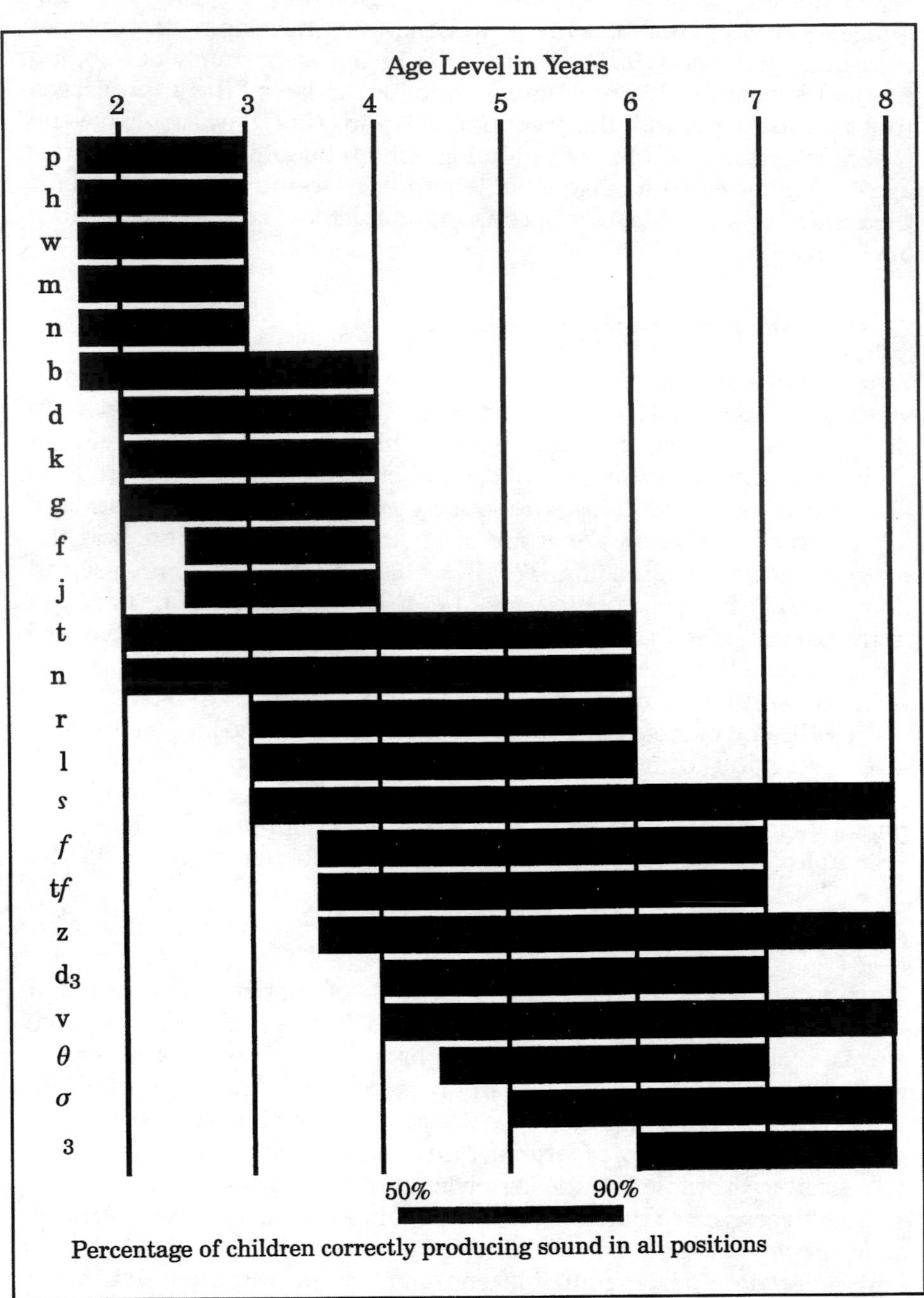

Figure 3–3. Phoneme acquisition for standard English speakers. (From *Assessing Children's Language in Naturalistic Contexts,* 3rd ed., by N. J. Lund and J. F. Duchan, 1993, p. 118. Englewood Cliffs, NJ: Prentice Hall. Copyright 1993 by Prentice Hall. Reprinted with permission.) Reprinted by permission of Allyn & Bacon.

they come to consciously know that words are units and that they are made up of sounds. These segmentation skills are necessary for syllabication, rhyming, and other types of sound analysis. These skills are examined more closely in Chapter 4 as they become most significant in implications for teaching.

As will be seen in Chapter 4, the development of the phonological system has direct implications for both speaking and academic skills in school. Knowledge of the developmental stages and particularly of the phonological processes will be needed in planning for both spoken and written language.

✓ SUMMARY CHECKLIST

- ☐ **Definition of Phonology**

  Phonology is the study of the sound system of a language, including what those sounds are and the system of rules underlying the pronunciations of words, that is, the rules of combining and sequencing these sounds.

  Phoneme

- ☐ **Phonemic Notation**

  Consonants
  Vowels
  Suprasegmentals

- ☐ **Phonemic Classification**

  Consonants
  - Place of Articulation
  - Manner of Articlation
  - Voicing

  Vowels
  - Tongue Height
  - Tongue Frontness
  - Lip Rounding
  - Tenseness

- ☐ **Acquisition of Phonology**

  Perceptual Discriminations
  Prelinguistic Vocalization
  - Crying and Cooing
  - Babbling

  Phonology of First Words
  Phonological Processes
  - Syllabic Structure
  - Assimilation
  - Substitution

- ☐ **Completion of Phonemic Inventory**
- ☐ **Morphophonemic Development**
- ☐ **Metalinguistic Knowledge**

CHAPTER

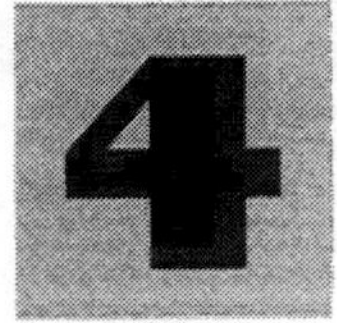

PHONOLOGY: ANALYSIS AND INTERVENTION

Phonology involves the sound system of language, including the classification system of sounds, ability to perceive and discriminate sounds, and knowledge of the rules related to the combination and sequencing of sounds. Disorders in phonology have been demonstrated to affect other aspects of language learning. When a preschool child is identified as phonologically delayed, there is a very high probability that he or she will also demonstrate delayed development of higher levels of oral language, as well as written language (e.g., Hoffman, 1997; Owens & Robinson, 1997). Specifically, Hoffman noted that children who are phonologically delayed are likely to experience delays in acquisition of morphology, syntax, and discourse structure of language, as well as difficulties in analyzing language into words, syllables, rhymes, and phonemes.

Knowledge and proficiency in the area of phonology also has an impact on academic areas. Phonological skills specifically related to reading and writing are described as phonological awareness skills. **Phonological awareness** is the general term used to indicate conscious knowledge that spoken words are composed of sounds (**phonemic awareness**), syllables, and subsyllabic units between syllables and sounds, composed of **onsets** and **rimes** (van Kleeck, 1995). The onset is the initial consonant or consonant cluster in a syllable and the rime is the remainder of the syllable. It always contains a vowel, and many rimes contain a final consonant or consonant cluster. For example, in *track*, *tr* /tr/ is the onset and *ack* /æk/ is the rime, in *tree*, *tr* /tr/ is the onset and *ee* /i/ is the rime. Phonological awareness also includes the ability to think about and consciously manipulate the sounds in words

(Ball & Blachman, 1991). The importance of this ability in reading has become more and more evident in the last few years (e.g., Blachman, 1994a, 1994b; Wagner & Torgesen, 1987) and is discussed in more depth in the section on reading.

ANALYSIS

Atypical Phonological Development

There are few descriptions of phonological development in children with language disorders. Children with problems in phonology may follow typical phonological development but at a delayed pace (Schwartz, Leonard, Folger, & Wilcox, 1980; Watson, Martineau, & Hughes, 1993) or utilize phonological processes that are not characteristic of typical development (Hodson & Paden, 1981; Leonard & McGregor, 1991).

Typically developing children begin to suppress the phonological processes (e.g., final consonant deletion) discussed in Chapter 3 by 4 years of age. Children who are using these processes past this age would be demonstrating a phonological delay. Children with phonological disorders do have rule-based phonological systems, however these systems are deviant from adult models (Hodson & Paden, 1991). How much intelligibility will be affected is dependent on the severity of the phonological disorder.

Related characteristics have been noted with children with phonological disorders. These students may have related problems in verbal short-term memory and rapid naming tasks (Torgesen, Wagner, & Rashotte, 1994). Many children with phonological disorders have a history of mild fluctuating hearing losses associated with middle ear infections (Hodson, 1994). Children with phonological impairments (both presently or in the past) perform more poorly than typical peers on phonological awareness tasks (e.g., Webster & Plante, 1992).

Phonological Awareness

Phonological awareness abilities are powerful predictors of later reading and spelling (Blachman, 1994a; Hodson, 1994). There is a correlation between phonological awareness and early reading abilities (Blachman, 1994a; Bradley & Bryant, 1978). Phonological deficits indicate problems with phonological coding, which may contribute to difficulty with the written code system (Ball, 1997). These difficulties have been noted mostly in young children. However, Apthorp (1995) found a correlation between phonological processing deficits and reading-related deficits in college students.

Three general areas of phonological awareness skills have been identified. These are abilities related to **rhyming**, **blending**, and **segmenting**. Difficulties in one or all of these areas may influence reading/writing difficulties.

Preschoolers (4- and 5-year olds) are generally aware of and play with rhyme and alliteration (Dowker, 1989). Young children should be able to recognize and produce rhymes. The level of awareness or sensitivity to rhyme is correlated with reading skills in the primary grades (Bradley & Bryant, 1991). A summary of research by Fazio (1996) indicated that children identified as having a specific language impairment (SLI) have been shown to have difficulty memorizing Mother Goose rhymes and songs. However, as children grow older the significance of the correlation between rhyming skills and reading ability appear to diminish (Yopp, 1988).

Blending is the ability to take individual phonemes and blend them into syllables and words. Most preschoolers can blend syllables into words (Yopp, 1988) and, conversely, break words into syllables. The ability to break syllables and words into smaller units (i.e., phonemes and syllables) is known as segmentation. Preschoolers have been known to clap or jump to the number of syllables in a word (Hodson, 1994). Students who have difficulty with such skills as identifying initial sounds, final sounds, and counting syllables would be showing deficits in segmentation skills.

A variety of tasks have been used to measure phonological awareness, including, for example, categorizing or matching words on the basis of common sounds, counting phonemes, segmenting words into phonemes, deleting phonemes, and manipulating phonemes (Blachman, 1991). Children who have difficulty with these types of tasks may warrant intervention. For a list of some of the numerous measures available for assessing phonological awareness in young children, see Catts (1996). Also, Jenkins and Bowen (1994) presented a checklist for phonological awareness progression ranging from rhyming to segmentation of words into three parts. With older children (e.g., by the end of third grade), it might be more useful to use a more complex task, such as phoneme deletion and/or phoneme manipulation (Blachman, 1991).

INTERVENTION

As models of language intervention focus more and more on functional communication, services in school are increasingly being provided in the classroom and involve the use of classroom curricula (Norris, 1997). Thus, use of collaborative-consultative models that include the teacher, the speech-language pathologist (SLP), aides, parents, and other professionals is increasing (Owens & Robinson, 1997). This is particularly important in light of the fact that many children who have language disorders may not be receiving services. For example, Gibbs and Cooper (1989) reported that in a population of 242 elementary school-age children with learning disabilities, language deficits were found in 90.5%, and 23.5% had articulation deficits or phonological delays. Only 6% of the children were receiving the services of a speech-language pathologist. With a collaborative-consultative model of delivery of services in the classroom, all students could benefit.

Speaking

Reciprocal teaching and scaffolding, first introduced to special education by Palinscar and Brown (1984), may be very useful for teaching phonological knowledge in context to individuals with problems in this area. **Reciprocal teaching** involves a dialogue between the teacher or SLP and the learners in which students and teacher or SLP interactively communicate, and the teacher or SLP provides support by taking the lead first and eventually turning responsibility over to the student, that is, **scaffolding**. A major strength of this approach is that it occurs within a context of meaningful use.

As preschool children are most often in need of intervention for a wide range of oral and written abilities, Hoffman (1997) recommended using oral language scaffolding techniques in the context of repeated storybook reading. This programming allows for simultaneous improvement in a range of language abilities, from speaking to reading. Effective communication serves as the motivation for changes in articulation and phonology.

Goals are organized from whole to part. For example, the first goal targets organizing discourse; the second goal targets some of the syntactic and morphological structures that will be acquired through achieving the first goal. The third goal specifies some of the phonological elements that the child will learn as parts of the story. The final goal includes some of the metalinguistic aspects of speech developed through discussions of the printed words and oral discussion of the story. Note that semantic understanding of a concept in context is required before metalinguistic levels are used.

Hoffman provided an example of an adult focusing on the child's production of fricatives by providing metalinguistic descriptions of the word *mouse*.

Adult: This hole is where the . . .
Child: mouse live /maʊ wɪv/
Adult: Yeah the mouse (extending the duration of /s/). Feel the air in that sound (putting the child's hand in front of her mouth to feel the air flow), mouse.
Child: mouse /maʊf/ the mouse /dʌ maʊf/
Adult: The little boy is trying to catch the . . .
Child: a mouse /ʌ maʊ/
Adult: catch the mouse
Child: the mouse /dʌ maʊs/ (Hoffman, 1997, p.86)

This example used a **cloze procedure**, providing part of the utterance which the child then completes. This allows the child to participate in the conversation in which the production of the sound is useful. The adult provides models and focuses on the characteristics of the sound, all in context.

The use of storybooks and other literature can be very helpful in providing context. Owens and Robinson (1997) provided an extensive list of popular children's books and suggested intervention uses for each. Examples include Rosen and Robins's (1993) *Little Rabbit Foo Foo* for initial /g, k, f/ sounds, Roddie and Cony's (1991) *Hatch Egg Hatch* for final /g, č / sounds, and Rosen and Oxenbury's (1989) *We're Going on a Bear Hunt* for initial /sk/ clusters. Suggested uses also include targets from morphology, syntax, semantics, and pragmatics.

More structured approaches to phonological intervention are also available. A phonological approach to speech deviations is based on the systematic nature of phonological development regardless of whether it is typical or atypical. Hodson and Padden (1991) recommended a cycles approach for intervention with children who are phonologically disordered. Emphasis is on discovering the rules or phonological processes that comprise an individual's system (Reed, 1994). Phonological patterns not mastered in the child's speech are presented, practiced, and recycled until 100% mastery is achieved. Several phonological patterns are included in each cycle; 2 to 6 hours of intervention will bc spent on each pattern. Each pattern will be practiced in several target words, with the assumption that generalization will occur. The use of amplification through earphones for presentation of target words is recommended to increase the child's focus and discrimination. For a complete description of this intervention program, see Hodson and Paden (1991).

Reading

Processing the complex language of many teachers may result in difficulty for children with immature language systems, and reading offers an even greater challenge (Owens & Robinson, 1997). Children learn to put sounds in words in their second year of life, but it is not until they begin to read that they must think of sounds as such and about how words are made up of sounds. Reading and writing depend on skills that go beyond speaking and listening (Jenkins & Bowen, 1994).

Phonological production affects phonological awareness (Webster & Plante, 1992), and the relationship between phonological awareness and reading and writing skills has been well established (MacDonald & Cornwall, 1995; Shafir & Siegel, 1994); however, other issues are still being debated. One issue is whether phonological abilities precede and lead directly to the development of word identification skills (e.g., MacDonald & Cornwall, 1995; Wagner & Torgeson, 1987) or whether the development of reading skills leads to the development of phonologic awareness (e.g., Strickland & Cullinan, 1991). These issues lead to questions of when and how to teach phonological skills most effectively. Phonological skills can be taught as a precursor to and along with instruction in letter-sound relationships (Ball & Blachman, 1991; Blachman, 1991; Yopp, 1992). Blachman (1994b) suggested that length of training, intensity, components of intervention, and timing of training need to be further examined.

Another debate in which one can get bogged down is the ongoing question of whole language versus phonics. This debate is much too intense to present here. Research has clearly demonstrated that training can increase children's phonological awareness and improve reading achievement (Catts, 1996). The decision to implement phonological awareness training need not become entangled with the issue of whether to teach using a whole language reading approach or a phonics approach. Moats and Lyon (1996) suggested that (1) inclusion of code-based instruction does not preclude well-designed instruction in comprehension and higher level language processing and (2) code-based instruction is not necessarily the largely workbook-oriented *phonics* of old. In fact, they pointed out that skillful implementation of phonological awareness training assumes the integration of decoding skills into meaningful contexts. The most promising strategies seem to be those that maximize effectiveness by teaching phonological awareness within the context of actual letter-sound correspondences as well as providing practice in reading meaningful text (e.g., Blachman, 1994a).

Blachman (1991) has reminded us that assessment should be used to decide who needs instruction in phonological awareness, not to eliminate anyone or place them in an alternative approach such as a whole word approach to reading. In fact, instruction in phonemic awareness may have the greatest benefit for those with low pretest scores.

Phonogical Awareness Training

Rhyming. As mentioned previously, the use of nursery rhymes and poetry provides children the opportunity to hear and practice rhyming skills. Repetitive stories such as the *Gingerbread Boy* offer students the opportunity to practice longer linguistic units with an increase in phonological complexity (Jenkins & Bowen, 1994). Activities such as matching games that use rhyming partners, either in picture or word representations, are effective, as is the traditional *word families* approach.

Examples:

It family	*Ot* family
sit	hot
fit	cot
bit	lot
kit	dot
hit	knot

A variation would be to include nonsense words.

In a study summarized by Fazio (1996), preschool children with specific language impairment (SLI) could better remember new poems if taught with hand motions. The children apparently used the hand motions as cues. It has been suggested that children with language deficits can learn nursery rhymes and poems but may need to hear and practice the target many more times than typical children (Fazio, 1996).

Blending. Activities that involve blending phonemes into syllables and words are appropriate. This should be done both in the oral production of phonemes and then later in the written production of graphemes. It has been suggested that initially words with continuous sounds (e.g., /s/, /f/, /n/, /l/) should be used followed by words that begin with stops (e.g., *bat* and *cup*). In conjunction with sound/letter correspondence training, the child will need to recognize the names and sounds of letters. The child must also be able to acknowledge that the same letter may have several sounds.

Segmenting. Syllable segmentation appears to precede word segmentation (the ability to identify word boundaries). For example, Jenkins and Bowen (1994) noted that young children will identify three words in Peter Pan (i.e., *Pe ter Pan*). Therefore, it may be wise to introduce syllable segmentation before word segmentation. Tapping or jumping to the number of syllables/words in a word or sentence is fun and involves motor stimulation and coding.

Sound categorization activities (Bradley & Bryant, 1985), identifying all words with the same initial sound, final sound, or medial sound, are recommended. Blachman (1991) suggested beginning with the initial sound in the child's name to make the activity a little more personal and familiar. *Odd one out* games where the student must find the one that does not belong are also useful.

Examples:

Initial Sounds: baby, bone, bacon, doll

Final Sounds: dog, big, bit, log

Segmenting phonemes in words could be practiced by token games, such as using tokens to move in boxes as one pronounces each phoneme in a word. When using written words, the student could move the token directly under the corresponding grapheme(s). Of course, one must keep in mind there is not always a one-to-one correspondence in English. Finally, the most difficult phonological awareness tasks are those involving the manipulation of phonemes or syllables.

Examples:

Say the word *backyard* without *back*.

Change the beginning sound of *hat* to /k/.

Training Program Example

Gillam and van Kleeck (1996) designed a two-stage intervention program in phonological awareness for preschool children with speech and language disorders. This program incorporates rhyming, segmenting, and blending skills in a progressively more difficult manner.

During the first stage, rhyming tasks are taught twice weekly for the first semester and segmentation/blending tasks twice weekly for the second semester. Rhyming activities are conducted with small groups of children and focus on different rhyme pairs each week with a series of increasingly difficult activities, progressing from recognition to imitation, to identification, to judgment, and finally to rhyme creation. In addition, teachers read aloud every day from a rhyming book (e.g., *Itchy, Itchy Chicken Pox*, Maccarone & Lewin, 1992) that contains the target rhyming pairs. Picture cards and a game board are also created for the rhyme pairs.

Teachers or SLPs stress the concept that the ends of rhyming words sound alike but the beginning sounds are different (rhyme **identification**). Next, the children practice saying the five rhyme pairs in response to picture cues and models (**imitation**). Finally a rhyme **identification** game is played in which half of a set of pictures representing one word from each pair are placed face-up in front of the children. As the other half of the pictures are presented one at a time, children select the face-up picture that completes the rhyme pair, say the pair, then place the pictures in a pocket on the game board. For example, children are shown the picture of a *nose* and asked, "Which word rhymes with *nose*?" After one child selects the picture of *toes*, everyone says, "*nose-toes*." One child puts the pictures together in a pocket on the game board.

Rhyming. During the second lesson of the week, children are reminded of the word pairs through an imitation activity. Then, the teacher or SLP plays a rhyme **judgment** game in which a picture of one target word paired with another word is presented. Children are to judge whether or not the two words rhyme. If not, the children provide the correct word. Finally a rhyme **production** game is played. The teacher or SLP selects a rhyme pair and says, "Let's think of some other words that rhyme with *tie* and *high*. I know one: *tie, high, by*. Let's all say those." Children are asked to suggest other words and all three words are said together; when children do not come up with a word, it is supplied and all three words are said aloud.

Segmentation. In the program designed by Gillam and van Kleek (1996), activities to help children acquire an awareness of sounds at the beginning and end of words are implemented during the second semester. Two target sounds are selected each week and a sequence of eight awareness activities is initiated for each phoneme.

The first 7 weeks focus on initial phonemes with five activities. The first is **initial sound-picture word relationships** in which the teacher and/or a puppet tell children about the initial sounds in the eight target words. The second is **initial position phoneme judgment and correction** in which the child is to identify when words are said correctly or incorrectly. The child is asked to correct the teacher's or a puppet's incorrect production. Third is **initial position sound matching** in which children pick pictures of words that begin with the sound that the teacher names. Fourth is **initial sound identification** in which the teacher selects a picture and the children tell the teacher what sound it starts with, or children choose pictures and sort them into sound bags. Fifth is **generating words** in which children select untrained pictures of words that begin with target sounds and think of words that begin with target sounds (no picture cues).

For the next 3 weeks, the first five activities are repeated for final sounds. During the final 2 weeks, the last two activities are initiated. Activity seven is **sound blending-synthesis** in which the teacher says the component sounds (one at a time) in previously trained words and children select the pictures. The teacher then says the component sounds in previously untrained words and the children select the pictures. The last activity is **sound analysis** in which the teacher shows a picture of a trained word and says the word; children say the sounds. Then the teacher will show a picture of an untrained word and say the word; children will say the sounds.

Emphasizing Form and Meaning Separately

Van Kleeck (1995) suggested that both meaning and form (sound-letter correspondence) are important but initially should be emphasized in separate activities. In her review of literature on the topic, Blachman (1994b) noted that children trained in both phonological awareness and letter names and sounds (in separate activities, not simultaneously) do better in reading than children trained only in phonological awareness.

Van Kleek (1995) offered a two-stage model of preliteracy development. Stage 1, the **meaning foundation stage**, establishes the understanding that print is meaningful and useful for many purposes and that interacting with print is enjoyable and rewarding. In many families, this is introduced as a book-sharing routine around age 5–6 months. Unfortunately, for some children this stage may not be initiated until formal schooling begins.

Stage 2, the **form foundation stage** of preliteracy development, includes the integration of phonological awareness of sounds in words and alphabetic awareness (knowing letter names, shapes, and sounds). Based on recent studies, Van Kleeck (1995) suggests that awareness of syllabic and subsyllabic units emerges before alphabetic instruction and is the first level of phonological awareness. Activities to foster awareness of the subsyllabic units of onset and rime can be informal (such as reading rhyming books, playing rhyming games) or more structured activities.

After syllabic and subsyllabic knowledge is established, instruction in alphabetic knowledge begins with letter names. Children often learn letter names by learning the "Alphabet Song." The tune seems to help with the memory load and even though children may not know the words in the song are letters, it provides an anchor for children to learn to associate letter names with shapes. After letter names are learned, letter sounds may be introduced, and activities should be fun, not worksheet drills. Learning sound-letter correspondence integrates letter knowledge and phonemic awareness. Treiman (1992) suggested that using onsets and rimes as a starting point allows for more consistent sound-letter correspondence and increased predictability of vowels.

In conclusion, Blachman (1991) pointed out that most phonological training activities require only 15–20 minutes, and, although they are crucial, do not provide a complete literacy program. They should be incorporated in a classroom with storybook reading, oral language activities, learning about basic concepts of print, the functions of reading and writing, and opportunities to talk and write about experiences. Gillam and van Kleeck (1996) recommended that children participate in language intervention for other form, content, and use interactions at the same time they receive phonological awareness intervention.

Furthermore, O'Connor, Notari-Syverson, and Vadasy (1996) have demonstrated that phonological awareness intervention can be successfully implemented by kindergarten teachers in regular whole-group activities with group sizes determined by existing class sizes and with assistance from other adults drawn from normally available personnel. The classroom populations in their study included children with behavior disorders, mild mental retardation, and learning disabilities, as well as transition students (repeaters), and general education kindergarten students. They found that type of disability does not necessarily inhibit phonological growth when instruction is provided. However, they did point out, as did Torgeson, Wagner, and Rashotte (1994), that large and lasting differences in future reading performance of children with disabilities may require much more intense instruction than that delivered to large classroom groups.

Writing (Spelling)

Development of spelling abilities appears to be closely related to the development of expressive phonology. Normally developing children (Hoffman & Norris, 1989; Read, 1975; Temple, Nathan, & Burris, 1982; Weaver, 1988), phonologically delayed children (Clarke-Klein & Hodson, 1995), and children with learning disabilities (Smiley, 1977) evidence the use of phonological processes in their spelling errors.

Read (1971) was among the first to present evidence that indicated that children tacitly categorize speech sounds according to perceived phonemic similarities. His evidence was obtained through naturalistic studies of preschoolers' invented spellings and supported by experimental studies (e.g., Beers, 1974; Gerritz, 1974; Read, 1975) using various tests to elicit phonemic judgments from kindergartners and first graders who had not created original spellings. These studies suggested that children analyze and categorize sounds based on articulatory information and therefore may assign spelling based on these phonemic feature categories, that is, they spell similarly those phonemes that are articulated similarly. Of course, in standard English orthography such a logical system does not exist; rather, phoneme spellings, or **grapheme-phoneme correspondences**, are based on historical relationships (e.g., silent letters that once were not silent) or meaning relationships (e.g., *muscle* and *muscular*). It seems likely that children in early stages of reading and writing assume that spelling is based on pronunciation, and no provision is made for having them revise this assumption. At some point, children must learn to reject their own system of logical spelling and embrace the illogical standard orthography of English in which there are numerous options for spelling all vowels and many consonant sounds (see, for example, Table 4–1).

Essentially, it appears from Read's (1971, 1975) data that children begin with a knowledge of the traditional names for the letters of the alphabet. They then learn that a letter may spell a phoneme in its name (e.g., A spells /e/, or B spells /b/), and they attempt to write messages with this information. An obvious shortcoming in this system is that not all phonemes of English can be represented in letter names. It appears that two strategies are adopted to overcome this shortcoming. One involves asking adults for a spelling, thus standard spelling enters. The other strategy involves pairing each missing phoneme with one for which a spelling is known, evidently based on articulatory features. For example, /e/ (A) is easy, but what happens when the child wants to write /ɛ/ as in *wet*? Well, it appears that he or she decides very systematically to use the letter name that is most closely articulated like /ɛ/, and that is the letter name for A, thus the spelling for *wet* is

TABLE 4–1. Possible spellings of some American English phonemes.

Segment		***Options Available***
	Vowels	
Tense		
/i/	(b<u>ee</u>t)	16
/o/	(b<u>oa</u>t)	16
/e/	(b<u>ai</u>t)	16
/aɪ/	(b<u>i</u>te)	14
Lax		
/ɪ/	(b<u>i</u>t)	22
/ɛ/	(b<u>e</u>t)	13
/ʌ/	(b<u>u</u>t)	14
	Consonants	
/k/	(<u>k</u>ite)	13
/n/	(<u>n</u>ight)	6
/s/	(<u>s</u>ight)	10
/m/	(<u>m</u>ight)	6
/l/	(<u>l</u>ight)	9

Source: Data from *Phoneme-grapheme correspondences as cues to spelling improvement*, by P. R. Hanna, J. S. Hanna, R. E. Hodges, & E. H. Rudorf, 1966. Washington, DC: U.S. Department of Health, Education & Welfare.

WAT. As the reader may recall from Table 3–4, /e/ and /ɛ/ are both mid front vowels. Similar pairings occur for other phonemes, for example /i/ (E) and /ɪ/ (b*i*t), both high front vowels, thus the spelling of *BET* for *bit*. A teacher's telling this child to *listen* to the sound in *bit* is not the solution; in fact, it appears that the child is the better listener. Rather, it would seem that the child needs to *see* how this sound is written.

Another example from Read (1975) was children's use of CH and J to represent the spelling of /t/ and /d/ before /r/, resulting in spellings of CHRIE for *try* and JRAGIN for *dragon*. These spellings again appear to be based on features of articulation, that is, before /r/ in English, /t/ and /d/ are affricated and are thus articulated much like /č/ and /ǰ/. Ask yourself, as many first-grade and preschool children were asked, which words begin with the same sound as *truck*: *train*, *turkey*, or *chicken*? If the reader attends to articulatory features and ignores his or her knowledge of standard written orthography, he or she must respond that *train* and *chicken* are most like *truck*.

In an analysis of 619 spelling errors of third and fourth graders with learning and spelling disabilities, Smiley (1977) found evidence that some of these and other phonological strategies described by Read as typical of preschoolers and first graders may have still been present and were now interfering. Examples of these follow.

Vowel sounds, which are the most difficult, accounted for the most errors made by the children with spelling disabilities. Interestingly, very few vowel segments were represented as consonants, indicating that all of the subjects demonstrated a knowledge of vowels as a distinct category of spelling. The largest category of errors in long/tense vowels consisted of the use of the letter name strategy when another spelling was required, for example, in *beet*, *bait*, and the ending of *twenty*. In short/lax unrounded vowels, although /ɪ/ is rarely ever represented by the letter E, this spelling accounted for 60% of errors in spelling of /ɪ/, for example, BELD for *build*, SKEN for skin, WEMMEN for *women*. Similar to Read's (1975) data, the largest category of errors in spelling unstressed vowels was omission,for example, BOTL for *bottle*, PEPL for *people*, and TRN for *turn*.

In consonants, Read (1975) reported some interesting data on children's affrication. Although only three examples occurred in Smiley's (1977) data, Read's explanation of representing articulatory information may apply: TLIE for *July*, LACH for *large*, and CHILDCHEN for *children*. Again supporting the existence of Read's strategy of spelling based on articulatory features, the largest category of incorrect spellings of nasals was that of omission. This could be considered phonetically correct, as nasalization of the vowel is most accurately descriptive of what occurs. Examples include NUBER for *number*, FID for *find*, and EVEING for *evening*. The other most common error in nasals was substituting one nasal for another, again indicating some feature categorization: CLOWM for *clown*, TINES for *times*, and CLINBED for *climbed*.

Although no cases of children's spelling the intervocalic /t/ with a D occurred in Read's data, Smiley reported six cases of intervocalic /d/ spelled with a /t/, for example, SUMBOTE for *somebody*, EVERBOTE for *everybody*, and EVREBATY for *everybody*. This representation may indicate an overgeneralization of the standard spelling of T for the intervocalic flap /D/.

Alternations involving voicing that are not represented in standard spelling are found in the past and plural morphemes. Although no errors occurred in Smiley's data for plural voicing errors, such errors did occur for the past tense, for example, LOOKET and LOOKT for *looked*, JUMPT and JUMP'T for jumped, CLIMBD for *climbed*, and SKARD for *scared*. These representations illustrate the stages of morphophonemic development of the past tense spelling presented by Read.

These examples and others indicate that some of Read's spelling strategies based on articulatory features are present in third and fourth graders with learning disabilities. Enough data exist to indicate a possible inference of this type, particularly in a younger sample and/or even in a more significantly disabled population.

However, it is interesting to note that the most consistent pattern (63%) of spelling errors overall was the substitution of another possible spelling in place of a standard spelling. These data suggest that most children with spelling disabilities are able to distinguish between phonological segments and have even learned appropriate possible spellings for these segments by the end of third grade. However, even by the end of fourth grade, these subjects are not able to accurately select from the possible spellings they have apparently learned. The majority of errors are, in fact, made on the segments with the largest number of options available. This has implications for a de-emphasis on phonemic information and the inclusion of a strong visual memory strategy, that is, remember what this word looks like. Indeed, further investigations with these children indicated a lack of knowledge in what American English words look like. This suggests a need for instruction in remembering what words look like, as well as some fairly consistent orthographic rules such as "i before e except after c," or the longer version, "i before e except after c, and in sounding like A as in neighbor, veil, and weigh." Weird, eh?

Phonological awareness is fundamental to spelling. Although the importance of the relationship of phonological awareness to spelling ability cannot and should not be denied, it alone does not appear to be sufficient for spelling proficiency. Spelling requires that words be represented in detail in the speller's mind to be retrieved during the act of spelling. In the absence of these representations, poor spellers resort to a purely phonetic spelling strategy, thereby increasing spelling errors (Clarke-Klein, 1994). See Figure 4–1 for an example of possible spellings as well as an illustration of the nasal omission rule described by Read (1975).

In conclusion, based on the literature on phonological awareness, Blachman (1994a) has urged professionals to continue supporting the inclusion of code-based strategies in beginning literacy programs. However, she has also pointed out that no one has suggested that code-based strategies preclude the use of meaning-based strategies and has noted that Vellutino (1991), in a summary of research on code-oriented versus whole language-oriented controversy, pointed out that "the

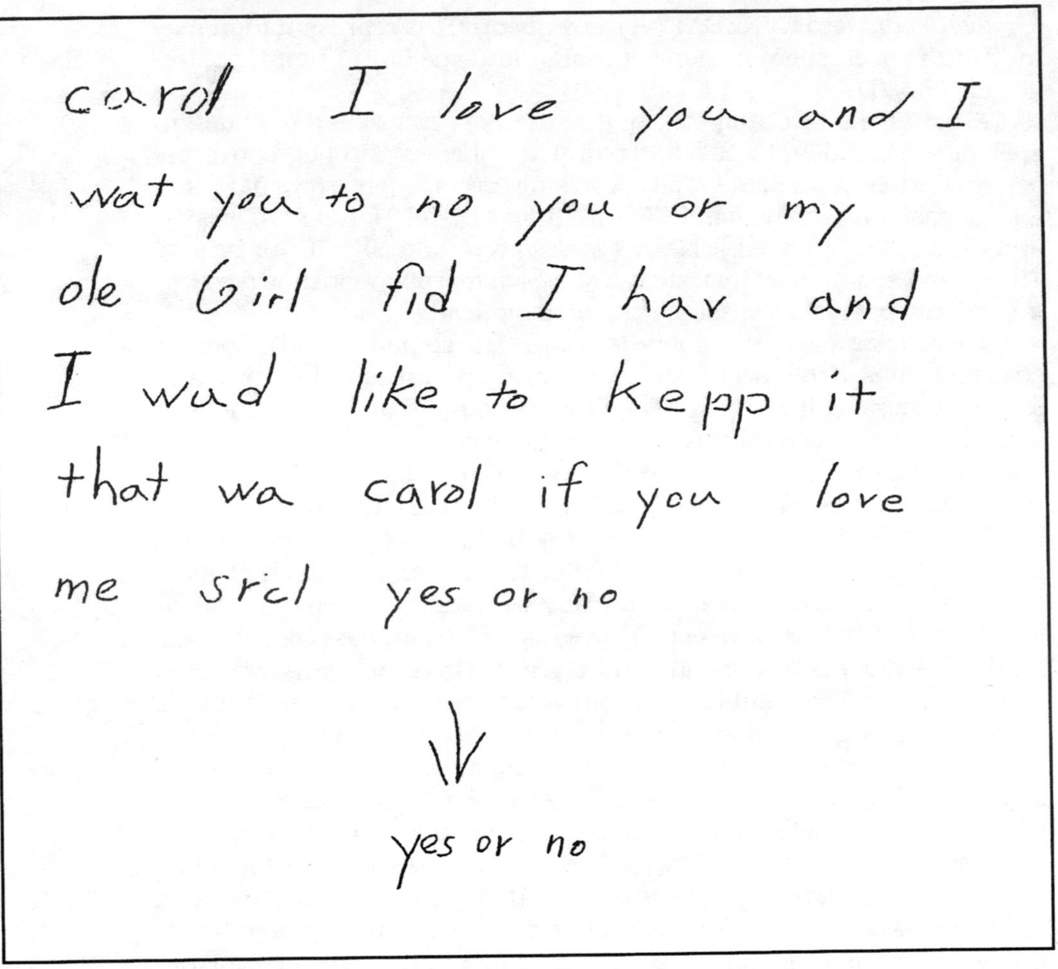

carol I love you and I
wat you to no you or my
ole Girl fid I har and
I wad like to kepp it
that wa carol if you love
me srcl yes or no

yes or no

Figure 4–1. An example of young children's spelling.

research supports a balanced approach" (p. 442). This is especially important when one considers that children with problems in the area of phonology are likely to have problems in the areas of content and use as well.

✓ SUMMARY CHECKLIST

☐ **Analysis**
Atypical Development
Phonological Awareness

☐ **Intervention**
Speaking
Reciprocal Teaching
Scaffolding
Cloze Procedure
Reading
Phonological Awareness Training
Rhyming
Blending
Segmenting
Writing (Spelling)
Grapheme-Phoneme Correspondence

CHAPTER

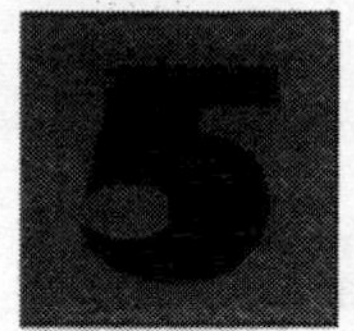

MORPHOLOGY AND SYNTAX: BASIC CONCEPTS

DEFINING MORPHOLOGY AND SYNTAX

Morphology is the study of minimal units of meaning, or **morphemes**, and the rules governing their use. **Syntax** refers to the rules of word function and word order; it encompasses the rules for forming phrases, clauses, and sentences with words. A morphemic analysis of language cannot be successfully concluded without at least stepping into its syntactic elements. At the lexical unit level where morphemes are words and their bound affixes, the process is fairly straightforward, as is seen in the following discussion. As we begin to consider word classes, or parts of speech, the demarcation becomes less clear. For example, it is only when syntactic rules for combining words are used that the unit of meaning *dog* functions as a noun that is the subject of the sentence *The dog drank a bowl of water*. Grammatical words such as prepositions, articles, and conjunctions are practically devoid of meaning without syntax. For this reason, we do not attempt to separate the following sections into morphology and syntax beyond the word level. This tack will also be apparent in Chapter 6 when we examine how children develop morphology and syntax.

Morphemes that have meaning and can stand alone are **free morphemes,** or words; others that have meaning only when they are attached to another morpheme are **bound morphemes.** A free morpheme may be more familiar to many readers as the **root** word, whereas bound morphemes take the form of an **affix**, that is, prefixes or suffixes. Although some languages have infixes, English does not generally insert a morpheme into the middle of other morphemes. Bound morphemes in English are of two types: **derivational,** which result in a meaning change ({un} + {happy}) or word class change ({happy} + {ness}), and **inflectional,** which add grammatical information ({cat} + {s}). (Braces are often used to indicate morphemes.) All inflectional affixes are native to English, however, many derivational affixes are borrowings from other languages, in particular Latin and Greek (Parker & Riley, 1994). The eight inflectional morphemes in English are used to mark plural, possessive, comparative, superlative, present, past, past participle, and present participle. Because morphemes are meaningful units having more or less constant meaning associated with more or less constant form (Parker & Riley, 1994), it is often useful to represent them by a category, for example, {PLU} rather than specific form, for example, {/s/}, {/z/}, or {/əz/}. The rules that govern which form is to be used are generally based on distinctive features of preceding or following phonemes. Note that the unvoiced {/s/} form of the plural follows {cat}, which ends in an unvoiced consonant, whereas the voiced form {/z/} follows {dog}, which ends in a voiced consonant. The use of a categorical representation also makes it easier to express irregular forms of morphemes that do not occur as affixes but rather change the form of the word to which they are attached, such as the plural of *woman*, that is, *women* = {woman} + {PLU}. Representations of inflectional morphemes and examples of each are shown in Table 5–1.

It should be noted that these inflections are also governed by word class. The plural and possessive are attached only to nouns, the comparative and superlative to adjectives, and the present, past, past participle, and present participle to verbs. All inflectional affixes are suffixes, except for irregular cases (as in *women*); derivational affixes may be either.

In isolating morphemes, it is important to recall that a morpheme recurs with more or less constant meaning and more or less constant

THE FAMILY CIRCUS
By Bil Keane
GOIN' TO GRANDMA'S IS A LOT FUNNER THAN GOIN' TO SCHOOL!
NOT FUNNER, BILLY. YOU MEAN "GOIN' TO GRANDMA'S IS A LOT MORE FUN THAN GOIN' TO SCHOOL." NOW LET'S HEAR YOU SAY IT CORRECTLY.
GOIN' TO GRANDMA'S WAS A LOT FUNNER BUT NOW IT SEEMS JUST LIKE SCHOOL.
4-17

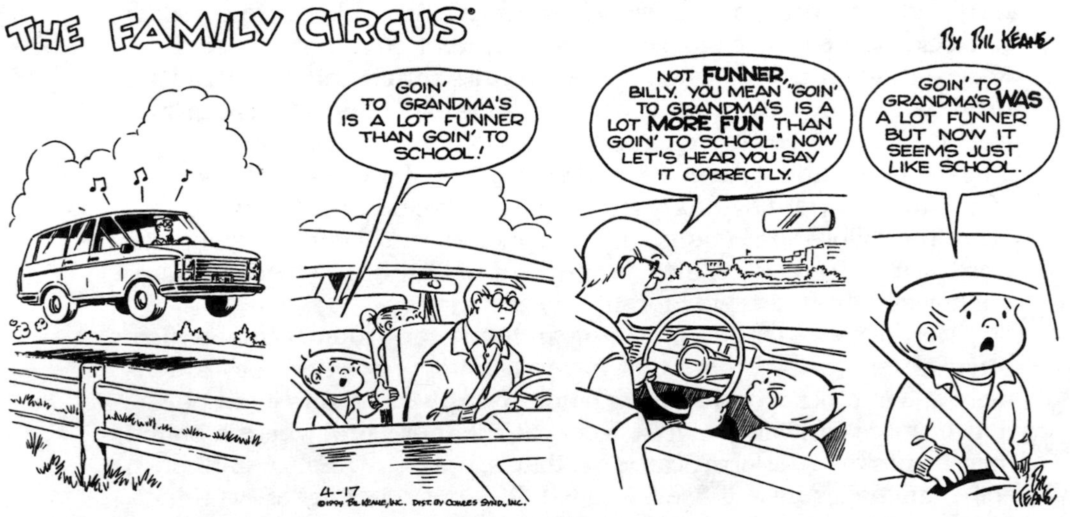

TABLE 5–1. Inflectional morphemes.

Inflection	*Representation*	*Example*
Plural	{girl} + {PLU}	girls
Possessive	{girl} + {POSS}	girl's
Comparative	{big} + {COMP}	bigger
Superlative	{big} + {SUP}	biggest
Present	{talk} + {PRES}	talks
Past	{talk} + {PAST}	talked
Past Participle	{give} + {PAST PART}	given
Present Participle	{give} + (PRES PART}	giving

form. This means that if a sequence of phonemes is a morpheme, we should be able find another word in which it occurs with the same meaning. For example, in the word *unhappiness*, {un} meaning "not" also occurs in *unlikely*, {happy} occurs by itself and in *happiness* with the same meaning, and {ness} meaning "a state of being" also occurs in *madness*. Thus, *unhappiness* consists of three morphemes: {un} + {happy} + {ness}. In isolating, or segmenting, morphemes, one should not be left with a uniquely occurring morpheme, or with a morpheme unrelated in meaning to its use in the present word. Although both *under* and *stand* occur elsewhere, they do not occur with any relationship to the meaning of *understand*, therefore *understand* is one morpheme.

Morphemes with common meaning may also take different forms, as noted in the forms of the plural inflection which has three phonological representations. This occurs with derivational morphemes as well. Although {ness} is used with both {happy} and {mad} to express "a state of being," consider "a state of being" for generous (*generosity*) or accurate (*accuracy*). However, these morphemes do recur in other words with the same meaning, as in *sincerity* and *democracy*. Knowledge of morphemes allows us to coin new words when needed, for example the increasingly familiar use of *wellness* for the "state of being well." And then there is "*with-it-ness*," a criterion used to evaluate beginning teachers in the state of Florida. And what about *clueless*?

To make morphology even more interesting, two different morphemes may have the same phonological representation. For example, the {er} in *teacher* is not the same as the {er} in *shorter*, the first use has the meaning "one who," whereas the second is the inflection for the comparative {COMP}. And of course, the *ers* in *butter* and *flicker* are not morphemes at all.

Compound words are another source of potential confusion. Some compound words have meaning derived from their parts, whereas others have meaning unrelated to their component parts. Although a *rattlesnake* is a snake that rattles, and a *girlfriend* is a friend who is a girl, a *hotdog* is not any kind of dog nor is a *mushroom* a room. Furthermore, the importance of sequence can be observed in *housecat* versus *cathouse*. And idioms are certainly more than the sum of their parts, for example, John *kicked the bucket*. The figurative meaning of these words as a whole indicate that John is now quite incapable of literally kicking a bucket for he has died.

Throughout a morphological analysis, it is important to keep in mind that a morpheme is not equivalent to a syllable. In fact, a morpheme may have one syllable as in {dog} or as many as five as in {hippopotamus}. Morphemes may have one sound, as {a} in *amoral* and *asexual* or as many as are in {hippopotamus}, and one syllable may contain two or more morphemes, for example, *cats* ({cat} + {PLU}) and *cats'* ({cat} + {PLU} + {POSS}).

The goal of a morphological analysis of words for the student of language development and language disorders is to determine the rules that speakers follow for forming words in English, in order to examine children's use of them. This is not to be confused with **etymology**, or history, of words. For example, Parker and Riley (1994) pointed out that although the word *hamburger* is historically derived from "a city in Germany," {Hamburg} + {er}, with the meaning "originating from" as in *New Englander* or *Southerner*, its structure may be different in the minds of today's speakers. This is illustrated by the use of *burger* alone ("burger and fries") or in combination with other words, for example, *shrimpburger*, *veggieburger*, *cheeseburger*, or even *Mexiburger*. Today's use may also lead to some confusion, as evidenced in this Family Circus cartoon.

THE FAMILY CIRCUS.
By Bil Keane
YES THEY ARE!
ARE!
AREN'T!
THEY ARE, TOO!
ARE NOT!
NOT!
BIL KEANE

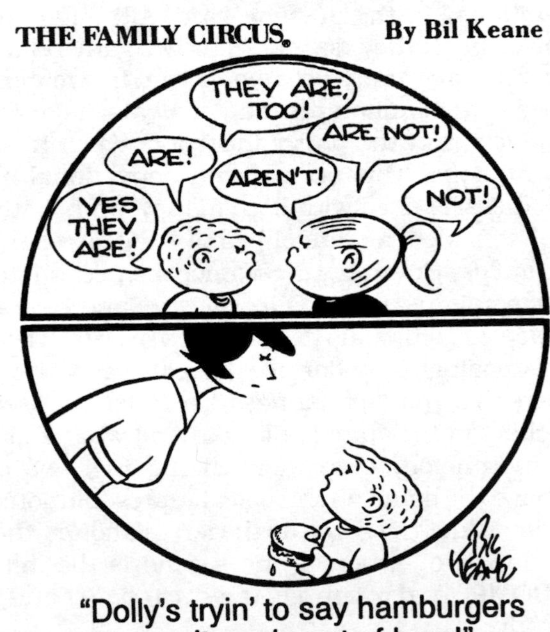

"Dolly's tryin' to say hamburgers aren't made out of ham!"

WORD CLASSES

As we have just seen, inflectional morphemes affect particular classes or functions of words (e.g., plurals are attached to nouns only), and derivational morphemes often change a word class (e.g., an adjective, *happy*, is changed to a noun, *happiness*). Also, in any language, a set of syntactic or grammatical rules dictate which word classes can fill which slots in sentences. Word classes are more traditionally known as parts of speech. In English, an ordinary simple sentence is made up of a noun phrase and a verb phrase (sometimes written as the Phrase Structure Rule S → NP VP). Following this procedure, a noun phrase may be made up of several elements or word classes; and a verb phrase may be made up of several elements. This noun phrase is sometimes called the complete subject and the verb phrase, the complete predicate.

Noun Phrase

Noun

A noun phrase may contain a noun (NP → N). A **noun** can be the name of a person, a place, a thing or animal, or an idea. There are **proper nouns** (specific persons, places, brand names, or creative works) and **common nouns** (nonspecific entities); nouns may vary in **gender** (masculine, feminine, or neuter), **number** (singular, plural or collective, i.e., a group that is considered singular such as *team* or *family*). **Count nouns** can be counted and pluralized (as in one *dog*, two *dogs*); **mass nouns**, on the other hand, are considered indivisible into smaller countable parts and cannot usually be pluralized (as in *salt* and *fruit*). **Noun inflections** which can be attached to nouns include the plural and the possessive markers.

Determiners

A noun phrase may contain a determiner with the noun (NP → Det N). Determiners may be placed before some nouns to indicate if the noun refers to a particular person, thing, animal, or object or if it refers to an unspecified one. One type of determiner is an **article.** Articles may be **indefinite** (*a, an*) or **definite** (*the*). Another type of determiner that can occur in a noun phrase is a **demonstrative,** which points out specific persons or things in relationship to location. Demonstratives also take different forms for singular and plural, for example:

this toy **these** toys
that toy **those** toys

One other determiner that may occur before a noun is a **qualifier**, which serves to qualify the noun in some way, as in:

some boys	**any** boys
all girls	**few** girls
many teachers	**no** teachers

Pronoun

A noun phrase may contain a pronoun (NP → PN). A **pronoun** is a word used in place of one or more nouns or a noun phrase, as in:

Paul likes to sing. **He** practices everyday.

There are various kinds of pronouns. **Personal pronouns** change in form based on number, gender, person, and the functions they have, that is, case (to be elaborated on in the next section).

Subjective Pronouns. These function as subjects: **I** love Paul.

1st person	singular: I	plural: we
2nd person	singular: you	plural: you
3rd person	singular: he, she, it	plural: they

Objective Pronouns. These function as objects: Paul loves **me**.

1st person	singular: me	plural: us
2nd person	singular: you	plural: you
3rd person	singular: him, her, it	plural: them

Reflexive Pronouns. These pronouns are used with reflexive verbs: I cut **myself**.

1st person	singular: myself	plural: ourselves

B.C. by johnny hart

pro·noun
WILEY'S DICTIONARY
4·14

A NOUN THAT HAS GIVEN UP ITS AMATEUR STATUS.
WILEY'S DICTIONARY
hart

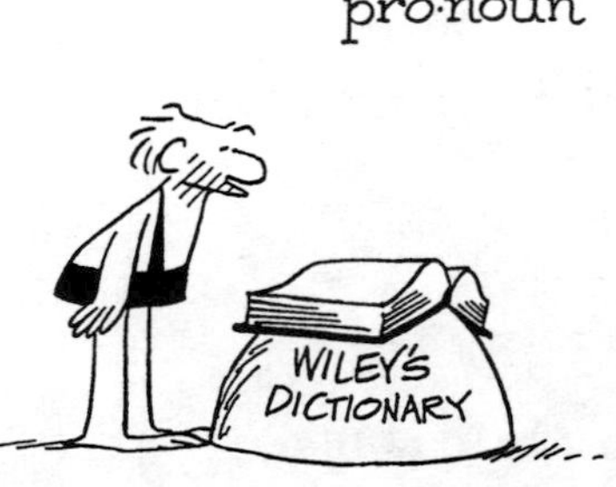

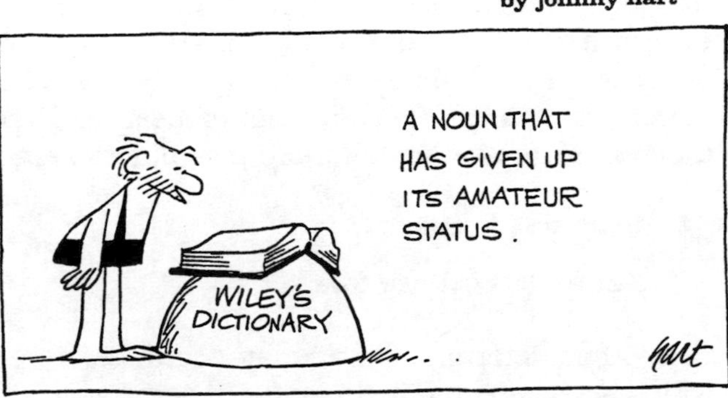

2nd person	singular: yourself	plural: yourselves
3rd person	singular: himself	plural: themselves
	herself	
	itself	

Possessive Pronouns. Possessive pronouns show possession: **Yours** is on the way.

1st person	singular: mine	plural: ours
2nd person	singular: yours	plural: yours
3rd person	singular: his, hers, its	plural: theirs

Another set of **possessive pronouns** (note the differences) are used before nouns (as adjectives) to tell whose: **My** book is new.

1st person	singular: my	plural: our
2nd person	singular: your	plural: your
3rd person	singular: his, her, its	plural: their

Interrogative Pronouns. These pronouns are used in questions and vary according to their referent. If the referent is a thing: **What** is that? or **Which** do you want? If the referent is a person, the pronoun is also marked for case: **Who** is that? **Whom** did you call? In informal use, the case marker for objective is often omitted: **Who** did you call?

Relative Pronouns. Relative pronouns are used in embedded clauses (to be elaborated on in a later section) and have many forms similar to interrogative pronouns.

The man **who** sang is my brother.

The dog **which** barked is mine.

The dog **that** barked is mine.

The book **which** I read is great.

The book I read is great.

The person to **whom** I spoke said so.

The person I spoke to said so. (Informal use)

Demonstrative Pronouns. These pronouns indicate a specific referent(s) without naming it (them). As with demonstratives, location and number are marked:

That is mine. **Those** are mine.

This is mine. **These** are mine.

Indefinite Pronouns. Indefinite pronouns refer to unknown or general referents:

Someone was here. **Nobody** was here.

Table 5–2 illustrates just how indefinite these pronouns can be.

Existential Pronouns. Existential pronouns consisting of *it* and *there* are referred to as sentence trappings, expletives, or even "dummy" subjects (Wardhaugh, 1995) as they do not operate in the usual manner of noun replacement. Their use is purely grammatical and they have no meaning.

It's raining, and **there**'s a child outside.

Adjective

A noun phrase may contain an adjective (NP → {Det} Adj N). The brackets here indicate that a determiner may or may not be present. An **adjective** describes (modifies) a noun. A **descriptive adjective** tells what kind: a **large** house. An **interrogative adjective** asks which: **What** book? **Which** book? **Whose** book?

Adjective Inflections. Adjective inflections include the comparative and superlative forms. Sally is nice, but Jane is nic**er**, and Jo is nic**est**.

Verb Phrase

Verb

A verb phrase must contain a verb (VP → V). A **verb** indicates an action, mental state, or condition. The action can be physical (*run, walk, hit*) or mental (*dream, think, believe*). Verbs are the most varied and complex

TABLE 5–2. Indefinite pronoun usage.

A LITTLE STORY

This is a story about four people named Everybody, Somebody, Anybody, and Nobody. There was an important job to be done and Everybody was sure that Somebody would do it. Anybody could have done it, but Nobody did it.

Somebody got angry about that because it was Everybody's job.

Everybody thought Anybody could do it, but Nobody realized that Everybody wouldn't do it.

It ended up that Everybody blamed Somebody when Nobody did what Anybody could have done.

Source: Unknown

of the word classes and are an excellent indicator of a child's mastery of the grammatical rules of language (Lund & Duchan, 1993). Several types of verbs and several inflections exist.

Verb Inflections. Verb inflections include markers for the past tense, present participle, past participle, and the simple present tense only for the regular third person singular (e.g., she run**s**).

Lexical Verbs. These are verbs that add content to the utterance. They indicate the action or mental state of the subject.

The dog **ran**.	The ball **hit** the wall.
I **think** too much.	The monkey **threw** the banana.

There are approximately 200 irregular verb forms in the English language, although many are archaic or used infrequently; however, irregular past tense verbs are among the most frequently used verbs in English (Bybee & Slobin, 1982).

Verb Particles. Some verbs have **verb particles** as part of the verb. Verb particles add further content to the verb. An interesting aspect of the verb particle is a rule that allows it to be placed before or after the noun (direct object) following it, but requires its movement when a pronoun is used. (An asterisk [*] marks structures that are not acceptable to the proficient English speaker.)

I **picked up** the kids. I **picked** the kids **up**.	I **checked out** the book. I **checked** the book **out**.
*I **picked up** them. I **picked** them **up**.	*I **checked out** it. I **checked** it **out**.

In 1996, James Kilpatrick, a nationally syndicated columnist, wrote of a gentleman in Washington state who made a list of 118 *up verbs* he had attained in a week. The list included: *start up, fill up, wake up, back up, do up, fix up, get up, give up, wash up*. You finish it. Note that the *up* is an integral part of the verb in all cases.

Copulas. This special class of verbs is also referred to as linking verbs (VP → Cop). The most common copula verb is the verb *to be* with its form depending on the subject and the tense.

Mary **is** a girl. Jeff **was** angry. The apples **are** rotten.

Pseudocopulas. Other verbs that operate as copulas are verbs of the senses (*feel, taste*), or appearance (*appear, look, seem*), or change of duration (*become, stay, remain*) (Lund & Duchan, 1993). By substituting the verb *to be*, it can be seen that only a subtle difference in meaning is present.

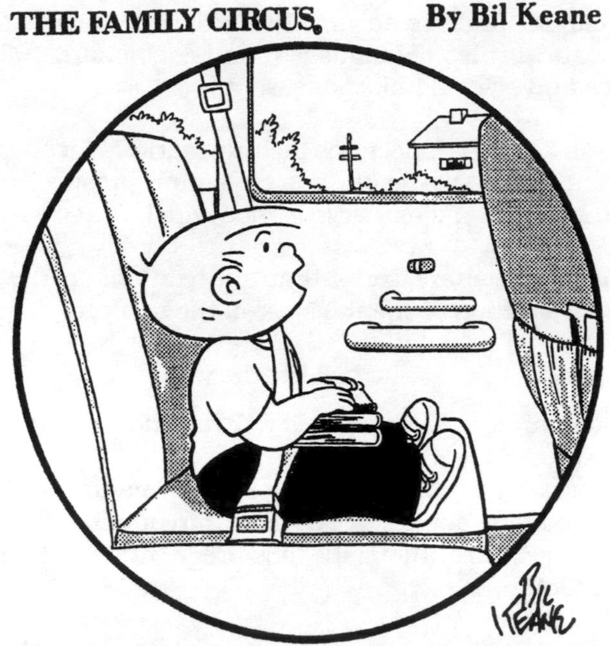

"In the car we buckle up, but at school I hafta buckle down."

This food **tastes** great.	This food is great.
He **looks** sick.	He is sick.
She **remains** the same.	She is the same.

Auxiliary Verbs. These verbs are also known as helping verbs, as they are used with another main verb and indicate tense or mood of the verb (VP → Aux V). The verbs *to be* and *to have* (in their various forms) are used to indicate tense change. The *emphatic do* is used to add emphasis.

Takemi **is** going to school.

Paul **has** lost his place again.

He **does** want to go.

All of these verbs can also be used as main verbs, but they are not then in the helping or auxiliary role. The emphatic *do* is also used in questions and negatives.

Do you want to go? I **do**n't want to go.

Modals. These are auxiliaries that are used to indicate the mood or attitude of the speaker.

We **should** go. We **can** go.

We **shall** go. We **must** go.

Wardhaugh (1995) declared that modal verbs are deficient in their inflectional morphology and are sometimes referred to as *defective verbs. Will, shall, may,* and *can* have irregular past forms (*would, should, might,* and *could*) and no other variants. *Must* and *ought* have only those forms.

Many auxiliary verbs can be contracted, or shortened. Most of these **contractions** involve the deletion of part of the auxiliary.

I am ⇨ I'm   you are ⇨ you're   she is ⇨ she's

I have ⇨ I've   you have ⇨ you've   we have ⇨ we've

Verb Tenses. Using auxiliary verbs, main verbs, and verb inflections, many tenses are possible in English, as can be seen by the sample in Table 5–3. Bill Bryson (1990), author of the best seller *Mother Tongue*, pointed out that English, instead of having a lot of verb forms (e.g., Latin has 120 inflections), has only five, but we employ them in lots of ways by making use of auxiliary verbs.

Adverbs

A verb phrase may contain an adverb (VP → Adv V). An adverb modifies a verb, an adjective, or another adverb. As an adverb may modify an adjective, it may also occur in a noun phrase (e.g., A *very* bright student). Adverbs may indicate:

Quantity: Mary sleeps **little**.

Time: He will come **soon**.

Place: He left his book **behind**.

TABLE 5–3. Verb tenses in English.

Mary **studies.**	Present
Mary **is studying.**	Present Progressive
Mary **does study.**	Present Emphatic
Mary **has studied.**	Present Perfect
Mary **studied.**	Past
Mary **was studying.**	Past Progressive
Mary **did study.**	Past Emphatic
Mary **had studied.**	Past Perfect
Mary **will study.**	Future
Mary **will be studying.**	Future Progressive
Mary **will have studied.**	Future Perfect

WHY DO WE HAVE TO LEARN THIS STUFF ANYHOW?
IT'S GOOD FOR YOUR MENTAL DISCIPLINE, SKYLER.
AND IT'LL HELP YOU IN LATER LIFE...
RIGHT.
IN CASE I LAND A JOB IN A VERB CONJUGATION PLANT.
9-27

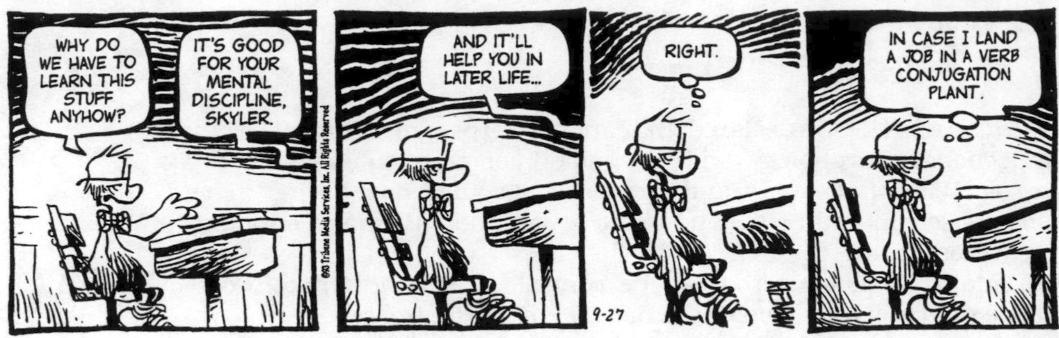

Intensity: Bob **really** wants the part.

Manner: Bill dances **beautifully**.

Adverb Inflections. Inflections for adverbs include the **comparative** and **superlative** forms. *Sally runs fast, but Jessica runs fast**er**, and Jo runs the fast**est**.*

Prepositional Phrase

A prepositional phrase may occur in a noun phrase (NP → {Det} N PP) and/or a verb phrase (VP → {Aux} V PP). A prepositional phrase is made up of a preposition and a noun phrase (PP → Prep NP): *The boy **on the hill** fell **in a hole**.*

Prepositions

A **preposition** shows the relationship between a noun and another word. It is often related to position or location. Information that prepositions may indicate include:

Spatial: The books are **on** the table.

Temporal: We will go **after** dinner.

Manner: We did it **with** good intentions.

Instrumental: I hit it **with** a hammer.

Accompaniment: He's **with** his friend.

A comprehensive list of prepositions is included in Table 5–4.

Noun Phrase

A prepositional phrase also contains a noun phrase, which has already been described.

TABLE 5–4. Prepositions.

about	
aboard	except
above	
across	for
after	from
against	
along	in
amid	into
among	
around	near
at	
	of
before	off
behind	on
below	
beneath	to
between	toward
beyond	
by	under
	up
down	upon
during	
	with
	within
	without

Source: Unknown

Other Word Classes

Two other word classes are traditionally included in a list of parts of speech.

Conjunctions

A **conjunction** joins words or groups of words and is not usually included in a description of a simple sentence, but will be discussed more in depth later.

Rashad plays basketball **and** tennis.

We can go now **or** later.

The children are happy **because** he is here.

Interjections

An **interjection** stands apart as an exclamation, starter, or filler: **Yes**, I want to go. It's, **like, you know**, over.

SIMPLE SENTENCE SYNTAX

Syntax includes the rules for the order of words as sentences are generated with the Phrase Structure Rule S → NP VP. Rules of syntax also include the possible functions of the word classes as they are included in our sentences. Simple sentences are constructed from a rather small set of basic structural patterns which include most of the functions of word classes. Table 5–5 outlines most of the basic structural patterns in English. The functions of the word classes are defined and further illustrated here.

Word Class Functions

Each word class may function in different ways in a sentence. A noun may function as a subject, direct object, indirect object, object of a preposition, or a noun complement; an adjective may function as a simple adjective or an adjective complement and an adverb as a simple adverb or adverbial complement. A prepositional phrase may function as either an adjective or an adverb.

Subject

The person, place, or thing that performs the action in a sentence is called the **subject.** The subject is a noun or pronoun and may occur in many different positions in the sentence. The subject answers the question "who or what?" about the verb in the sentence. For example, in the first sentence below, *Karl* is the answer to the question, "***Who speaks*** French?"; therefore, *Karl* is the subject of the sentence.

Karl speaks French.

Tom and Mary Lou are coming tonight.

Did **the game** start on time?

Looking in the window was a little **girl**.

The **boys** were talking while Jerryll was performing.

Direct Object

The **direct object** receives the action of the verb or shows the result of that action directly. A direct object is a noun or pronoun and answers the question "what" or "whom" asked after the subject and verb. In the first sentence below, *the book* is the answer to the question, "Paul ***reads what***?"; therefore, *the book* is the direct object of the sentence.

Paul reads **the book**.

They invited **Beverly and Mike**.

TABLE 5–5. Basic simple sentence patterns.

Word Classes	*Word Class Functions*
noun + verb 1. Ice melts.	Subject, predicate
noun1 + verb + noun2 2. Horses eat oats.	Subject, predicate, direct object
noun1 + copula + noun2 3. Oranges are fruit.	Subject, copula, noun complement
noun + copula + adjective 4. Oranges are sweet.	Subject, copula, adjective complement
noun + copula + adverb 5. Oranges are here.	Subject, copula, adverbial complement
noun + copula V + adjective 6. Oranges taste good.	Subject, copula verb, adjective complement
noun + verb + adverb 7. Oranges cost alot.	Subject, predicate, adverb.
noun1 + verb + noun2 + noun3 8. Dave gave Cathy oranges.	Subject, predicate, indirect object, direct object
noun1 + verb + noun2 + noun3 9. FAU named Kamal president.	Subject, predicate, direct object, object-noun complement.
noun1 +V + noun2 + adjective 10. Exams make LePing nervous.	Subject, predicate, direct object, object-adjective complement.
noun1 +V + noun2 + adverb 11. Meg made LynnEllen late.	Subject, predicate, direct object, object-adverbial complement
noun1 +V + prep + art + noun2 12. Becki ran down the hall.	Subject, predicate, preposition, object of Prep.with PP (Adv)
N1 +V + Art + N2 + Prep + N3 13. Lois spilled a cup of tea.	Subject, predicate, preposition, object of Prep. with PP (Adj)

Indirect Object

The **indirect object** also receives the action of the verb; however, it receives the action indirectly. The indirect object is a noun or pronoun and generally occurs before the direct object. It answers the question "to whom" or "to what" asked *after* the verb. In the first sentence below, *Lewis* is the answer to the question, "Rick ***wrote to whom***?"; therefore, *Lewis* is the indirect object of the sentence.

Rick wrote **Lewis** a letter.

Martha gave **her** the answer.

Nahomie mailed **the customer** a receipt.

Object of a Preposition

The **object of a preposition** receives the action of the verb indirectly through a preposition. It is a noun or pronoun and answers a question made up of the "preposition + what or whom" asked *after* the verb. In the first sentence below, *tree* is the answer to the question, "Ron hid ***behind what***?"; therefore, *tree* is the object of the preposition.

Ron hid behind the **tree**.

Lou came with **Nadaige**.

The dog ran after **the cat**.

Complements

A **complement** is a word or group of words that completes a predicate by describing, or complementing, the subject, or sometimes the object. A complement generally occurs after a copula or implied copula. Complements may be nouns, adjectives, or adverbs.

Subject Complements. These complete the subject and add new information about the subject.

Nehemiah is **happy**. (adjective complement)

The coach was **a science teacher**. (noun complement)

Michael is **here**. (adverb complement)

He seems **happy**. (adjective complement)

Object Complements. These complete the object and add new information about the object. It is as if a copula were between the object and the complement as in "It made his fingers *to be* dirty."

It made his fingers **dirty**. (Object-adjective complement)

I'd call him **a hero**. (Object-noun complement)

Sonia made him **late**. (Object-adverb complement)

When subjects/objects and complements are reversed, there is no change in the meaning, although it may not always sound right. For example, the sentence *John is happy* could be reversed to read *Happy is John* with no meaning change.

Prepositional Phrases

Prepositional phrases (PP), made up of a preposition and a noun phrase, can function as adjectives or as adverbs.

He dropped a box **of books**. (PP as adjective)

Tiffany ran **to the store**. (PP as adverb)

SIMPLE SENTENCE MODIFICATIONS

What we have discussed thus far is a simple sentence formation that contains a basic subject-verb-object (S-V-O) order. In fact, what simple Phrase Structure Rules (S → NP VP) generate are **SAAD sentences**, that is, simple, affirmative, active, declarative sentences. The competent speaker of English is aware that there are more complex sentences used within the language, and these more complex variations of the simple sentences will be discussed later in this chapter. First, there are also related variations of these affirmative, active, declarative simple sentences that can be formed through the use of specific syntactic rules.

Negative

Simple sentences can be either affirmative or negative. The purpose (i.e., the pragmatic use) of the negative is to deny or reject an affirmative statement. The simple syntactic negative usually involves the insertion of *not* into the sentence and may also require the insertion of an emphatic-*do* auxiliary verb (in the negative and past tense forms) and the movement of past and present markers.

The cat is cute. ⇨ The cat is **not** cute.

The cat runs fast. ⇨ The cat **does not run** fast.

The cat is running fast. ⇨ The cat is **not** running fast.

The cat ran fast. ⇨ The cat **did not run** fast.

Negative forms of the verbs may also be contracted, or shortened. The regular form of **contractions** involves deleting the vowel in the not, as in *don't, doesn't, isn't. Will not,* however, becomes *won't.*

Passive

Simple sentences can be either active or passive, referred to as active and passive voice. A sentence is in the **active voice** when it expresses an action performed by the subject. The purpose of the **passive voice** is to place the emphasis on the receiver of the action by moving it to subject position. The passive is a complicated syntactic structure in English, requiring considerable rearrangement of the elements within the basic sentence (Lee, 1974). The passive requires the movement of the object, the addition of an auxiliary verb with the past participle form of the verb, and the addition of a prepositional phrase with the subject as the object. The speaker also has the option of deleting the prepositional phrase if the information is not needed in the context of its use.

The dog chases the ball. ⇨ The ball **is chased by the dog**.

The dog lost the ball. ⇨ The ball **was lost**.

To quote one of Richard Lederer's (1987) students, "A passive verb is when the subject is the sufferer, as in "*I am loved.*" (p. 4)

Interrogative

A simple sentence can be declarative or interrogative. The **declarative** form is used to make a statement; the **interrogative** is used to ask a question. There are several types of questions in English.

Yes/No Question. The **Yes/No Question** simply calls for a yes/no response. One way to ask a Yes/No question is through rising **intonation**, that is, suprasegmentals or paralanguage, as in *It's a brown dog*?

The Yes/No Question may also require syntactic changes involving an interrogative reversal of the subject and the auxiliary verb. This may require the addition of an auxiliary verb, again the emphatic-*do*, and the movement of the present or past tense markers.

Andie will finish. ⇨ **Will Andie** finish?

The dog likes cats. ⇨ **Does the dog like** cats?

Tag Questions. Tag questions also require a yes/no response in the form of verification of a statement. Tag questions may simply add a tag such as *right*, *huh*, or *okay* to the end of a statement (You have a new dog, **huh**?). Other tag questions involve an auxiliary verb that is either affirmative or negative in contrast to the statement.

You do have a dog. ⇨ You do have a dog, **don't you**?

You don't have a dog. ⇨ You don't have a dog, **do you**?

Ernie has a son. ⇨ Ernie has a son, **hasn't he**?

OR (more likely)

Ernie has a son. ⇨ Ernie has a son, **doesn't he**?

WH-Question. The **WH-Question** asks for more information. Generally, the question begins with a word that specifies the type of information that is being requested. These words include *who, what, where, when, why,* and *how*. Again the emphatic-*do* is often added, and past and present markers are moved.

Roxanne wants someone. ⇨ **Who does** Roxanne want?

Troy wants something. ⇨ **What** does Troy want?

Lois went somewhere. ⇨ **Where** did Lois go?

Ebony goes sometimes. ⇨ **When** does Ebony go?

Carolyn did it for a reason. ⇨ **Why** did Carolyn do it?

Cody plays the game somehow. ⇨ **How** does Cody play?

Imperative

Simple sentences may be imperative instead of declarative. The **imperative** is used to make a command and omits the subject (2nd person) to do so. The reader may remember these as "you-understood" statements.

You do it. ⇨ **Do** it.

You go first. ⇨ **Go** first.

You take the test. ⇨ **Take** the test.

With all of the preceding variations, we still have only simple sentences. In most communication, the speaker combines simple sentences in a variety of ways to make his or her intentions known. Each of these combinations of sentences is generated through a set of syntactic rules, which will be examined next.

COMPOUND AND COMPLEX SENTENCE SYNTAX

The combination of simple sentences into more complex structures involves reduction, addition, and rearrangement of information similar to some of the processes already observed. For example, contractions involved a reduction of information, negatives and WH-Questions involved the addition of words, and questions sometimes required the rearrangement of sentence elements (interrogative reversals). Some of the most common structures are discussed here.

Conjoined Clauses

Conjoining involves making one sentence out of two or more.

Coordination

Coordination is the conjoining of similar syntactic elements, such as words, phrases, and clauses. Clauses may be conjoined by the addition of coordinating conjunctions resulting in clauses of equal status. Traditional grammar texts refer to these clauses as independent clauses as they can both stand alone. Common coordinating conjunctions include *and, but, or,* and *either/or.*

Iris works days. Rufus works nights. ⇨

Iris works days and Rufus works nights.

She is sound asleep. She is dead. ⇨

Either she is sound asleep or she is dead.

Comparative

The comparative consists of adding conjunctions and sometimes reducing redundant information. The comparative and superlative morphemes are sometimes included. Common conjunctions include *than, as . . . as,* and *that* used with the adverbs *so/such.*

Bill is tall. John is tall. ⇨

Bill is as tall as John.

Ramado is tall. Jeremy is taller. ⇨

Jeremy is taller than Ramado.

The registrar is slow. The student is frustrated. ⇨

The slower the registrar is, the greater the student's frustration.

He was slow. We left. ⇨

He was so slow that we left.

Embedded Clauses

Relative Clause

The relative clause is embedded into another clause and functions as an adjective describing a noun in that clause. The embedded clause is a dependent clause, that is, it cannot stand alone. Relative clauses are typically headed by the relative pronouns or conjunctions *who, which,* or *that.* However, the speaker may chose to omit the conjunction.

The book is new. The book is on the table. ⇨

The book **which is on the table** is new.

The book is new. Junelle read the book. ⇨

The book **that Junelle read** is new. OR

The book **Junelle read** is new.

Noun Complement Clause

The noun complement clause is sometimes referred to as simply a noun clause, or a subject or object clause. It is a clause that is embedded in a sentence and functions as a noun. It may function as the subject of the sentence, the direct object, or as a noun complement to the subject. It involves the addition and reduction of sentence elements. Common noun complement clauses begin with the conjunction *that* or *for* with an infinitive form of a verb. It may include a **gerund**, which is an *-ing* form of the verb used as a noun.

Janet loves snow. I am surprised. ⇨

That Janet loves snow is surprising. OR

I am surprised **that Janet loves snow**.

They laughed. It was difficult. ⇨

It was difficult **for them to laugh**.

Diane left. I was amazed. ⇨

Diane's leaving amazed me.

Subordination Clause

A subordination clause, sometimes referred to as an adverbial clause, is a clause embedded in another clause adding a subordinating conjunction such as *because, when, since, if,* or *so.* The subordination clause is a dependent clause and is subordinate, not equal to, the main clause.

I was not home. She arrived. ⇨

I was not home **when she arrived**.

You go. I will go. ⇨

If you go, I will go.

Participles and Infinitives

The **participle** is the present or past participle used as an adjective or adverb. An **infinitive**, or full verb form, is used as the object of the main verb or as the main verb of the second clause. Infinitives may also be adjectives or adverbs. The *to* element of the infinitive may be deleted in some structures. Both participles and infinitives involve the reduction of redundant information.

I saw a giraffe. The giraffe was running. ⇨

I saw a **running** giraffe.

I know a girl. The girl is named Ruby. ⇨

I know a girl **named Ruby**.

Nick died. Nick was laughing. ⇨

Nick died laughing.

They start. They run immediately. ⇨

They start **to run immediately**.

I heard. The baby cries. ⇨

I heard the baby **cry** (to cry).

Remember that if the present participle {ing} form is used as a noun, it is a gerund not a participle. A gerund is always a noun. A participle is never a noun.

Once again, to make language more interesting, these constructions are often used in various arrangements and combinations. Consider: *When you get ready to go, let me know so I can alert the kid wearing the red hat.* This structure contains two subordination clauses, an imperative, and a participle.

Although these are not all of the possible structures used in English, they are the main structures and have all been studied in terms of how children learn them. Chapter 6 will include much of what we have learned about the acquisition of these structures.

✓ SUMMARY CHECKLIST

☐ Definition

Morphology

Morphology is the study of minimal units of meaning, or **morphemes**, and the rules governing their use.

Free Morpheme

Bound Morpheme

Derivational

Inflectional

Syntax

Syntax refers to the rules of word function and word order; it encompasses the rules for forming phrases, clauses, and sentences with words.

- ☐ **Word Classes**
  - **Noun Phrase**
  - **Verb Phrase**
  - **Prepositional Phrase**
  - **Other Word Classes**
- ☐ **Simple Sentence Syntax**
  - **Word Class Functions**
  - **Simple Sentence Modifications**
    - Negative
    - Passive
    - Interrogative
    - Imperative
- ☐ **Compound/Complex Sentence Syntax**
  - **Conjoined Clauses**
    - Coordination
    - Comparative
  - **Embedded Clauses**
    - Relative Clause
    - Noun Complement Clause
    - Subordination Clause
    - Participles and Infinitives

CHAPTER

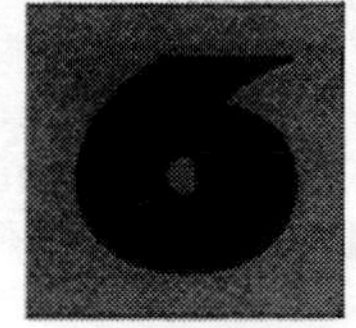

THE DEVELOPMENT OF MORPHOLOGY AND SYNTAX

Children begin to express meaning very early, as indicated in the phonology of the first 50 words, discussed in Chapter 3. Indeed, because of the variety and richness of meanings that appear to be expressed by these single words, this one-word stage is sometimes referred to as **holophrastic**. That is to say, these one-word phrases operate somewhat as holograms.

At about 18 months, children begin to string together two, or occasionally more, words in what has been referred to as **telegraphese**, due to the heavy emphasis on content and the lack of functional words such as articles and prepositions. However, from this point on, children begin to connect words to meaning in ever-increasingly adultlike syntactic forms. It is at this point that evidence of syntactic development can be noted.

Researchers between 1965 and 1970 focused investigations solely on sentence structures with no concern for how children connect meaning, resulting in some elegant but essentially empty formal descriptions of the syntax of children (Hopper & Naremore, 1978). In the early 1970s, research began to take into account how children connect words to meaning. Rechecking a decade of research, taking into consideration semantic relations and adding functional elements, Roger Brown and his colleagues at Harvard presented one of the most elaborate descriptions of early syntactic development in terms of stages. These stages are presented and elaborated on throughout this chapter, along with additional data on each stage and beyond.

Although many studies in other languages were considered as they appeared, Brown's stages were developed primarily from longitudinal studies of the development of grammar in three now renowned preschool subjects, Adam, Eve, and Sarah (Brown, Cazden, & Bellugi-Klima, 1968, 1971), Adam was the son of a minister in Boston and Eve was the daughter of a graduate student. Sarah was the daughter of a man who worked as a clerk in Somerville, MA. The parents of Adam and Eve had college degrees; Sarah's parents had high school diplomas. Observations were based on transcriptions of the children and their mothers, and occasionally fathers, in conversations at home. For each child at least 2 hours and up to 6 hours of speech were transcribed for each month over a period of several years. At the beginning of the study, Eve was 18 months old; Adam and Sarah were 27 months old. Children were selected on the basis of matched initial performance, not age. The measure of performance was based on utterance length, as were the stages of development. In fact, the data indicate that a **mean length of utterance** (MLU) is more reliable than age at the earliest stages of development, as rate of development may vary greatly. For example, consider the following data from Brown (1973):

	Adam	Sarah
AGE	MLU	MLU
30 months	2.5	1.75
35 months	2.5	2.5

As can be seen, although at 30 months of age Adam's utterances were longer than Sarah's, 5 months later they were equivalent. Adam remained at 2.5 MLU, whereas Sarah's utterances increased. To make matters even more interesting, Eve's MLU was 3.0 at 24 months! Data collection began at approximately 1.75 MLU for each and was terminated at 4.0 MLU. Eve reached this point at 28 months, Adam at 42 months, and Sarah at 48 months. Although rates of development varied, the stages of development were consistent for each subject. In other words, the three subjects varied widely on the age and rate at which they mastered specific features of language, but each followed a similar sequence of development. The introduction of MLU made it possible to search for commonalities in grammatical development among children who were, regardless of age, at the same MLU stage. The MLU has become a popular standard measure by which to assess young children's progress in language development (Shatz, 1994).

Brown found the MLU to be a better index than age for comparison in the earliest stages. Brown's (1973) method of calculating MLU included counting the morphemes in 100 fully transcribed utterances, excluding fillers such as *mm* or *uh* and counting all cases of compound words, ritualized reduplications, and diminutives (e.g., doggie) as only one morpheme each. Irregular pasts of verbs were also counted as only one morpheme as there was no evidence to indicte that any of these forms function in other way at this point in time. Grammatical inflections such as possessive, plural, and regular past were counted separately, as were auxiliaries. All catenatives (e.g., *gonna, wanna, hafta*) were counted as one morpheme for they appear to function as such for children. The total number of morphemes was then divided by the total number of utterances included to arrive at the MLU. Brown suggested 100 utterances be counted; no fewer than 50 should ever be used. It is important to keep in mind that this is an average length and therefore utterances beyond the MLU will occur. In other words, at a MLU of 2.0, utterances of less than 1 and greater than 3 may occur, but the average length is 2.0. The use of MLU has been recommended by Brown as a reliable measure only up to a MLU of 4.0; others (e.g., Lund & Duchan, 1993) have suggested an upper limit of 3.0. Shatz (1994) noted that children are fairly similar in the structures and forms they use and the sequence in which they use them up to MLU 3.0, but divergences become more common thereafter.

Brown's (1973) stages based on MLU can be seen in Table 6–1. The name of each stage and the features of language that are included in each stage are indicative of features that are particularly evident at that time; some of these features may appear before the stage and continue to develop after the stage. Brown's stages, as well as stages of other researchers using different criteria, indicate that children learn syntax incredibly fast and that a general progression in syntactic development does exist. This progression is presented here, using the descriptive names of Brown's stages as a guideline for discussion, but other re-

TABLE 6–1. Brown's stages of syntactic development.

Stage and MLU	*Developmental Level*	*Characteristics*
Stage I MLU 1.75	Semantic Roles and Grammatical Relations	Semantic roles such as agent and locative expressed by linear order; syntactic relations
Stage II MLU 2.25	Grammatical Morphemes and Modulation of Meaning	Semantic modulations such as inflections for number, tense, aspect, articles
Stage III MLU 2.75	Modalities of the Simple Sentence	Yes-no and WH-interrogation, negation, imperative
Stage IV MLU 3.50	Embedding of One Sentence Within Another	Object noun complements, embedded WH-questions, relative clauses
Stage V MLU 4.00	Coordination of Simple Sentences and Propositional Relations	Compound sentences, subordination

Source: Adapted from *A first language: The early stages* by R. Brown, 1973. Cambridge: Harvard University Press.

search findings are also included. Thus, as not all researchers have used MLU as a measure, age may be included when appropriate.

SEMANTIC ROLES AND GRAMMATICAL RELATIONS

Brown concluded that, in early word combinations, children show mainly an awareness of a small set of semantic relations. Although terms may vary among researchers, most agree that these early word combinations reflect the ability of children to categorize the world in terms of "roles" assumed by the words. In fact, Brown (1973) and his colleagues, in examining their data as well as those of other researchers and in other languages, found that early multiword utterances are probably governed more by semantic than syntactic rule systems. The use of pronouns is uncommon, except in the first person, and frequently occurs in the objective case first, that is, *me*. In the early two-word stage, there are few or no inflections, such as markers for tense, number, or plural, and there are no function words, such as prepositions, articles, copulas, and auxiliary verbs. This maintains in spite of the fact that most function words occur more frequently than most content words such as nouns and verbs. This telegraphic characterization of early two-word utterances, that is, retaining content words and omitting function words, seems to be universal. This characterization has also been shown to hold true for imitation tasks (e.g., Brown & Fraser, 1963). For example, when asked to imitate the sentence, *Read the book*, both Eve and Adam responded *Read book*. For *I am drawing a dog*, Eve responded *Drawing dog*, and Adam, *I draw dog*.

Maintaining normal linear order of words was also found to be important in imitation, as can be noted in previous examples, and in spontaneous production. Interestingly, in English declarative sentences, order typically will distinguish roles such as subject from object, modifier from modified, possessor from possessed. Thus, maintaining order will aid in communicating meaning in telegraphic utterances using content words only. Maintaining word order also seems to be universal even in languages in which general word order is much freer, for example, Russian (Slobin, 1965, 1971b).

With evidence that the child's semantic intentions include certain semantic roles and grammatical relations, several categories of Stage I speech have been described by many (e.g., Bloom, 1970; Schlesinger, 1971) as being characteristic of children's earliest word combinations. The basic relations of a sentence include the subject, the predicate, and the object of the verb. Semantic roles indicate that the noun phrases used for subject and object may take several roles, including agent, patient, instrument, and beneficiary. (See Chapter 2 for a description of each.) Examples of major semantic roles and grammatical relations expressed by children in Brown's Stage I are presented here (Brown, 1970). These characterize the majority of two-word sentences in Stage I.

Operations of Reference

The first set of two-word utterances contains instances of constant words in conjunction with various nouns, verbs, or adjectives to express specific semantic relations or meanings. At this point, children are limited to two-word combinations with which to express themselves and are thus limited in the range of meanings in their first sentences. Children learning different languages, including Samoan, German, French, Hebrew, Luo (in Kenya), and Russian, seem to express the same set of meanings in their first sentences (Brown, 1973). DeVilliers and deVilliers (1979) reported that children with mental retardation combine words into sentences at a later age and slower rate than usual, but express the same set of meanings in their first sentences.

Nomination

Nominative sentences are used to name or label something and occur in the presence of the referent that is pointed at, looked at, or picked up, as in:

That book.

There cat.

It should be noted that, although *this-that* and *here-there* are used quite frequently and appropriately as demonstratives or adverbs, the distinction in terms of locative requirements, that is, *this/here* for a nearby object and *that/there* for a faraway object, may not yet be mastered. This will be examined further in the area of semantics.

Notice

Bloom noted that children do not use *hi* as a greeting when someone arrives, but are likely to suddenly say *hi* to someone, some animal, or something that has been there all along. This seems to be simply an expression of attention or notice.

Hi, spoon.

Hi, plane.

Adam once asked *How are you, belt?* Apparently the pragmatic rules for use have not been totally mastered as yet.

Recurrence

Recurrence (again Bloom's category) of a referent includes the reappearance of something recently seen, a new instance of the same category, an additional quantity of a substance, and repetition of an action.

More milk.

'Nother nut.

More read.

Bloom found no semantic distinction between *more* and *'nother*, although *another* was not used before verbs (Brown, 1973). In adult English, *more* is limited to pluralized count nouns or mass nouns. Brown noted that children's early use of *more* occurs with unmarked count nouns, mass nouns, proper nouns, verbs, and even adjectives.

Nonexistence

Another of Bloom's categories, nonexistence, means that a referent that was previously present or was expected to appear is not now seen. It is most often expressed with the use of *no more* or *all gone*.

No more soup.

All gone egg.

Although nonexistence was the predominantly occurring negative, both rejection and denial, further discussed in Stage III, also occurred in this stage. It will be noted that the use of nonexistence precedes the use of the rejection and denial negatives.

Relations

Beyond these basic operations of reference, more abstract semantic relations are expressed. Particular words are no longer relevant as both initial and final words are varied.

Attributive

This construction expresses a specific attribute of an entity by combining a noun and an adjective.

Big train.

Red book.

Possessive

Children express the concept of possessor and possession without the syntactic inflection. Children typically divide objects in the house among family members.

Mommy chair.

Adam checker.

Entity and Locative

This construction is the expression of the location of a person or thing. In syntactic terms, it is equivalent to a noun and a prepositional phrase describing where that object is without the use of verbs or prepositions, or to a noun and a complement without the inclusion of the copula verb.

Baby table (for *Baby is eating at the table*).

Lady home (for *The lady is home*).

Action and Locative

This relation is expressing location or locus of an action. However, in syntactic terms, the verb is present with a noun expressing location without the occurrence of a preposition or object.

Go store (in response to *Where did Mommy go?*).

Put table (in response to *Where did you put your socks?*).

Early two-word utterances also begin to express various components of agent + action + object. Although, as pointed out earlier, other types of subjects do exist, they are not typically expressed at this early stage. Also, as utterances are limited to two words, one of these three components is absent. However, it is interesting to note that order is maintained in these productions.

Agent-Action

These constructions include a verb (involving perceived movements) and the initiator or performer of the action (most often animate).

Eve read (for *Eve reads a book*, turning pages).

Adam push (for *Adam pushes the bear*).

Daddy go

Action-Object

These constructions include the verb and the recipient or target of the action.

Hit ball (for *Mommy hits the ball*).

Eat cookie (for *Kathryn is eating the cookie*).

Agent-Object

In context, these constructions appear to be sentences without verbs.

Mommy lunch (for *Mommy is having lunch*).

Kathryn ball (for *Kathryn throws the ball*).

Thus, at this stage, as DeVilliers and DeVilliers (1979) pointed out, a child typically has three options for reporting the collision of a car and a truck when it is the truck's fault: *truck bump*, *bump car*, or *truck car*. Brown and his colleagues, as well as others, have further demonstrated the child's awareness of order in sentences through experimental tests of comprehension. For example, they asked 30-month-old Adam to act out with toys different agent-object contrasts: Show me *the duck pushes the boat* and, later on, Show me *the boat pushes the duck* (Brown & Bellugi-Klima, 1964, 1971). Lovell and Dixon (1965) asked 2-year-olds and older subjects to select the correct picture from agent-object contrast pairs such as *the dog bites the cat* and *the cat bites the dog*. These and other studies lend support to the conclusion that children in Stage I have the semantic meanings required for these relations.

At the end of Stage I, as children are moving into Stage II (MLU 2.25), there is an increase in complexity and several kinds of three-term relations become frequent. Examples include the following:

Agent-Action-Object

Children begin stringing together all three components of the simple sentences they had previously reduced to two components.

I dump trash out.

Action-Object-Locative

Again, an increase in length and complexity is noted as more components previously used in two-word utterances (action-object *put cabbage* or action-locative *put here*) are occurring together (Lindfors, 1987).

Put cabbage here.

Another occurrence that increases the child's utterance to a MLU that is characteristic of Stage II is the addition of grammatical morphemes.

GRAMMATICAL MORPHEMES AND MODULATION OF MEANING

In English, modulations of meaning include word endings such as tense markers and plurality, articles, and prepositions. The modulations studied in Stage II by Brown and his colleagues were not exhaustive but met criteria of being obligatory in certain contexts and therefore could be measured for 90% accuracy as mastery. This mastery did not necessarily occur within Stage II, but it began in Stage II. Overgeneralizations also occur as learning is acquired. Although the average order of acquisition reported has been supported or closely matched by many other studies (e.g., deVilliers & deVilliers, 1973), the 14 morphemes studied may occur at different ages and rates of development for individuals. For example, for Sarah, 16 months elapsed from the time the present progressive morpheme was used 50% of the time correctly until it reached the 90% criterion for mastery. Development of these grammatical morphemes will be discussed here in the order suggested by Brown's (1973) data and presented in Table 6–2. The order of difficulty appears to be a function of the linguistic complexity of the forms rather than their frequency. However, determining the order in which these morphemes appear in children's speech and are finally mastered is not as important as tracing their changes over time (Lund & Duchan, 1993).

Present Progressive

The progressive inflection indicates actions that are in progress at the time of mention. The adult speaker produces the present progressive tense by the use of an auxiliary verb and the addition of the *-ing* inflection at the end of the verb. Not all verbs take the progressive form, but children rarely use it incorrectly. Brown (1973) suggested that the dis-

TABLE 6–2. Brown's acquisition order for 14 morphemes.

Morpheme	*Example*
1. Present Progressive (-ing)	Adam eat**ing**.
2–3. Prepositions in, on	Put **in** you coffee. Doggie **on** sofa.
4. Plural (Regular and Irregular)	Kitt**ies** eat my ice cream.
5. Past Irregular	Mommy's balloon **broke**.
6. Possessive	I sit Adam**'s** chair.
7. Uncontractible Copula	He **is**. (response to Who's sick?)
8. Articles	I have **a** fingernail.
9. Past Regular	Mommy pull**ed** the wagon.
10. Third Person Regular	Mommy eat**s**.
11. Third Person Irregular	Just like Mommy **has**.
12. Uncontractible Auxiliary	He **is**. (Who's wearing your hat?)
13. Contractible Copula	That**'s** mine!
14. Contractible Auxiliary	Mommy**'s** eating bread.

Source: Adapted from *A first language: The early stages* by R. Brown, 1973. Cambridge: Harvard University Press.

tinction is between voluntary actions (e.g., *play, look, sleep*), which take a progressive inflection, and involuntary actions (e.g., *need, want, believe*), which do not. Thus, *I am playing a game* is possible, but not *I am needing a game.* However, the progressive form is completely regular, marked at the end of a word, and indicative of ongoing action. Perhaps these features account for its early appearance in children's language acquisition.

The child first produces the present progressive by use of only the *-ing* on the main verb; no auxiliary is used in the earliest formations. The earliest form is thus:

Adam eating.

Prepositions

The only prepositions used frequently by most children in early speech occur during Brown's Stage II. These prepositions are *in* and *on* and generally occur at about the same time. Most prepositions relate to fairly abstract spatial and temporal concepts, for example, *behind, above, before, after.* Considering children's early experiences, *in* and *on* are probably fairly concrete prepositional relations and this may explain their early occurrence. Furthermore, movement has been shown to be a very salient feature in children's language development, particularly in semantics, and children's experiences with *in* and *on* are related to movement. Children spend much of their early lives being placed on or in something, for example, *on* the bed, *on* the changing table, *in* the crib, *in* the highchair. Children also spend much of their time placing things on or in something, for example, toys *on* a table, shoes *on* the floor, socks *on* the bed, blocks *in* a box, toys *in* other toys.

Eve sit on couch.

Owens (1992) reported that the development of prepositional concepts and use continues throughout the preschool years with most spatial or locational prepositions (e.g., in order of development: *under, next to, behind* and *in front of, above, below, at the bottom of*) preceding temporal terms (e.g., *before* and *after*). Even in school-aged children, development continues with complex terms such as *in a week*, which places a spatial preposition in a temporal expression and the more precise locational directive referencing the body (*left* and *right*).

Plural

Both the regular and the irregular forms of the plural occur early in Brown's Stage II. Miller and Ervin (1964, 1971) noted that plurals develop in four stages (see Table 6–3) beginning with an uninflected distinction in number in Brown's two-word Stage I, for example, *two duck.* In other words, the semantic concept of number has been acquired at Stage I. At Stage II, children begin to use the grammatical marker for plural in contexts some of the time, *two duck* and *two boys*

TABLE 6–3. Sequence of plural development.

Stage	***Characteristics***	***Examples***
Period 1	Distinction without inflection	two duck
Period 2	Marked in some contexts, not all	two duck two boys
Period 3	Use more consistent, rules for regular overgeneralized	two ducks two boys two mans
Period 4	Distinction made and marked for regular and irregular	two ducks two men

Source: Adapted from The development of grammar in child language, by W. R. Miller & S. M. Ervin, 1971. In B. A. Bar-Adon, & W. F. Leopold (Eds.), *Child language: A book of readings* (pp. 321–339). Englewood Cliffs, NJ: Prentice-Hall. (Original work published 1964.)

occurring in the same time period. In a report on plural development at this stage of inconsistency, Brown and Bellugi (1964, 1971) report experiencing both the delights and limitations of working with preschoolers. Because Adam sometimes pluralized nouns and sometimes didn't, they directly questioned his knowledge of correct form by asking, "Adam, which is right, 'two shoes' or 'two shoe'?" His enthusiastic response to that question? "Pop goes the weasel!"

Miller and Ervin (1964, 1971) noted that following this inconsistency in use of plural inflections, children become more consistent in applying the plural, but they also overgeneralize the regular rule to irregular plurals, resulting in *two ducks, two boys, two mans* or even *two mens*. Finally, a distinction is made between regular and irregular plurals and most plurals are formed correctly, *two ducks, two men.*

There are still plurals to be mastered. In her experimental test of morphology, which has since become a model for testing morphology, Berko Gleason (1958, 1971) demonstrated preschoolers' lack of mastery in nonsense words ending in affricates and fricatives (e.g, *tasses* and *gutches*), as well as real words (*glasses*). Graves and Koziol (1971) found that many third graders still had not acquired the /əz/ form of the regular plural and words ending in /sk/ as in *desks*. Some irregular forms still indicated ongoing development, with the final /f/ words such as *leaf* becoming correct only between first and second grade.

Past Irregular

Most high-frequency verbs in English are irregular. For Brown's children, these included *came, fell, broke, sat,* and *went.* It is likely that as children first use the past tense irregular forms, they are simply learning these as separate words and not relating them to the past tense, that is, *go* and *went* are at first used with no connection between the two forms. Eventually, children will discover the relationship, but this probably does not occur until the use of the regular past tense is acquired and overgeneralization begins. This occurs later in Brown's Stage II and verbs such as *went* will be replaced with *goed*. The child does return to correctly producing these irregular past tense forms by Stage V.

Possessive

The concept of possession was indicated in Brown's Stage I by word order and context (*Daddy chair*). Pronouns are also used to mark possession before an inflection is added, as in *my baby*, but in Stage II the grammatical marker is added. Brown (1973) noted that early constructions are usually attached to an animate noun who possesses an inanimate entity, as in *Mommy's dress* in a temporary or optional relationship, as opposed to body parts, for example.

As with the plural, mastery of the /əz/ forms may take some time to fully develop. However, it should be noted that the possessive marker does not develop at the same time as the plural, indicating that this is the development of a morpheme and all its forms, not just phonemes.

Uncontractible Copula

Brown found that the first forms of the copula as the main verb show up in contexts where contractions are not allowed, that is, as uncontractible copulas. For example, in response to the question "Who is good?" a full form is required as in *Adam is* or *I am*. Or in response to "Where are you?" *Here I am* is required in full form. *What is that*? can be produced as *What's that*? but no contraction is possible for *What is it*? Children first learned copulas (and auxiliaries) in contexts in which contractions are not allowed. Although forms such as *it's went* and *it's will go* did show up in Adam's speech, this has been explained as a segmentation problem, not a contraction occurrence, that is, *it's* has been learned as a single word. In general, the copula is not fully mastered until Stage V (Miller, 1981). There are many variations to learn when person, number, and tense are considered.

Articles

The articles *a* and *the* appear in Brown's Stage II, but may take some time to master in terms of full usage. According to Lund and Duchan (1973), the common finding is that children first master the indefinite article in situations in which the referent has already been identified, as in *That's a hot dog*. Somewhat later, they use the definite article to introduce unidentified referents, as in *The kitty went meow*.

What appeared at first to be unusual occurrences of function words such as articles after demonstrative pronouns and verbs, for example, *this-a*, *have-a*, on further examination could also be explained as segmentation problems. In the production of *have-a pants, have-a* represents one word with the article incorporated in it as a word-final sound. Another example of segmentation problems was demonstrated by Adam, who, after producing sentences such as *it's raining* and *it's funny*, went on to produce *it's went* and *it's was working*, indicating that *it's* was a single segment for him. We find it amazing that such occurrences of segmentation problems are not much more common than they are, as children are learning words and morphemes by listening to a constant stream of sound as we saw in Chapter 3.

Other semantic and pragmatic considerations add an additional complexity to the use of articles. In referential expressions, for example in telling a story, the first time an entity is introduced it is indefinite, but thereafter it becomes definite, as in "Once upon a time there was *a cow*. *The cow* was big and healthy." Maratsos (1976) found that children are not proficient at this until at least age 4, and Warden (1976) suggested that children may not fully master this usage until between the ages of 5 and 9. This use requires children to take the listener's knowledge into full account.

Past Regular

As discussed earlier, the regular past marker is acquired after the child has already demonstrated the use of some irregular past tense forms. However, as the regular past tense rule is acquired, he or she overgeneralizes it to the previously occurring irregular forms, thus producing *comed, eated,* and *falled.*

Third Person Singular Marker: Regular and Irregular

Although the regular and irregular forms appear in Stage II, they are not fully mastered until Stage V as would be expected based on their level of abstraction. Trantham and Pedersen (1976) reported a long period of inconsistent use. Again, it should be noted that children distinguish this morpheme (*she run**s***) from its phonologically similar, but less abstract, plural (*two dog**s***) and possessive morphemes (*dog'**s** bowl*).

Uncontractible Auxiliary Verbs

The uncontractible form of the auxiliary occurs in contexts similar to those requiring the uncontracted or full form in the copula. For example, in response to "Who is going?" the full form *He is* or *I am* is required; *He's* or *I'm* is not acceptable. Note that the copula and auxiliary are developed as different morphemes at different times even though in these instances they are both forms of the verb *to be.*

Contractible Copula and Contractible Auxiliary

Next in Brown's Stage II, the copula is contracted, followed shortly by the contracted form of the auxiliary. As previously mentioned, full proficiency of these forms may not be acquired until Stage V.

The order of acquisition reported by Brown in describing Stage II might be explained by syntactic complexity of the structures being acquired. Syntactic markers required for a particular structure seem to be added one by one, not all at once. For example, in the present progressive formation, a child first says *Daddy go*, then increases length and complexity to *Daddy going* for a while, and finally adds the auxiliary resulting in *Daddy is going*. After full forms are acquired, contractions may be added, as in *Daddy's going*. This step-by-step mastery of adult syntactic forms has been observed in other stages of development, as will be seen.

The sequence of development of these forms also supports an explanation of semantic complexity, that is, meaning expressed and the amount of information required to express it. The developmental order of plural, possessive, and third person singular markers can be viewed as most concrete to most abstract in terms of meaning and information required. Plural, indicating more than one, is certainly more concrete than the relationship of ownership, and the information required to know when to mark third person singular is certainly more abstract than either of the others. The earlier developing expression of tense, present progressive, is the expression of an ongoing activity as opposed to the past tense which indicates something that has already occurred, making it a more abstract concept than present progressive.

It is important to keep in mind that many months may pass between the time that a particular form first emerges and the time that it is used consistently whenever required. As children progress through increasingly longer utterances, these utterances become more complex, but errors and inconsistencies are still displayed. Berko Gleason (1958/1971) also found that, although Standard English speaking children can apply most of these morphological rules to new words by at least 4 years of age, their knowledge is still developing at age 7.

Comparative and Superlative

In addition to Brown's studies, there have been numerous experimental and naturalistic studies of morphological development. A few studies have investigated the development of the comparative and superlative markers. Children's production of these forms was tested by Layton and Stick (1979) by asking children 2½ to 4½ years old to complete sentences (This truck is big, but this car is _______). Before age 3, children simply used the uninflected form, for example, *big*. Between ages 3 and 4, children tended to add the inflections {er} and {est}, but they made no distinctions between them. Between the ages of 4 and 4½, children used both with the appropriate distinction made. Wales and Campbell (1970) found that the distinction for superlative was understood earlier than for comparative. Donaldson and Wales (1970) noted that the use of true comparatives is often in competitive discourse situations (e.g., *I've got a bigger one than you . . . up to my ceiling*).

Gitterman and Johnston (1983) found that some comparisons were easier than others. Contrasts based on visual comparisons (tall, short) were made correctly more frequently than tactile comparisons (light, soft), and the least frequently made were those that required a combination of visual and tactile (smooth, rough).

MODALITIES OF THE SIMPLE SENTENCE

Up to this point, the sentences most in evidence in children's production are simple, active, affirmative, and declarative, that is, SAAD sentences. At Brown's Stage III, MLU 2.75–3.49, sentence types other than affirmative declarative develop. Miller and Chapman (1981) reported that about two thirds of middle-class children in the United States reach Stage III sometime between 24 and 41 months of age, and at this young age, imperatives, questions, and negatives emerge. The majority of children possess the basic sentence types in English by age 5 (Wells, 1985).

Imperatives

It is difficult to recognize imperatives in English because there are no morphological markers, simply the deletion of the subject. Although children have been producing subjectless declarative sentences and continue to do so, evidence of conscious imperatives appears in Brown's Stage III. This evidence is mainly the children's use of the words *please* (*Get it, please*) and *gimme* (*Gimme book*) (Brown, Cazden & Bellugi-Klima, 1968, 1971). Subjectless sentences are increasingly restricted to imperatives.

Negatives

The acquisition of negatives actually begins before Brown's Stage III and continues after, but sentential negatives, that is, negatives as part of a sentence, are much in evidence in Stage III. The beginning of this development can be seen even in the one-word, or holophrastic, stage with the appearance of *no* as a single utterance. By closely analyzing the context of children's utterances, Bloom (1970) was able to describe several subcategories of negatives being used in the two-word stage, that is, Stage I. The semantic categories of negatives which she described included **nonexistence**, *no hat* for "hat doesn't exist"; **rejec-**

...AND THEN THERE WAS YOUR FIRST WORD....
ELIZABETH! NO!!
NO-NO!
©1989 Universal Press Syndicate
7-5
NO, NO, HONEY!!
NO!
LYNN

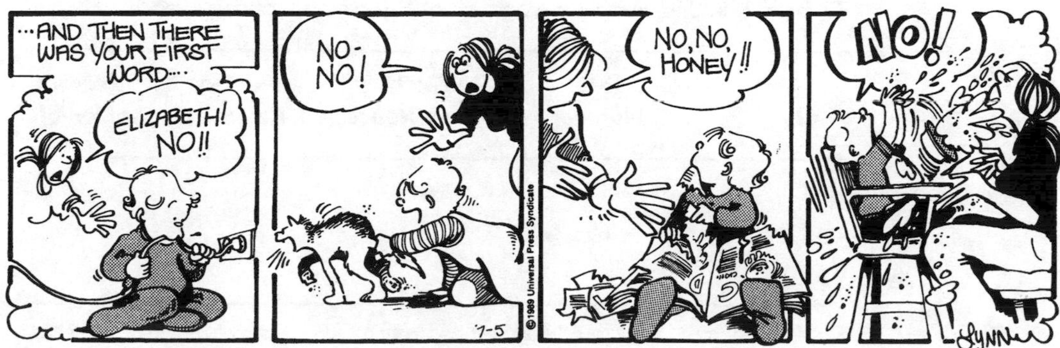

tion, *no soup* for "I don't want soup"; and **denial**, *no dirty* for "I am not dirty." Examples from Kathryn at 21 months of age can be seen in Table 6–4. Bloom also noted examples of disappearance as in *Soup all-gone*. By comparing these subcategories of negatives at different points of development, Bloom further noted, as is demonstrated in Table 6–5, that these categories developed in a sequence: nonexistence, rejection, then denial. Considering that children practice what they are learning and that there are so many negatives to learn, one may want to reconsider the label "the terrible twos."

The semantic categories described by Bloom (1970) developed at

TABLE 6–4. Examples of Kathryn's use of negatives at 21 months.

Nonexistence	*Rejection*	*Denial*
no pocket	no dirty soap	no dirty
no pocket in there	ə no chair	no (3 times)
no sock	no sock	
no fit (7 times)	no (24 times)	
no zip		
no turn		
no close		
no window		
ə no		
no (11 times)		

Source: From *Language development: Form and function of emerging grammars*, by L. Bloom, 1970, p. 185. Cambridge: MIT Press. Copyright 1970 by MIT. Reprinted with permission.

TABLE 6–5. Sequential development of Kathryn's use of negatives.

Phase	*Total Number*	*Percent Nonexistence*	*Percent Rejection*	*Percent Denial*
Time 1	19	.79	.16	.05
Time 3 (12 weeks later)	65	.38	.17	.45

Source: Data from *Language development and language disorders* by L. Bloom & M. Lahey, 1978. New York: John Wiley.

different rates for her three subjects (Kathryn, Eric, and Gia), but all developed in the same sequence. This sequence has been supported in other languages as well (e.g., McNeil & McNeil's 1967 studies of Japanese, as cited in Brown, 1973). This development continued to be observed as utterance lengths increased and sentential use of negatives occurred. For example, Kathryn later produced *no driver in the car* (nonexistence), *no put in there* (rejection), and *no Daddy hungry* (denial).

As children begin to use negative sentences, an occurrence that is very characteristic of Stage III, three substages occur (Brown, 1973). As children progress, they add more conventional adult aspects of language.

Substage 1

As children begin to add negative markers to utterances that are two words or longer (MLU approximately 1.75), they often simply attach *no* or *not* to the front of their simple sentences (Klima & Bellugi-Klima, 1966, 1971).

↘No money.

↘No want stand head.

↘No sit there.

Occasionally, the marker appears as the last word, *wear mitten no,* but the markers are not placed within the sentence.

Shatz (1994) described Ricky, who added an intensifier with strong stress to the ends of his negative utterances: *No I like it e-der* (either). *Either* became a standard addition to his negatives: (indicating his stuffed animals in a crib) *All the animals is sleeping,* (taking one out) *No dis sleeping e-der.*

Substage 2

As the child progresses (MLU approximately 2.25), he or she next places *no,* or sometimes *not,* within a clause.

That ↘not O, that blue.

I ↘no want envelope.

I ↘no taste them.

That ↘no fish school.

The child also begins to use *can't* and *don't* interchangeably with *no* and *not.* These words are used as if they were single words rather than contractions as their positive forms do not appear until later. Furthermore, no distinction is made between *don't* and *can't,* thus *I don't eat it* and *I can't eat it* may mean the same thing (Owens, 1992). *Won't* appears in late Stage III and is also used interchangeably.

↘Don't leave me.

I ↘don't want it.

I ↘don't sit on Cromer coffee.

By the age of 3 or 4, however, children usually have a whole range of auxiliaries, both positive and negative: *would/wouldn't, was/wasn't,* and others. DeVilliers and deVilliers (1979) reported that at this age, children can play a game with puppets which requires that they speak for an argumentative puppet by negating any statement used by another puppet, for example, "He must buy socks" is responded to with *He mustn't buy socks.* Children successfully negated all auxiliaries.

Substage 3

Children's negative utterances become much more adultlike (MLU between 3.4 and 3.9) and *no* within a clause is replaced by *not.*

I am ↘not a doctor.

This ↘not ice cream.

I ↘don't want cover on it.

Although the child has mastered the basic principle for adult forms which places *not* internally within the sentence, deviations still occur (Reich, 1986). Children sometimes produce double tense markers, indicating that they have not yet mastered the adult rule requiring that only the emphatic *do,* inserted for the formation of negative past tense, is marked for past:

I didn't caught it.

I didn't did it.

Double negatives may occur:

No one didn't come.

I didn't see nothing.

It is many years before the use of indefinites such as *some, none,* and *any* are mastered (deVilliers & deVilliers, 1979).

I didn't see something.

Don't let someone touch this.

You don't want some supper.

It is important to note that children move through orderly, systematic, and predictable stages (Parker & Riley, 1994), and children learning other languages (e.g., French, German, and Italian) appear to go through similar stages (Reich, 1986).

Interrogatives

Several different interrogatives also exist and must be learned. Some of these are comprehended early and even produced early. These include the Yes/No question (*Sit chair?*) and information or Wh-question (*Where kitty?*). Still other, more complicated questions exist. Polar questions (*Did you talk to Mary or to John?*) require a more complex two-sentence combination. There are also tag questions (*You are going, aren't you?*) and requests for action (*Can you reach my pencil?*). As with negatives, the acquisition of questions actually begins before stage III and continues beyond this stage, but it is very much in evidence in Stage III.

There is general agreement on the sequence of question acquisition (e.g., Ervin-Tripp, 1970). What, where, and yes/no are the earliest comprehended and produced. These are related to object and locative relations produced earlier. Who, Whose, What-do occur next. These are related to agent, possession, and action relations. Why, How, When are more complicated and are mastered much later. Three stages of children's question development have been reported (Klima & Bellugi-Klima, 1966, 1971).

Substage I

In this first phase (MLU of 1.75 to 2.25), the question function is performed and the meaning gets across, but the question form is very simple. The child's first questions are typically Yes/No questions marked by rising intonation added at the end of a sentence in its normal order. Children also use *what* and *where* attached to a noun phrase to ask for the names of objects (nomination), actions, or locations.

Daddy going?	What that?
Taste it?	What cowboy doing?
You like this?	Where horse?

During this stage, children do not respond appropriately to Wh-questions. For example, Ervin-Tripp (1970) reported that children may answer complex *Who* questions as if they were *What*, *What-doing*, or *Where* questions.

Who's eating? Meat.

Who's watching Daddy? Shaving.

Who put the car in? In that hole.

Substage 2

During this phase (MLU 2.25-2.75), children begin to put some verbal machinery into place, although they still haven't mastered adult use of pronouns and auxiliaries. Yes/no questions are still indicated by rising intonation, but may be longer. The child continues to ask *What* and *Where* questions but uses both a subject and predicate. The first subject-verb inversion may appear at the end of this phase in Wh-questions with the copula.

Do like grapefruit?	What doggie eat?
Daddy go work?	Why you smiling?

At this point, children may produce Why questions, but do not understand meaning. Adults may find that children easily lose interest in their long involved responses to the many Why questions they produce. However, What and Who questions may be understood and answered appropriately. There also appears to be a *because* stage parallel to the *why* stage. Once children learn to respond to Why-questions with *because* . . . , it also becomes a common answer for When and How questions (Ervin-Tripp, 1970).

Substage 3

At this point (MLU 2.75-3.5), most necessary auxiliary verbs and pronouns are present, although they may disagree in number and case and sometimes appear out of adult order. The more difficult When and How questions may appear, although the child may still have difficulty with the temporal aspects.

Who took them all down?

Did you drink your coffee?

How can he be a doctor?

Does lions walk?

Occasionally when the auxiliary first appears, it does not occur at the beginning of the sentence as it would in an adult question, but in the middle (deVilliers & deVilliers, 1979).

We can go home?

You will bathe me?

As with negatives, development of question forms continues far beyond Stage III. Although tag questions begin early with tags such as *okay*, *huh*, and *eh*, adult tag questions do not appear until much later and begin without the addition of negation, for example, *You want cookies, do you?* Full adult tag forms are acquired during early school age and negative interrogatives do not appear until after age five (Owens, 1992).

Reich (1986) pointed out that, just as in the case of negation, there are still a number of other grammatical details to be worked out. Sometimes there is double tense marking as children have not yet learned the adult rule of marking past tense only on the inserted emphatic auxiliary verb.

Did I caught it?

What did you doed?

There may also be problems marking number and case.

Does lions walk?

Why me going?

Questions in full adult form take years to master, but, once again, a systematic, predictable sequence of stages exists in development.

EMBEDDING OF ONE SENTENCE WITHIN ANOTHER

Brown's Stage IV, MLU 3.5, is characterized by more complex sentences in which one clause is embedded in another. In English, three major options for embedding clauses exist, including noun complement clauses, relative clauses, and infinitives. Again, although the development of these highly complex structures may have begun earlier and will continue beyond Brown's Stage IV, they are very evident at this stage.

Noun Complement Clauses

Limber (1973) reported on data from three children between 2 and 3 years of age with MLUs of 3.5–4.0. Limber noted that the first type of complex construction observed was noun complement clauses functioning as objects (but not as subjects).

I want **mommy do it**.

I don't want **you read that book**.

Wh-clauses, or embedded questions, were used adverbially or appeared as object complements (Limber, 1973):

Do it **how I do it**.

I remember **where it is**.

I show you **what I got**.

Subject-complements modifying the subject are the last to appear (Menyuk, 1977). The use of embedded questions as subject complement clauses may be the earliest to occur.

Whoever gets touched first is the loser.

Relative Clauses

Relative clauses, that is, clauses modifying nouns, appear next. The first relative clauses also appear at the end of a sentence, thus modifying the object, not the subject, of the sentence (Brown, 1973; Limber, 1973).

I show you the ball **I got**.

That is the way **Mommy talks**.

Now where's a pencil **I can use**?

Bever (1970) reported that in comprehension studies on cleft-sentence constructions, that is, those with ending embedded relative clauses, children perform better if the subject-object relationship is maintained without disrupting the subject-verb order. For example, *It's the cow that kisses the horse,* which maintains the subject-verb-object (SVO) relationship, is easier than *It's the cow that the horse kisses.* Note that in the first sentence *the cow* is the subject of the verb in the following clause (cow kisses the horse); however, in the next sentence *the cow* is the object of the second clause (the horse kisses the cow) interrupting the SVO relationship or flow.

Menyuk (1977) reported that relative clauses modifying the subject, as in *The boy* ***who hit the girl*** *ran away,* may not occur until after 5 years of age and are rare at age 7. Center embedding (subject position) is particularly difficult in that it too disrupts the SVO format that children prefer. In such cases, the child may resort to a SVO interpretation, that is, the object in the relative clause (e.g., *the girl* in the previous sentence) is interpreted as the subject of the verb in the main clause (i.e., *the girl ran away*). However, if the object of an embedded clause is inanimate, it is less likely to be misinterpreted than one in which the object is animate and therefore could be the subject of the following verb (Maratsos, 1974).

The boy, who broke the window, ran away.

The boy, who hit the girl, ran away.

A window cannot run away, but a girl can, allowing for easier misinterpretation of the second sentence by use of a SVO strategy. Bever (1970) stated that such semantic constraints may allow the syntactic factors to be bypassed entirely. In other words, children's use of real world knowledge helps in interpreting complex syntax.

Using some very complex sentences, Schlesinger (as cited in Bever, 1970) supported this by showing that center embedded sentences are easier to comprehend when the SVOs are semantically constrained. In the following sentences, the first is easier than the second, because as syntactically complex as they both are, the first is more semantically constrained.

The question the girl the lion bit answered was complex.

The lion the dog the monkey chased bit died.

Fodor and Garrett (as cited in Bever, 1970) demonstrated that center embedded sentences with relative pronouns present are simpler to paraphrase than the same sentences without the relative pronouns. Menyuk (1977) reported that deletion of relative pronouns is a late-developing construction for children.

The normally developing child's use of complex syntax may begin at an early age, but full control is not apparent until 10 or 11 years of age. First graders rely heavily on word order for interpretation and are confused by subject-object reversals in clauses. It is not until seventh grade that the child can interpret these sentences with little difficulty (Abrahamsen & Rigrodsky, 1984). Naremore and Dever (1975) pointed to the use of such complex constructions as distinguishing between normal learners and children with mental retardation. B. Warde (personal communication, May 14, 1997) reported that college students with learning disabilities demonstrate problems with complex center embedded relative clauses in textbook reading.

Infinitives and Participles

Infinitives

Often early developing infinitives occur before children are even producing complete sentences and seem to function as modal verbs: for example, *wanna go, gonna fall down, gotta get it.* Limber (1973) cautioned that it should not be inferred that these are simpler than other noun complement clauses. Laura Lee (1974) indicated that the development of infinitives listed in her Developmental Sentence Scoring is probably equivalent to Brown's Stage IV. Lee described these early developing infinitives as occurring first as objects in sentences.

I wan**na go home**.

I'm gon**na go**.

I got**ta see**.

Other infinitives are added that also occur most commonly in conversational English, that is, as objects of the sentence with the same subject:

He stopped **to play**.

I'm afraid **to look**.

The next developing usage is infinitives with different subjects, but are still used as object complement clauses:

I told him **to go**.

I want you **to come**.

These are followed by obligatory deletions (or bare infinitives), and infinitives with Wh-words.

Make it (to) **go**.

I'd better (to) **go**.

I know what **to get**.

I know how **to do** it.

Later developing are passive infinitival complements:

I have **to get** dressed.

I want **to be** pulled.

Although infinitives may be used as subjects, this does not occur in young children's language; this structure is used rarely by adults, but it still would be understood: *To do this for you is no big deal.*

Participles

According to Laura Lee's Developmental Sentence Scoring, children are considered to produce true participial structures when their sentences contain two verbs with one functioning as an adjective as in describing a picture as *That's a man washing his car* and *I see a dog lying on the floor*. This occurs at the same time as later developing infinitives.

COORDINATION OF SIMPLE SENTENCES AND PROPOSITIONAL RELATIONS

Coordination

Brown's Stage V, MLU 4.0, is characterized by the use of conjoining two clauses. The earliest connective structures begin with the use of conjunctions *and* and *and then* used for conjoining equal phrases and clauses. The conjunction *and* is also found to be the first in studies involving children learning languages other than English, for example, Swedish, Italian, and German (Bloom & Lahey, 1978). The most common conjoining of phrases occurs in the object position as opposed to the subject position (Reich, 1986).

He still has milk and spaghetti.

He was stuck and I got him out.

In general, *and* becomes the all-purpose conjunction and is used for temporal, causal, and adversative functions in place of *when*, *then*, *because*, *but*, and others (Bloom, Lahey, Hood, Lifter, & Fiess, 1980; Scott, 1988).

We left *and* mommy called. (meaning *when*)

She went home *and* they had a fight. (*because*)

Later, redundant sentence units may be deleted, resulting in more complex coordinated clauses. This reduction generally occurs first as forward reductions and later as backward reductions (Ardery, 1980; Lust & Mervis, 1980). In **forward reductions**, the clause is stated first, followed by a conjunction, and then the deletion of redundant information, *Reggie took his toy to school and left it on the bus. Reggie* would be redundant in the second clause. In backward reductions, the full clause appears after the conjunction, *Reggie and Jeremy left their toys on the bus.* Ardery's (1980) examples in Table 6–6 illustrate how complex coordination can be and the late age of acquisition should be noted. These are ages at which comprehension occurs. **Intransitive verbs** are those that take no direct object; **transitive verbs** take an object.

Subordination

In Brown's Stage V, MLU 4.0, children also learn to use more complex kinds of conjoining with the use of subordinating conjunctions to give prominence to one clause over another. Children now use conjunctions such as *because, so,* and *but* to signal subordinate relations that they previously conjoined as equal clauses with coordinating conjunctions.

I hit him *and* he cried. ➪ He cried *because* I hit him.

You have toast, *and then* I have toast. ➪

After you have toast, I'll have some.

Bloom and Lahey observed a gradual decrease in the use of *and* as other connectives formed to express different meanings, and the use of *and* came to be cued for coordination primarily.

Clark and Clark (1977) reported that the earliest subordinating conjunctions include *when, 'cuz,* and *if.* Eve Clark (1971) further noted that, when two events are mentioned in a sentence, young children assume that the one mentioned first occurred earlier in time than the event mentioned second (order-of-mention strategy). Later emerging conjunctions include *before, until,* and *after,* as would be expected based on cognitive demand.

Full development of subordination in conjoining does not occur until school age. For example, comprehension of *because* does not seem to develop until age 7 and may not be consistently correct until around age 10 or 11. This is particularly important to note as "cause and effect" are often taught in reading in elementary school before this development is complete.

Pragmatic constraints are also found to play a part in the development of conjunctions (Owens, 1992). Owens illustrates this with *because, although, unless,* and *if.* The conjunction *because* expresses strong belief and a positive relationship; *although* expresses certainty, but a negative relationship.

TABLE 6–6. Coordinate sentence types and age of acquisition.

Coordinated Constituents	***Example***	***Mean Age Correct (in years)***
Intransitive verb	The frog ran and fell.	3.11
Object noun phrase	The giraffe kissed the tiger and the cat.	4.0
Sentential intransitive	The dog ran and the cat fell.	4.3
Verb phrase	The dog kissed the horse and pushed the tiger.	4.5
Subject noun phrase	The tiger and the turtle pushed the dog.	4.9
Sentential transitive	The turtle pushed the dog and the cat kissed the horse.	5.0
Gapped verb with particle (preposition phrase)	The horse bumped into the cat and the dog into the turtle.	5.0
Transitive verb	The turtle kissed and pushed the frog.	5.2
Gapped verb, no particle	The giraffe kissed the horse and the frog the cat.	5.7
Gapped object	The cat kissed and the turtle pushed the dog	5.9

Source: Adapted from "On coordination in child language," by G. Ardery, 1980, *Journal of Child Language*, 7, pp. 313–314. Copyright 1980 Cambridge University Press. Adapted with permission.

It is a block because it is cubical.

It is a block although it is made of metal.

On the other hand, *unless* and *if* presuppose uncertainty, with *if* being positive and *unless* negative.

It is a block if it is wooden.

It is a block unless it is round.

In general, the more positive the belief and the relationship, the easier it is to comprehend. Thus, *because* is learned before *if* and *although*, which are followed by *unless*. Even fifth graders have difficulty understanding *unless* (Wing & Scholnick, 1981).

Passive Sentences

Production of passives begins in late preschool years with short sentences such as *It got broken*, but children do not fully comprehend passive constructions until age 4 or 5 or even later (deVilliers & deVilliers, 1979; Owens, 1992). Fraser, Bellugi, and Brown (1963, 1970) found that the predominant error in interpreting passive sentences was to interpret them as active. In other words, *the cat is chased by the dog* was interpreted as *the cat chased the dog*. The children apparently filtered out the auxiliary and the preposition and chose to maintain a subject-verb-object (SVO) order interpretation. These errors have been noted as being more likely if the sentence is a semantically well-formed passive which is reversible (Strohner & Nelson, 1974; Turner & Rommetveit, 1967). In **reversible sentences**, either noun could logically be the subject or the object, as in *the dog was bitten by the cat*. The dog could bite the cat, or the cat could bite the dog, thus, this sentence is reversible. In a **nonreversible** sentence, such as *the hot dog was bitten by the boy*, the nouns cannot be so plausibly reversed, resulting in an easier and earlier learned correct interpretation. DeVilliers and deVilliers (1979) reported that, in testing the reversible passive, they presented a child with the passive *The truck is bumped by the car* and she took the truck and bumped the car. Then when told, "Now make the truck bump the car," she looked at them and asked, "Again?"

At age 5, only about 50% of children can correctly interpret reversible passives (Bridges, 1980). Furthermore, the semantic nature of the verb plays a role in the emergence of the reversible passive (Maratsos, Kuczaj, Fox, & Chalkley, 1979). Action verbs such as *shake* and *kick* are correctly interpreted earlier than nonaction verbs such as *remember, know*, and *hear*. Several studies have reported a sharp, but temporary, drop somewhere between the ages of about 4 and 5 in the progress of developing understanding of the full passive (Bever, 1970; deVilliers & deVilliers, 1973). This temporary decrease in correct responses has been explained by overgeneralization errors, that is, the children interpreted active sentences as passive.

There are actually three cues to indicate a passive interpretation of a sentence. There is the presence of an auxiliary (*to be*), the use of the past participle inflection on the main verb, and the presence of a preposition, usually *by*. Some investigators have contended that the preposition is the salient feature of the passive sentence. Maratsos and Abramovitch (1975) demonstrated that preschoolers who showed comprehension of passive sentences would misinterpret them when the preposition was removed and replaced by a pause but not when the preposition *of* was used in place of *by*. In other words, *the bear is bitten*

* *the lion* was interpreted as active, but *the bear is bitten of the lion* was still interpreted as passive. The presence of a preposition was found to be necessary for a passive interpretation. Maratsos and Abramovitch had intentionally selected *of* due to its membership in the same semantic class of neutral prepositions as *by*. Shorr and Dale (1981) investigated replacing *by* with the locational prepositions *to* and *from* and found that, although the use of *from* still resulted in a passive interpretation by preschoolers and kindergartners, the use of the preposition *to* resulted in an active interpretation. For example, preschoolers and kindergartners interpreted *the lion is tickled from the bear* as passive and *the lion is tickled to the bear* as active. Although the auxiliary and preposition are not in conflict in the *from* sentences, they are for the *to* sentences, and in most cases the preposition prevailed. Children's performance with passive sentences varied depending on the semantic aspects of the preposition.

Shorr and Dale (1981) noted that both elicited imitations and spontaneous production of passives containing *from* as the preposition have been reported. Horgan (1978) reported such productions in both preschool and school-age children (e.g., *they got shot from the Japanese*). She also noted occurrences, although infrequent, of *of* in passive productions. Bowerman (as cited in Shorr & Dale, 1981) also reported the use of *from* in early productions of the passive. The development of passives has been noted to continue into school age. Approximately 80% of 7½- to 8-year-olds produce full passive sentences (Baldie, 1976). Some passives do not appear until 11 years of age (Horgan, 1978).

DeVilliers and deVilliers (1979) noted that comprehension is much better in situations in which a particular grammatical form is naturally used. Parents tend to use elaborate nonverbal signals to help their children understand directions, so in natural circumstances it is difficult to tell how much language is contributing to the child's response.

Although its beginnings can be seen in 3-year-olds, and by age 4 or 5 at the latest, children have acquired most of the basic principles of syntax, these and other constructions are not fully developed until adolescence. In fact, language development continues into adulthood, and school-age years are much more important than was first recognized. Increase in size and complexity of repertoire and in use within different contexts continues.

LATER-LEARNED EXCEPTIONS TO THE RULES OF SYNTAX

Carol Chomsky's 1969 study was one of the first to demonstrate that some rules are not acquired until age 10 or 12. In a very creative dissertation, C. Chomsky demonstrated that specific exceptions to the rules of syntax are learned late. Some of her investigations and replications of them are detailed here.

SVO Order Violations

In specific constructions, C. Chomsky noted that true grammatical relations that exist among words in a sentence are not expressed directly in its surface structure. Note the SVO direction of the following examples.

John is eager to see Mary.

BUT

John is easy to see.

In the first statement, *John* is the subject of both verbs, but in the last statement, *John* is the subject of the first verb, but the object of the second. In fact, the subject of the second verb is not included in the statement. A similar construction reported by Bever (1970) is ambiguous: *The missionary is ready to eat.*

To test the understanding of the unambiguous construction, Chomsky placed a blindfolded doll in front of the child and asked, in a conversational manner,

(1) Is this doll easy to see or hard to see?

(2) Would you make her easy/hard to see?

If the child were using a SVO order strategy, he or she would misinterpret (1) as the doll doing the seeing and consider the blindfold as making this difficult (or hard). Almost all 5-year-olds answered incorrectly and all 9-year-olds answered correctly. In between these ages, the answers were mixed. Those who answered that the blindfolded doll was hard to see removed the blindfold when told to make the doll easy to see. Those children who responded correctly, that is, said that the blindfolded doll was easy to see, when asked to make her hard to see, put the doll under the table, covered her up, or covered their own eyes. For example, consider the following illustration from Chomsky (1969).

Displaying a blindfolded doll,

Experimenter: Is this doll easy to see or hard to see?

Peter (aged 6.9): Hard to see.

Experimenter: Why?

Peter: 'Cause she got a blindfold.

Experimenter: Will you make her easy to see?

Peter removes the blindfold.

In a similar study, Kessell (1970) eliminated the possibility of the influence of the blindfold by using Peanuts dolls playing hide and seek.

The children were shown two dolls and told, for example, "Lucy was easy to find" and then asked "Who is hiding?" and "Who is seeking?" A similar rate of acquisition to that reported by Chomsky was found. Reich (1986) reported further support for Chomsky's rate of acquisition in a similar study (Cambon & Sinclair, 1974) of French-speaking children using the counterpart word *facile* (easy).

Minimal Distance Principle

Syntactic structures associated with a particular word may violate the minimal distance principle (MDP), which states that the noun closest to a verb is the subject of that verb.

John wanted to leave.

John wanted Bill to leave.

John begged Bill to leave.

BUT

John promised Bill to leave. (John leaves, not Bill)

Promise Constructions

To test children's understanding of this construction, Chomsky placed a book and two dolls in front of the child. After establishing the child's knowledge of the word *promise*, and explaining the game, sentences such as the following were presented to the children.

Bozo tells Donald to hop up and down. Make him do it.

Donald promises Bozo to hop up and down. Make him do it.

In this situation, success was found to be very independent of age. The age range of children getting all correct was from 5.2 to 10. However, stages were noted and overgeneralization in learning this exception was observed. The first stage of development consisted of responding to all statements with a minimal distance principle interpretation; therefore all of the *tell* constructions were correct and all of the *promise* constructions were incorrect. In the next stage, as children learned the exception to the MDP, they overgeneralized, resulting in inconsistent responses for both *tell* and *promise*. Next, the children returned to correct responses to *tell*, but continued responding to *promise* inconsistently. Finally, all responses were correct. The order of development is very similar to that of other exceptions in syntax, for example, irregular past and plural morphemes.

Ask Constructions

Another exception may occur when conflict exists between two of the potential syntactic structures associated with a particular verb. The *ask* construction is such a verb and is even more complex than *promise*. The verb *ask* has more than one meaning.

John asked Bill what to do. (John asks and John will do.)

John asked Bill to leave. (John asks and Bill will leave.)

The first statement violates the minimal distance principle as the noun closest to the second verb (Bill) is not the subject of that verb. However, the second statement does not violate the MDP, as the noun closest to the second verb, *Bill*, is the subject of that verb. On closer examination of the verb *ask*, it becomes apparent that it has different meanings in these two statements. The first statement is a question (ask-Q); the second is a request (ask-R). However, the second statement could have an interpretation that does violate the MDP. The alternative interpretation is a request for permission as in *John asked Bill (for permission) to leave.*

Ask-R Constructions. Thus, the verb *ask*, meaning a request in the same construction, sometimes violates the MDP and sometimes does not, depending on the meaning of the construction. To check children's understanding of the complex ask-R verb, Chomsky gave children dolls and told them, for example, *Suppose Mickey Mouse asks Bozo to stand up, what does Mickey say?* Ask-R responses were correct for all children with only 1 child, the most advanced, assigning the less likely interpretation of a request for permission.

Ask-Q Constructions. Although Ask-Q has only one interpretation, it is even more complex in that it has several different possible syntactic constructions. To investigate this construction, Chomsky set up situations with two children, dolls, and other manipulatives. The following constructions were used by Chomsky and are presented here in order of complexity. Compare the responses required by *ask-Q* with the responses for the simpler *tell* constructions which follow the MDP consistently.

CASE 1: WH-CLAUSE, SUBJECT SUPPLIED
Ask X what her name is. [What is your name?]
(Tell X what her name is. [X])

CASE 2: NOUN PHRASE ONLY
Ask X her name. [What is your name?]
(Tell X her name. [X])

CASE 3: WH-CLAUSE, SUBJECT OMITTED
Ask X what to feed the doll. [What do I feed the doll?]
(Tell X what to feed the doll. [the name of a food])

Chomsky found that the ability to respond correctly to the different cases of Ask-Q constructions was not totally age dependent, but developed in a definite order made up of five sequential stages.

STAGE A Interpreted ask and tell both as tell in all constructions, (Cases 1,2, and 3). All 5-year-olds operated at this level.

Experimenter: Ask Eric his last name.
Child: Handel. (Eric's last name)

Experimenter: Ask Eric this doll's name.
Child: I don't know.

STAGE B Success was demonstrated on Case 1, failure on Cases 2,3.

Experimenter: Ask Joanna who this is?
Child: Who's that?

Experimenter: Ask Joanna the color of Mickey's trousers.
Child: Blue.

STAGE C Success was demonstrated on Cases 1, 2, failure on 3. Almost all children who were successful were beyond age 6.

Experimenter: Ask Joanne what color this book is.
Child: What color's that book?

Experimenter: Ask Joanne her last name.
Child: What's your last name?

Experimenter: Ask Joanne what to feed the dog.
Child: The hot dog.

STAGE D Success was demonstrated on Cases 1 and 2 and Case 3 was partially right in that a question was asked, but the wrong subject was used, indicating that the exception to MDP had not yet been learned.

Experimenter: Ask Lynn what to put back in the box.
Child: What are you going to put back in the box?

STAGE E Complete success on all cases was demonstrated.

Chomsky found no regular progression by age. For example, one child aged 5 years 10 months was in Stage E and one 10-year-old was in Stage C. There was also no correlation with success and the teacher's rating of ability. In the Case 3 construction (Ask X what to feed the doll), it was found that many 9- and 10-year-olds could not respond even with prodding. Consider the number of times a teacher tells a student "Ask Ms. X what to do with your paper" and then is reprimanded for telling Ms. X what to do with his or her paper.

Through informal questioning, Chomsky found that this structure is a problem for many adults. Owens (1988) reported that the ability to comprehend and generate ask/tell utterances increases until seventh grade and then changes little. Some adults may still use some this form incorrectly.

In general, Chomsky found through all of these investigations that stages of development are much more reliable than ages of children. Children's use of syntactic structures related to SVO relations were evident in all of her investigations.

It appears that there are definite stages of development in morphology and syntax, many of which also indicate semantic constraints. This development begins very early and continues into school age for normally developing children. It can be expected that children with problems in language will demonstrate even later ages of development.

✓ SUMMARY CHECKLIST

☐ **Developmental Studies**
Holophrastic Stage
Telegraphese
Mean Length of Utterance (MLU)
Developmental Stages
Semantic Roles And Grammatical Relations
Operations of Reference
Nomination
Notice
Recurrence
Nonexistence
Relations
Attributive
Possessive
Entity and Locative
Action and Locative
Agent-Action-Object Relations
Action-Object-Locative

☐ **Grammatical Morphemes and Modulation of Meaning**
14 Morphemes
Comparative and Superlative
Modalities of the Simple Sentence
Imperatives
Negatives
Interrogatives
Embedding of One Sentence Within Another
Noun Complement Clauses
Relative Clauses
Infinitives and Participles
Coordination of Simple Sentences and Propositional Relations
Coordination
Subordination
Passives

Later-Learned Exceptions

SVO Order Violations

Minimal Distance Principle

Promise Constructions

Ask Constructions

CHAPTER

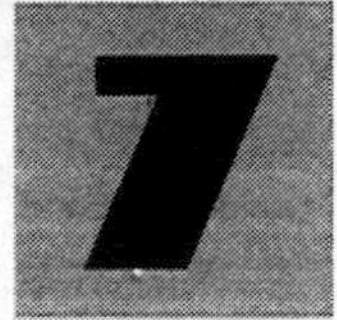

MORPHOLOGY AND SYNTAX: ANALYSIS AND INTERVENTION

As discussed in Chapter 1, a valid analysis of language needs to be made in a naturalistic context; however, most formal language tests designed to assess morphology and syntax are lacking in naturalistic context and do not show how children will respond when they can choose the topic and ask questions (Lund & Duchan, 1993). The purpose of analysis is to determine and evaluate goals for intervention programming, and thus, the importance of having a true picture of the child's language abilities cannot be stressed enough. Suggestions about how to obtain a representative sample of language and transcribe it are given in Appendix A. This chapter focuses on the analysis of morphology and syntax from the language sample and includes typical errors displayed by children with language delays or disorders. Some suggestions for intervention are included.

ANALYSIS

Preparing the Sample Transcript

Although the transcription of the language sample includes everything said by the subject of the analysis, for purposes of analyzing morphology and syntax, all fillers, repetitions, reformulations, and self-corrections should be removed. This allows the final formulation of the subject's structures to be evaluated for word functions and grammatical complexity. The use of parentheses may be helpful in segmenting the utterances for analysis. However, all of the information removed at this point will be important for later analysis in the area of semantics and pragmatics, where pauses and disruptions will need to be considered. The structures remaining for the analysis of morphology and syntax typically include at least one subject and verb. For example, the following structure, for purposes of syntactic analysis, becomes much shorter and simpler: **(the doctor s/c) the hospital (I mean) was (um it was oh gosh) (I forgot what hospital was) Albert (something like that)**. In the end, the statement that **"the hospital was Albert"** is syntactically correct; the embedded statement "**I forgot what hospital was**" is not (Smiley, 1991a). Long run-on sentences may be separated for syntactic analysis according to Lee's (1974) "AND" rules in Table 7–1. Only one AND conjunction is allowed per sentence *when it connects two independent clauses.* This does not apply to other conjunctions nor to AND in a series or in compound subjects, verbs, or objects. AND as an initial conjunction is discounted. For example, the following run-on sentence becomes four separate sentences, as indicated: #1-**my brother and I like to ski and my sister skis too** #2-**(and) my mom cross-country skis and my father skis downhill** #3-**(and) I got some new boots and poles and skis and we're going to Vail for a week during spring vacation** #4-**(and) we'll stay at my aunt and uncle's condo** (Smiley, 1991a).

After segmenting utterances for analysis, it may be helpful to transfer them to a worksheet, numbering each utterance and using two lines for each. The first line contains the segmented and num-

TABLE 7–1. Rules for sentences connected with conjunctions.

1. **Initial Conjunction.** Sentences that begin with conjunctions are counted as complete simple sentences.
2. ***And* joining independent clauses.** Only one *and* conjunction per sentence is allowed when the *and* connects two independent clauses.
3. ***And* with series and compound functions.** The conjunction *and* used in a series, a compound subject, or a compound predicate does not require the sentence to be broken up.
4. **Conjunctions other than *and*.** Internal conjunctions other than *and* do not require a sentence to be broken up. Others are seldom used in long strings because the semantics of the sentence do not often allow it.
5. **Other overused conjunctions.** At the teacher or clinician's discretion the rules for *and* may be applied to any other overused conjunction. For example, sometimes a child may use *so* in the same way as *and*.

Source: From *Developmental sentence analysis: A grammatical assessment procedure for speech and language clinicians* by L. L. Lee, 1974, pp. 74–77. Evanston: Northwestern University Press. Copyright 1974 by Northwestern University. Adapted with permission.

bered utterance; the second line may be used to expand the utterance based on the meaning derived from the context in which it occurs. Tyack and Gottsleben (1977) recommended that expansions should be made only within utterances, not to the left or right. Exceptions include only morphological endings or verb particles at the end or articles at the beginning. The teacher or clinician should not assume too much and should use his or her knowledge of development in making these expansions. For example, *Doggie eat* may be expanded to *The doggie is eating* as the present progressive is learned before the third person singular marker. If it is necessary to insert a semantic expansion, it should be placed in parentheses and referred to as the part of speech in a summary. For example, *And then go to school* may be expanded to *And then (the girl) will go to school*, indicating that the subject was omitted. It may be useful to circle or underline incorrect forms and use carets for omitted forms in the child's utterance.

Lund and Duchan (1993) suggested that once the teacher or clinician becomes familiar with the regularities in the use, misuse, and omissions of forms in the sample, it will become possible to choose the aspects of syntax that are most relevant for a particular subject and find shortcuts for carrying out the analysis. Interest should focus on the areas in which there are problems noted and targeted for intervention. A more comprehensive analysis might be desirable to show development of language over time as new structures emerge.

Analysis of Morphology

In assessing the use of a particular form in language, it is generally considered mastered if correct adult form is used 90% of the time. Table 7–2 illustrates a format that might be useful in the analysis of morphology. Markings that may be useful in calculating the mastery of each morpheme include: + for adult Standard American English (SAE) form, – for omission, and × for a substitution, noting the utterance number where each occurs. Substitutions will need to be further noted, for example, *him* for *he*. This substitution indicates a possible problem in the use of case in pronouns as opposed to number or gender in pronoun use, for example. Based on studies of typical and atypical language development, it becomes apparent that, at a minimum, the morphemes presented in Table 7–2 may need to be assessed. Each of these is discussed along with examples from students with disabilities. Some of the examples are from Smiley (1991a). Possible dialect differences which should be further evaluated are indicated by an asterisk (*).

Plural Markers

The use of both regular (*rats*, *dogs*, or *cheeses*) and irregular (*children*, *wolves*, *deer*) plural markers should be noted. For example, from the language samples of 6-year-old Kelly: **I counted six *peoples* in this room** and 9-year-old Brian: **I saw *mouses*.**

TABLE 7–2. Analysis of morphology.

	Adult SAE +	*Omission* –	*Substitution* X	*Mastery Level**
Plural Regular Irregular				
Past Tense Regular Irregular				
3rd Person Singular Regular Irregular				
Articles				
Copula				
Auxiliary To be To have				
Modals				
Emphatic do				
Pronouns				
Prepositions				
Verb Particles				
Comparative/ Superlative				

*Mastery Level = Number Correct/(Omissions + Substitutions)

Source: From "Informal language assessment, Part I" by L. R. Smiley, 1991, p. 25. *Learning Disability Forum, 16*(4). Copyright 1991 by Council for Learning Disabilities. Adapted with permission.

Past Tense Markers

Note the use of both regular (*jumped*, *called*, or *sorted*) and irregular (*gave*, *found*, *hit*) past tense. Markers may be omitted or the regular past tense marker may be overgeneralized to the irregular past. For example, 10-year-old Brooke: **So he *cutted* the plants and *make* them into anything he *like*** and **She saw a scissors so she *ranned* out**, and 9-year-old John: **The alligator *drowneded* him.**

Third Person Singular Markers

Both regular ([he/she/it] *hits*, *runs*, or *sneezes*) and irregular (*says*, *has*) use should be examined. 16-year-old Joe: **That pencil *have* teeth mark on it**. Omissions* should also be noted.

Articles

Articles (*a, an, the*) should be checked for use of the appropriate article* (Bret, age 13: **You're *a* idiot!**), omission of the article (Rebecca, age 7½: **I don't have ^ camera**), and insertion of an unnecessary article (Joe, age 16: **I am writing on a man who is in *the* politics**). Other analysis would include appropriate use of articles in context.

Copula

The copula is probably better known as the linking verb "to be." These verbs need to be checked for tense and number (Robert, age 6: **Cause my dad *are* one at Ohio**—referring to his dad being a policeman). Other problems could include the omission* of the copula (Gary, age 9: **It ^ pink**) or the use of an uninflected form* (Doris, age 12: **He *be* good**).

Auxiliary

Commonly known as helping verbs, the auxiliary includes *to be* and *to have*. Errors in auxiliary use may occur in tense, and number* (Ellyn, age 9: **Two people *was* running**), as well as omission* (Chris, age 13: **You should ^ been working more**) and uninflected form of *to be** (Tanya, age 14: **We *be* winning and we ^ going to beat you**).

Modal

The modal auxiliaries (*will, can, could, may, might, must,* and *should*) need to be checked for tense and omission (Marilyn, age 7: **I wanted to give my mom a valentine today, but I ^ give it to her tomorrow**). Corona, age 9, was having trouble with the modal use in forming a Wh-question: **What *could* a leopard *can* eat?**

Emphatic

The emphatic auxiliary (*to do*) should be checked for number (**How *does* you spell 'excellent'?**), tense, and omission (Doris, age 12, arguing a point: **It ^ make him happy**!) The misuse of the emphatic *do* in the interrogative and negative may also be included in the analysis of syntax.

Pronouns

Pronouns should be checked for correct case (Michael, age 8: **I don't know where them are**), number (Chris, age 8, while pointing to one pencil: **You hafta count these** and Chad, age 9: while discussing the movie *Home Alone*, **The whole family forgot about *them* on the trip**—him), and person (Kelsey, age 7, in trouble with her teacher: **Are you gonna call *your* father?**). Ambiguous referents and gender errors should also be noted.

Prepositions

Sheldon, age 9, demonstrates the omission of a preposition: **I left it ^ the bus stop**, and Chrissy, age 7, inserts an unnecessary preposition: **I gaved my mommy kisses and hugs *in* this morning**. Substitutions should also be noted for further examination in the area of semantics (Shannon, age 5: **Ebony buries her bones *inside* the dirt**).

Verb Particles

The wrong verb particle may be used or the required particle movement may not occur (Fran, age 10: **They took *away it*.**)

Comparative and Superlative

An error may occur in the use of these markers on adjectives and adverbs. Errors particularly occur with irregular forms as with Fred, age 6: **Frogs are my *bestest* friends** and John, age 7: **You think The House of Pancakes is the *most best* place to eat pancakes**? Colleen, age 9, used the superlative form for the comparative: **Is an alligator *biggest* than a crocodile?**

Analysis of Syntax

In the previous section, linguistic structures were identified from a language sample in order to evaluate morphology. The same structures should be considered when analyzing syntax. The development of syntax begins in preschool; school-age children who use only simple active affirmative declarative sentences may be exhibiting problems in language competence. Therefore, the first question that should be asked is whether the level of complexity of the student's sample is appropriate for his or her age. For students who are attempting more complex formations, several structures should be analyzed, addressing the following questions: (a) Is the structure present in the sample? (b) Is it in adult SAE form? (c) How often does it occur? (d) If it is not in adult SAE form, what specific errors are evident? A sample format for recording the analysis can be seen in Table 7–3.

Table 7–3 can be completed by placing an utterance number under (a) the Adult SAE + column when a linguistic structure is produced accurately, (b) the Omission – column for an omission of the required structure, and (c) the Substitution × column for the occurrence of a structure substitution (e.g., *he's is* . . . would be noted under the substitution column for contractions). As in analyzing morphology, mastery level for more complex syntax is also considered to be 90% accuracy and is calculated by dividing the number of adult SAE structures by the total number of required structures. A description of the specific structural errors should be noted for intervention programming.

Based on studies (e.g., Berko Gleason, 1989; Owens, 1992; Reich, 1986) of typical and atypical language development, the following section describes linguistic structures of complex syntax that should be

TABLE 7–3. Analysis of complex syntax.

	Adult SAE +	**Omission** –	**Substitution** X	**Mastery Level***
Single Sentence Unit				
Contractions				
Negatives				
Imperatives				
Passive				
Infinitives and Participles				
Questions				
Embedded or Conjoined Clauses				
Coordination				
Subordination				
Relative Clauses				
Noun Complement Clauses				

*Mastery Level = Number Correct/(Omissions + Substitutions)

Source: From "Language assessment, Part II" by L. R. Smiley, 1991, p. 18. *Learning Disability Forum, 17*(1). Copyright 1991 by Council for Learning Disabilities. Adapted with permission

assessed to aid in instructional planning. These structures include some incorporated in single sentence units as well as embedded and conjoined clauses. Examples of errors in each area from language samples of students with disabilities are provided. Some of the examples are from Smiley (1991b). Possible dialect differences will again be indicated by an asterisk(*).

Single Sentence Unit

The following structures require additions, deletions, and rearrangements within a single sentence unit, thus making them more complex than simple active affirmative declarative sentences (e.g., *Is the dog running down the street?* is more complex than *The dog is running down the street*).

Contractions. These should be analyzed to determine how the contracted form is used. One common type of error is the use of the contracted form along with the full form (Louis, age 8, **I'*ve have* lots of books** and Joey, age 8: **I'm am eight**).

Negatives. Errors in negatives might include the use of *no* for *not* (Jason, age 9: **I *no* have my thing**), a negative contraction plus full form (Morris, age 15: **I did*n't not* ask the teacher anything about this**), auxiliary confusion* (Frank, age 11, **I *might won't* be here**), double negative* (Amelia, age 8: **I *don't* want *no* bonuses today**), or word order (Sonya, age 9: **They're doing stuff that they *not should be* doing**). Phillip, age 5: used the wrong qualifier with the negative: **I can't find *some* eggs**.

Imperatives. Errors may be most evident in the negative imperative form (Rodney, age 8: ***No* hit me!**)

Passive. Passive constructions should be evaluated for errors in comprehension as well as for confusion in production. Courtney, age 9: **The wilabeast got ate** and Daniel, age 9, referring to a sea turtle: **One got crashed by a boat**.

Infinitives and Participles. The use of the infinitive (uninflected verb form as in *to eat* or *to have*) may result in errors such as the omission of *to* (Danielle, age 8: **And then a bear came and tried *eat* him**), or omission of the infinitive itself (Kirk, age 11: **He look around the city ^ if there are any bad guys**).

The use of the participle (*-ing*) form of the verb used to complement another verb or as a gerund may also cause confusion (Nathan, age 9, **She's keeping looking at my paper**—She keeps looking at my paper confused with She's looking at my paper? and Latoya, age 13: **I don't enjoy to call people names**—used infinitive instead).

Questions. There are several types of questions and many errors may occur within them. The Yes/No question formulation may show substitution errors with the emphatic DO (Micha, age 8: ***Is* your person have white hair?**), omission of the DO* (Rodney, age 8: **School end tomorrow?**), lack of a reversal (Robert, age 8: **I can now sharpen my pencil?**), or confusion with another form (Victor, age 6: **Please may I give me some glue?**—question and imperative forms confused).

The Wh-questions may show omission of the verb* (Corey, age 10: **How come it small?**), or of the auxiliary or emphatic DO* (Arthur, age 8: **How you open it?**), confusion in tense use (Tyrone, age 9: **Why should I did them?**), or the lack of interrogative reversals* (Johnny, age 8: **How much you can buy Snicker bar for?**). In both comprehension and production, the wrong word may be used or understood (Brian, age 9: **When can't I eat this now?).** Tag questions may also cause a problem (Mike, age 13, seeing a man carrying a plant: **He got a tree, he does?**).

Ask/tell constructions cause confusion not only in interpretation or use of the command (Jimmy, age 7: **Will you go *tell* her for a cookie?**), but also in the pronoun demands: When the teacher asked JJ, age 7, to tell Emily what she is supposed to do, he told Emily: ***I'm* supposed to take out *my* book to read**.

Embedded or Conjoined Clauses

The following structures require the joining of more than one clause, either through embedding or conjoining another clause.

Coordination. When two equal clauses are to be joined with a conjunction, errors may involve omissions (Drew, age 7: **You get finished fast but ^ could have an accident**), or confusion in the conjunction (Wendy, age 13: **You better hurry up Andre *and* you will be late.**). Kelly, age 7, shows difficulty with the comparative: **I hit ^ hard that the ball almost got over the fence**.

Subordination. When dependent clauses are embedded with a conjunction in an independent or main clause, the variety, if any, of subordinating conjunctions should be noted. Errors may include omission (Erin, age 10: **The boy fell off the donkey ^ it kicked**), confusion in conjunction use (Robert, age 6: **I was using a metal fishing line then it wouldn't break**), or confusion in order (John, age 8: **My sister is more older than me because she stays up past me**).

Relative Clause. Errors may occur when a clause that starts with a relative pronoun as the subject or a relative conjunction is embedded to modify a noun. Errors may include use of both the pronoun and its antecedent (Robert, age 8: **Mario Two has a face *that it opens a mouth***), *omission of the relative pronoun (Anthony, age 11: **My teacher wrote me a note ^ *said I could go***), verb confusion (Brooke, age 10: **The boy *that really did loved her* got killed**), use of the wrong word (Brooke, age 10: **Edward Scissorhand had fingers *but except they were scissors***), or confusion with the rules of embedding (Brooke, 10: **Edward Scissorhand saw a little boy *that the girl with the red hair it was her brother***) or placement of the clause (John, age 7: **Who put the drawing in the garbage *that I did*?**). If relative clauses are used, even correctly, it should be noted whether they are embedded in the center of the sentence or only attached to the object at the end of a sentence.

Noun Complement Clauses. When clauses are used to function as a noun, that is, as the subject, object, or complement of the sentence, errors may include omission where it is not allowed (Allen, age 9, **I know *you mean***—for *I know who you mean*), reversals (Chris, age 13: **I'm not sure *what was it* that I should put for the sun** or Noel, age 9: **It tells *how many is it***—confusion with interrogative), confusion in the formation of the clause (Skippy, age 14: **I used to tell him my scary things *like what was that felt bad about me***—for *like what I felt bad about*), or use of the wrong word (Tyrone, age 9: ***Who was cooking* get in front of me**—for *whoever was cooking*). It should be noted whether noun complement clauses are used in various functions or simply as the earliest developing object clauses.

Formats such as those in Tables 7–2 and 7–3 should serve as organizational supports from which a description of a student's language can be summarized. Questions should also be asked about the complexity level and variety of the sample. For example, some variations in conjunction use should be evident in the school-age subject. Overuse of the immature form *and* may indicate an immature level of language use.

Analysis of Comprehension

Before intervention on production of a form or structure begins, comprehension of that form should be evaluated. The technique used by Berko-Gleason (1958, 1971) in her Experimental Test of Morphology (e.g., This is a wug. Now there are two of them. There are two _______) may be adapted to check production/expressive ability of morphemes by using pictures or objects and real words (This is a dog. Now there are two of them. There are two _______). It may also be adapted for comprehension/receptive ability by using pictures and asking students to "Point to two dogs."

Other structures can also be checked for comprehension by using pictures and objects or, with younger children, dolls and puppets. For example, comprehension of relative clauses may be tested by telling the student that these are pictures of a boy and a girl on the playground and then asking him or her to point to the picture of *The boy who hit the girl is running away*. Included will be a picture of a boy running away and a picture of a girl running away.

INTERVENTION

The importance of context has become increasingly clear and must be considered when intervention planning occurs. However, Kirchner (1991) reported that contexts for language instruction, particularly for children with more severe disorders, continue to be "dydactic and drill oriented rather than dyadic and interaction oriented" (p. 84). This may be particularly true for morphology and syntax. Owens (1995) referred to linguistic cues such as "What do we say?" and "Now, tell me the whole thing" as examples of pseudoconversational cues.

The much documented development of morphological forms and syntactic structures provides a guideline for intervention, but more needs to be taken into account. Intervention should be provided in context and, whenever appropriate, in conversation, thus involving pragmatic skills as well. Forms and structures to be taught should not be selected solely on the basis of syntactic complexity and place in developmental sequence, but also for their position or function in discourse (Kirchner, 1991). Training using discourse can occur in both the oral and written mode (Owens, 1995).

Spoken Language

Supported Language Intervention

Kirchner (1991) suggested that intervention approaches do not have to be unstructured to be interactive and conversationally driven. She described an interactive approach to intervention that uses **verbal scaffolding**, or borrowing from the preceding dialogue, and verbal repetition, or imitation. The teacher or clinician, with a series of preplanned dialogues, uses **forced alternative** questioning or commenting strategies (Crystal, Fletcher, & Garman, 1976) to provide models while restricting the possibilities of response. In other words, the child is given the model required for the answer, thus minimizing recall and formulation. Examples of each provided by Kirchner include *Do you need shoes or a hat for the baby's feet?* as a forced alternative question and *Let's see we can draw, paint, or color* as a forced alternative comment. Thus, the child may produce a borrowed part of the dialogue in order to participate in a meaningful context. All teaching is conducted in a dialogue allowing the child to learn conversational skills as well as specific linguistic forms simultaneously.

Conversational Contingencies

To enhance language stimulation and facilitate language learning, Owens (1995) recommended a hierarchy of contingencies that require a response during a naturalistic conversation with the child. This hierarchy, illustrated in Table 7–4, may be used from initial training through practice after acquisition. Teachers or clinicians may already use many of these contingencies but may not be aware of the hierarchical nature of the responses. As with other areas of learning, for example, decoding, no more information than is necessary should be provided at a particular point in learning. In Table 7–4, the contingency farthest down in the list provides the least amount of information and the correction model at the top of the list provides the most information, that is, a full model. The contingency farthest down the list that can ensure success should be used. Only if a full model is needed, for example in initial acquisition, should it be provided. All of the contingencies should be used in conversational tones that indicate more concern with comprehension of the message than with correctness of the message. Use should be limited so as not to disrupt communication and frustrate the speaker. Turnabouts should be used to keep the conversation going and support the student's efforts to maintain the topic.

General Procedures

Bos and Vaughn (1994) pointed out that opportunities abound for teaching language in school and provided some general procedures for teaching oral language to students with learning and behavior problems. These procedures are presented in Table 7–5. Note that their first recommendation is that **language should be taught in context**. Use needs to be taught along with form and content. Dramatic play using a story that contains many examples of plurals in the lines may be appropriate for JJ, age 7, who needs practice in plurals. In deciding on a targeted form or structure to teach or focus on, the **normal language development sequence should be followed**. However, as

TABLE 7–4. Hierarchy of conversational contingencies.

Conversational Contingency	***Example****
Correction model/Request	He *gave* me two ponies. Can you tell me again? (Cue to say it again is used if the child does not repeat spontaneously)
Incomplete correction model/Request	*Gave*. Can you tell me again? (Cue is again optional)
Reduced error repetition/Request	*Give?*
Error repetition/Request	He *give* you a pony?
Self-correction request	Was that right?
Contingent query	I didn't understand you. Say it again please. (Other options include *Huh?* and *What?* or in this example *What did he do?*)
Expansion request (Used if the targeted response is correct but in a smaller unit than desired)	Tell me the whole thing again. (or *Gave? Gave* you what? I didn't get it. You'd better tell me again.)
Repetition request (Used with complete, correct responses)	Tell me again (or Could you say that again?)
Turnabout (Used with complete, correct responses)	Wow! A pony? Your grandpa sounds great! What did he do for you at Christmas?

*In a conversation about his grandpa, Jose, a 16-year-old with moderate retardation, has told the teacher that "He give me a pony for my birthday." (Sample provided by Becki Paynor).

Source: From *Language disorders: A functional approach to assessment and intervention* (2nd ed.) by R. E. Owens, 1995, p. 307. Boston: Allyn & Bacon. Copyright 1995 by Allyn & Bacon. Adapted with permission.

Kirchner (1991) noted, discourse needs must also be considered and may sometimes take precedence. All too often, language comprehension is slighted; **both understanding and expression must be taught**. The teacher should make an effort to use a form or structure that is being taught (or is the next to be taught) frequently in class. For example, if the present perfect tense is being practiced, the teacher could make many comments such as Julio *has finished* his work; Kamal *has gone* to speech class. To practice production, he or she could incorporate many questions or comments throughout the day or class period, such as, *Where have you been?* or *Tell me if you have already had a turn.*

Effective teaching strategies should be used when presenting a new concept or skill. Many effective teaching strategies that are already

TABLE 7–5. General procedures for teaching oral language.

1. Teach language in context.
2. In most cases, follow normal language development sequence.
3. Teach comprehension and production.
4. Use effective teaching strategies when presenting a new concept or skill.
5. Use self-talk to explain what you are doing or thinking.
6. Use parallel talk to describe what others are doing.
7. Use modeling for practice and feedback on a specific language skill.
8. Use expansion to demonstrate how an idea can be expressed in a slightly more complex manner.
9. Use elaboration to demonstrate how more information can be expressed.
10. Use structured language programs for intensive practice and feedback.
11. Reinforce language learning by using intrinsic reinforcers and naturally occurring consequences.
12. Systematically plan and instruct for generalization.

Note: From *Strategies for teaching students with learning and behavior problems* by C. S. Bos and S. Vaughn, 1994, p. 80. Boston: Allyn & Bacon. Copyright 1994 by Allyn & Bacon. Reprinted with permission.

being used in other areas of study in the classroom may be applied to oral language, for example, brainstorming, reciprocal teaching, metacognitive strategies. One of these strategies that should be used is **self-talk to explain what you are doing or thinking**. Self-talk is simply self-instruction or thinking aloud. For example, if the future tense is being worked on, the teacher may think aloud statements such as, *Let's see, I will need paper for the printer to finish my last draft. Where did I put my paper? Oh yes, I will have to go to the supply closet. That's where I put it yesterday.* This example also made use of the past tense, which was an earlier goal. A similar effective strategy is parallel talk. The teacher or clinician should **use parallel talk to describe what others are doing** or what is occurring to the student in his or her environment. For example, if subordinating clauses are being focused on, *Syrynthia will put two tablespoons of butter in because we are doubling the recipe.*

Teachers or clinicians should also **use modeling for practice and feedback** on a specific language skill. The forced alternative questions and comments (Crystal et al., 1976) described earlier could easily be incorporated into the school routine. Also, **expansion should be used** to demonstrate how an idea can be expressed in a slightly more complex manner and **elaboration should be used** to demonstrate how more information can be expressed. An example of an expansion to demonstrate the use of a relative clause might be used following Amber's simple sentences, *I like this pencil. I like the red pencil. Oh, you* *like this pencil which is red.* The teacher or clinician may follow Andrew's comment that *Wilbur was Charlotte's friend* with the elaboration, *Yes, Wilbur was Charlotte's friend and Templeton, Avery, and Fern were Charlotte's friends, too.*

Students with learning problems may need extra practice, and so, in addition to context, the teacher or clinician may **use structured language programs for intensive practice and feedback**. Materials such as *Fokes Sentence Builder* (Fokes, 1976) may be used to train sentence structure, or games and activities may be developed to focus on particular forms or structures. For example, playing the game Jeopardy in Social Studies is an excellent way to practice Wh-question development. Plural Bingo or a game board requiring the conjoining of two sentences in order to move can be both fun and beneficial.

Reinforce language learning by using intrinsic reinforcers and naturally occurring consequences. "Good talking" or "I like the way you said that" may disrupt communication and create awkwardness leading to decreased participation. The job interview that goes well after the role-playing activities is the naturally occurring consequence. Teachers and clinicians should **systematically plan and instruct for generalization**. Collaboration on the part of the special education teacher, the general education teacher, and the speech-language pathologists is an obvious route to generalization. The use of these procedures should also foster both intrinsic reinforcement and generalization.

Written Language

Using Written Language as Context

Norris (1991) has recommended that written language be used as the basis of language intervention. Whereas oral language is a rapid and temporary transmission of information, written language presents a stable expression of language that can be repeatedly and carefully examined. Norris suggested that good children's literature can provide meaningful contexts that are ideal for helping children recognize and use abstract, complex, and subtle aspects of language. She recommended the use of such techniques as **scaffolding** to turn reading into an interactive communicative exchange which proceeds more as a conversation than oral reading. The teacher or clinician may point to specific structures and point out what it tells or ask the student to find what it relates. For example, consider the sentence *Many years ago there was a handsome frog who lived by a rather nice pond,* from *The Strange Story of the Frog who Became a Prince* (Horwitz, 1971). Norris suggested the teacher may point to the main clause and say, "This tells us what the frog looked like." He or she may then point to the relative clause and ask the child to "find out where the frog lives." The relative pronoun can be associated with the frog to create awareness of the clause and how it functions to link concepts. A variety of embedded and conjoined clauses can be used to help the student learn how to combine the same ideas into different relationships. Metalinguistic knowledge about words can be developed in a meaningful context. For example, the adult can point to the word *handsome* and state, "I wouldn't use an adjective like handsome to describe him. I might use an adjective like homely. What adjective would you use?"

Reciprocal Teaching

Reciprocal teaching is a method of teaching that ties cognitive and metacognitive strategies directly to an academic task and turns reading into a conversational interaction. Teaching involves a dialogue between the teacher and the learner in which students and teacher take turns leading and for which the learner eventually takes full responsibility (Palincsar & Brown, 1984). The teacher provides support, or scaffolding, until the student is ready to assume control. Initially the teacher takes major responsibility for explaining and modeling, gradually turning this role over to students as they become experts. Modeling, feedback, and practice are provided by the teacher as indicated by student needs. During the dialogue, students are trained in four strategies that enhance both comprehension and self-monitoring: summarizing the main content in the form of self-review, formulating potential questions, clarifying any ambiguities, and predicting future content. An example of a beginning dialogue with a seventh grade student with a third grade reading equivalent is provided below (Brown & Palinscar, 1987). The focus of this dialogue between the student and teacher is on question-asking and occurs on Day 1 after Charles has read (silently) a passage on the water moccasin. He is trying to formulate a question about what he has just read.

S: What is found in the southeastern snakes, also the copperhead, rattlesnakes, vipers—they have. I'm not doing this right.

T: All right. Do you want to know more about the pit vipers?

S: Yeah.

T: What would be a good question about the pit vipers that starts with the word "why"?

S: (No response)

T: How about, "Why are the snakes called pit vipers?"

S: Why do they want to know that they are called pit vipers?

T: Try it again.

S: Why do they, pit vipers in a pit?

T: How about, "Why do they call the snakes pit vipers?"

S: Why do they call the snakes pit vipers?

T: There you go! Good for you.

By Day 15, Charles was able to perform his part unaided, immediately producing the following appropriate question after reading a passage on the South Pole: *Why do scientists come to the South Pole to study?*

A major strength of this approach is that strategies are taught during regular content instruction; all activities are undertaken when appropriate in the context of actual reading. This approach has been implemented with much success in actual classroom situations across the curriculum at many different ages, including with first graders on listening comprehension (Brown & Palincsar, 1987).

Children's Literature

Owens and Robinson (1997) have developed a list of young children's books and specified their potential uses in the classroom to target specific language skills, including prepositions, past, present progressive, and future tenses, interrogatives, noun-verb agreement, pronouns, possessive markers, adjectives, and relative clauses. They suggested that the literature be selected based on language goals of the classroom and individual children with communication impairments. An abbreviated list is presented in Table 7–6. The complete list is a very comprehensive list for use in all the components of language and can be found in the February, 1997, issue of *Topics in Language Disorders* (Vol. 17, No. 2). For those classrooms that adhere to a whole language approach to teaching, themes for each of the storybooks are also included.

The use of narratives in oral and written instruction with students who have language learning disabilities is increasing. See Hoggan and Strong (1994) for a description of 20 different narrative strategies from the literature.

Table 7–7, reprinted from Goodman (1986), summarizes what makes language very easy or very hard for children to learn in school. These points underscore the need for contextually based language lessons.

TABLE 7–6. Story books and uses within the classroom.

Book	***Language Use***
Allen, *A Lion in the Night*	Predicting, present progressive & future tense, sequencing
Baker, *The Third Story Cat*	Prepositions, past tense
Banchek, *Snake In, Snake Out*	Prepositions
Barton, *Airplanes*	Vocabulary, noun-verb agreement, categories
Brown, *Arthur's Nose*	Possessive marker, pronouns
Brown, *The Runaway Bunny*	Prepositions, pronouns, present progressive tense
Burningham, *Skip, Trip*	Verb Vocabulary, to elicit SVO structures
Charoa, *Kate's Box*	Pronouns, possessive, prepositions, present progressive & past tense
Gibbons, *The Season of the Arnolds' Apple Tree*	Regular plural, possessive, third person marker
Ginsburg, *Good Morning, Chick*	Past tense, chanting, predicting, demonstratives (this, that)
Hutchins, *Rosie's Walk*	Prepositions, present progressive & past tense, sequencing
Keats, *Over in the Meadow*	Singular/plural contrast, present progressive & past tense
Krauss, *Whose Mouse Are You?*	Possessive, interrogatives
LeSaux, *Daddy Shaves*	Verbs, third person marker
Marsollo & Pinkney, *Pretend You're a Cat*	Verbs, adjectives, questions
Numeroff, *Dogs Don't Wear Sneakers*	Negatives, verbs, noticing the ridiculous
Porter-Gaylord, *I Love My Daddy Because*	Causal phrases, discussion
Sendak, *Alligators All Around*	Present progressive tense, noun-verb agreement
Wood, *Silly Sally*	Initial /s/, relative clauses, chanting
Zukman & Edelman, *It's a Good Thing*	Verbal expression, discussion, "because . . ." structures

Source: From "Once upon a time: Use of children's literature in the preschool classrom" by R. E. Owens & L. A. Robinson, 1997, *Topics in Language Disorders, 17*(2), pp. 35–48. Copyright 1997 by Aspen Publishers. Adapted with permission.

TABLE 7–7. What makes language very easy or very hard to learn?

It's Easy When	*It's Hard When*
It's real and natural.	It's artificial.
It's whole.	It's broken into bits and pieces.
It's sensible.	It's nonsense.
It's interesting.	It's dull and uninteresting.
It's relevant.	It's irrelevant to the learner.
It belongs to the learner.	It belongs to someone else.
It's part of a real event.	It's out of context.
It has social utility.	It has no social value.
It has purpose for the learner.	It has no discernible purpose.
The learner chooses it.	It's imposed by someone else.
It's accessible to the learner.	It's inaccessible.
The learner has power to use it.	The learner is powerless.

Source: From *What's whole in whole language?* by K. Goodman, 1986, p. 8. Portsmouth, NH: Heinemann. Copyright 1986 by Kenneth Goodman. Reprinted with permission of Scholastic Canada, Ltd., 123 Newkirk Road, Richmond Hill, Ontario. L4C365 Canada.

✓ SUMMARY CHECKLIST

☐ **Analysis**
- **Morphology**

Syntax
- ***Single Sentence Units***
- ***Embedded or Conjoined Clauses***

Comprehension

☐ **Intervention**

Speaking
- ***Supported Language***
  - Verbal Scaffolding
  - Forced Alternative
    - ***Conversational Contingencies***
    - ***General Procedures***
      - Self-Talk
      - Parallel Talk
      - Expansion
      - Elaboration

Written Language
- ***Scaffolding***
- ***Reciprocal Teaching***
- ***Children's Literature***

CHAPTER

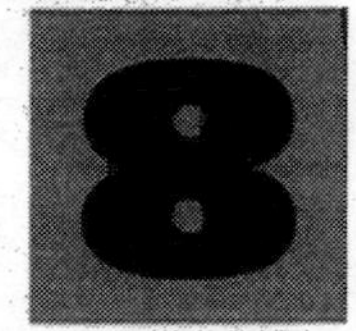

THE DEVELOPMENT OF SEMANTICS

As previously noted, the components of language have been discussed separately in this text. However, in reality, during the acquisition of language, all components are interrelated in both typical and atypical development. This is particularly relevant to the area of semantics, because semantic development and semantic problems are so intertwined with the other component areas (Camarata & Schwartz, 1985; Norris & Damico, 1990). Language is used to transfer a message and to translate meaning. Meaning is delivered through and derived from individual words and word combinations, language form (syntax and morphology), and context (pragmatics). Likewise, language form and language use are dependent on the meaning one intends to express.

DEFINING SEMANTICS

Berko Gleason (1993) defined semantics as the study of the meaning system of language. Unlike syntax, where the application of rules can be seen on the surface level, semantics is less tangible, less easily understood. Semantics involves the translation of one's cognitive representation of life experiences into language (Bloom & Lahey, 1978). In other words, as an individual interacts with the world, these events are cognitively processed and stored as mental images, which then must be translated into language for the purpose of communication, problem-solving, and social relations.

Receptively, semantics involves the comprehension of language. It requires an accurate delineation of meaning from our linguistic symbol system. Expressively, semantics is the appropriate choice of vocabulary and language structure to transfer meaning and is dependent on the content and purpose, that is, what and why one wants to communicate. Semantic study explores this process of encoding meaning into language and decoding meaning from language. This process includes the **lexicon**, that is, words/vocabulary, the relationship of these words to the concepts they represent, and the organization of these words (Cromer, 1988). This process of learning to encode and decode meaning (i.e., semantic acquisition) can be studied at the word level, at the multiword/sentence level, and at the discourse level.

SEMANTIC DEVELOPMENT AT THE WORD LEVEL

The process of attaching meaning to words is one part of the cognitive process of organizing and categorizing information learned about the world. The categories and classes that the child generates to understand the world are given names or labels. These linguistic symbols, conversely, help the child to become more efficient at assimilating and accommodating new information about the world (Owens, 1996). This interrelationship between cognition and language demonstrates the internal overlap and spiralling process that occurs in learning, across developmental domains.

Referential Meaning

One of the most interesting areas in the study of semantics is the attachment of meaning to a single word. This is known as **referential meaning**. Referential meaning is the ability to use a word as a sign or symbol to represent a referent, which may be an object, an event, or a concept. In general, assignment of a word, or symbol, to a referent is arbitrary. There is no particular reason why a certain word represents a certain object. The referent itself is not the meaning of the word; one's cognitive representation of that object is the meaning. For example, in *bird*, the actual bird is the referent, but not the meaning, of the word *bird*. It is one's concept or cognitive representation of *bird* that is the meaning. If the bird flies away, the word *bird* still has meaning.

As Shames and Wiig (1986) stated, "words and symbols do not represent reality but rather each language user's ideas and concepts of reality" (p. 42). Concept formation occurs through interaction with the environment and is never identical for any two individuals. In other words, I can say *cat* and you can say *cat*, and because we have had very different experiences with cats, our meanings may be different. In terms of the core concept of *cat*, our representations are probably the same, but there may be slight variations in meaning. Let us further consider the example, *cat*. If your experiences with a cat included an event where you had been badly scratched, you may associate pain and fear with the concept of *cat*. Another individual who has not had such an experience would not include these associations.

Variation in the meaning of vocabulary will be much greater with young children, because they have not had the wealth of experiences that an adult has had. Consider the following:

> My 2-year-old daughter and I were having a discussion about girls/boys; men/women. She was a girl, mommy was a girl, mommy was a woman, but when we got to daddy there was a problem. I said "daddy is a man" and she emphatically stated "Daddy no man!" She was quite insistent and finally stated "Daddy no man, daddy no fix things." I then realized the context in which she had heard the word *man* during her young life. "The man is coming to fix the washer today." "We have to wait, the man will be here to fix the oven." "I need to call the man to fix the toilet." And you know, according to the mental image or cognitive representation she had developed for the word *man*, she was right; Daddy no fix things, daddy no man.

Variation will also occur across children, depending on the quantity and quality of experiences the children have had with the environment and the strength of their cognitive abilities to process those experiences. A child's knowledge of the world will be demonstrated in word knowledge (Crais, 1990). Children growing up in poverty or experiencing an impoverished environment will obviously be delayed in concept formation, concept refinement, and referential meaning (i.e., vocabulary development).

Three primary hypotheses have been offered as explanations for the attachment of referential meaning (Owens, 1996; Valletutti, Mcknight-Taylor, & Hoffnung, 1989). These consist of the semantic feature hypothesis (Clark, 1973), the functional-core hypothesis (K. Nelson, 1974), and the prototypic complex hypothesis (Bowerman, 1978).

Semantic Feature Hypothesis

The semantic feature hypothesis suggests that the attachment of meaning to words (vocabulary development) occurs through a process of abstracting or recognizing attributes or features. Clark (1973) suggested that children initially identify perceptual features, or some combination of perceptual features, to generate a word meaning. The child attaches one or two features to a word and then adds other features over time. These features tend to be polar.

For example: **+ human** **+ nonhuman**

As the child's interaction with the environment continues, he or she gradually adds more features until adult meaning is eventually reached. It is during this process that the child learns that an addition of feature or features may mandate a new name or linguistic label.

For example, it is highly likely that a child will first categorize a zebra as a horse. Upon additional experience, the child will come to realize, with the addition of a combination of features such as black and white, striped, and wild, that the more appropriate label is *zebra.*

Generally, the perceptual features of shape, size, and movement are the first to be attached.

For example:	**Horse**	**Zebra**
	+ living	+ living
	+ animal	+ animal
	+ four-legged	+ four-legged
	+ mane	+ mane
		+ black and white
		+ wild
		+ striped

Words that have identical or very similar features are known as **synonyms**, for example, *happy* and *glad*; *beautiful* and *lovely*.

Words with similar features except for one opposite or polar feature are known as **antonyms**, for example, *heavy* and *light*; *night* and *day*.

The features attached to a word impose certain restrictions on word combinations. These are known as **selection restrictions**. These restrictions prohibit feature conflicts that result in confusion, conflict, or redundancy, as is illustrated by Shames and Wiig (1986) in the following examples.

A bachelor's wife
This word combination is not acceptable because one of the features of bachelor is + *unwed*, therefore this combination is contradictory in meaning and unacceptable.

An unwed bachelor
This word combination is unacceptable because it is redundant, as one of the features of bachelor is + *unwed*.

Functional Core Hypothesis

Another explanation for the attachment of word meaning is the functional core hypothesis described by K. Nelson (1974) and based on the Piagetian theory of development. This theory suggests a process by which a child organizes experiences with the world through structures Piaget referred to as **schemes** (Berk, 1994). It is through these schemes that a concept develops. Because the earliest stage of development (according to Piaget) is the sensorimotor stage, it is hypothesized that early schemes are built on motor actions. Concepts will be built on the basis of how something acts or can be acted upon. K. Nelson (1974) offered this example for the development of the concept of *ball*, or "ballness."

	*in living room, porch
	*Mother throws, picks up, holds
Ball (1)	*I throw, pick up, hold
	*rolls, bounces
	*on floor, under couch

(Nelson, 1974, p. 277)

These schemes are based on the functional relations experienced by the child and the ball. These functional relations then form the core of understanding of the concept. Additional experiences will cause addition, deletion, and modification of the concept.

Ball (2)

*on playground
*boy throws, catches
*rolls, bounces
*over ground, under fence . . .

(Nelson, 1974, p. 277)

A mature scheme will eventually form:

Ball (1,2)

*Location of activity: living room, porch, playground
*Actor: Mother, I, boy
*Action: throw, pick up, hold, catch
*Movement of ball: roll, bounce
*Location of object: on floor, under couch, under fence

(Nelson, 1974, p. 277)

In order for the child to eventually recognize this concept in pictures and in static situations, the child must begin to recognize the attributes or characteristics of the object. The concept at this point will possess functional and perceptual information. These concepts may then be labeled after the child notices that there is a relationship between a word and a concept. The word or object is embedded in an experience or a schema and is not identified in isolation (K. Nelson, 1974). Therefore, word meaning is generated by a scheme of events and routines. Some concepts that the child develops may not be the same as an adult's and therefore are left unnamed.

The child develops concepts or preconcepts that organize objects that are acted on in similar ways (K. Nelson, 1974). With Piagetian theory, the child attempts to translate dynamic experiences into relationships between objects, animals, people, activities, and so forth and into cognitive and linguistic meaning. Linguistic representation (i.e., the word) is dependent on the experiences and the different relationships that the child observes with the object.

Prototypic Complex Hypothesis

In contrast, the prototypic complex hypothesis suggests the child develops a **prototype** or *best example* of a concept or category (Rosch, 1973). The prototype is normally learned by first experience with a referent from the category (Rosch & Mervis, 1975) or from the frequency of use by an adult caregiver (Valletutti et al., 1989). Additional examples within that category are introduced and added. Again, this is dependent on the child's experiences. Referents that resemble the prototype will be included in the category, and those most similar to the prototype will be central, leaving those with less similarity on the periphery. See Figure 8–1 for an example of a prototype (Owens, 1992). In support of the prototypic theory, adults appear to categorize by the use of prototypes (Bowerman, 1978; Lund & Duchan, 1988).

The Development of Early Expressive Vocabulary

Expressively, children will begin using their first words at approximately 12 months of age. Vocabulary development will slowly progress to about 50 words or more by about 18 months. Studies of language development reveal that early vocabularies consist of **substantive words** and **relational words** (e.g., Bloom & Lahey, 1978).

Substantive words are objects or classes of objects. A substantive word can be a single or solo object such as *Mommy* or *Daddy*, or a class of objects that share perceptual and/or functional features such as *car*

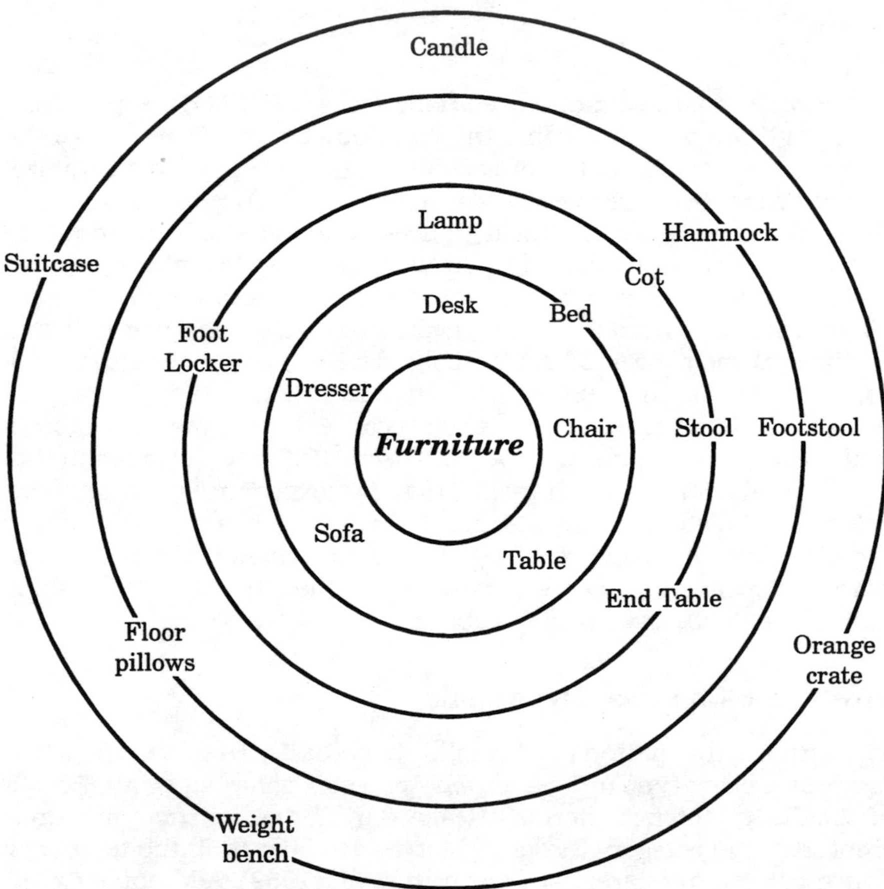

Figure 8–1. Possible prototypic concept of *furniture* with exemplars. (From *Language Development: An Introduction,* by R. E. Owens, 1992, p. 268. New York: Merrill. Copyright 1992 by Macmillan Publishing Co. Reprinted with permission.)

or *dog*. Substantive words have as referents objects or object concepts (Bloom & Lahey, 1978). Typically, first words tend to be objects or concepts that are important and familiar to the child such as family, pets, food, drink, animals, or animal noises (Nelson, 1974). Not surprisingly, children's first words are related to their daily activities (Nelson, Hampson, & Shaw, 1993).

Relational words describe the relationships that a referent has with him- or herself or other referents, including movement (Reed, 1986). The most frequently used relational words are reflexive (Bloom & Lahey, 1978). **Reflexive relational words** are words that refer to a relationship a referent has with itself. These relationships are expressed in four general meanings: existence, nonexistence, disappearance, and recurrence (Bloom & Lahey, 1978). These are very useful words, they enable the child to express what he or she wants and needs. As can be seen from Table 8–1, these first terms are the same as those in

TABLE 8–1. Reflexive relation words in single-word utterances.

Type	*Explanation*	*Examples*
Existence	Child's attention gained by entity, especially a novel one: notes that it exists	May point and say *this, that, here*, or *what's that?*
Nonexistence	Child notes that an entity is not present although expected	*No* or *gone* or name of object with rising intonation
Disappearance	Child notes that an entity that was present has disappeared	*Gone, allgone, away, bye-bye*
Recurrence	Child notes that an object appears after an absence or that another object replaces an absent one	*More, again*, or *another*

Source: From *Language development: An introduction*, (3rd ed.) by R. E. Owens, 1992, p. 273. New York: Merrill. Copyright 1992 by Merrill. Adapted with permission.

Chapter 6 in Brown's Stage I, Semantic Relations, as children begin to string together words.

Other relational words include action, attribution, location, and possession. **Attribution relational words** indicate attributes, features, or characteristics of objects, for example, *little* or *dirty*. **Action relational words** are associated with verbs. In fact, these are sometimes described as *protoverbs* (Clark, 1979). They are words used by the child to indicate an action without using the verb, for example *in*, *down*, or *bye bye*. These words serve the purpose of indicating an action or some kind of movement. **Locational relational words** indicate direction or spatial relationship. For example, the child might say *chair* indicating the cat is on the chair. **Possessive relational words** indicate possession, an important aspect of a young child's life. For example, the child learns early to say *mine*.

Initial vocabularies are predominantly made up of nouns, that is, substantive words (Gentner, 1982; Nelson et al., 1993). Children initially comprehend and produce more nouns than any other class of words. Nelson et al. (1993) suggested this could be due to the fact that there are more nouns than verbs in language. On the other hand, Gentner (1982) suggested that action words are more semantically complex, and therefore, nouns are easier to learn. Research appears to indicate that objects that have a greater variety of actions performed on them are more easily learned (Ross, Nelson, Wetstone, & Tanouye, 1986). However, in terms of usage, the relational words may occur more frequently. In other words, although there may be more nouns in their vocabulary, the frequency of use may be higher for relational words (Bloom, 1973).

Interestingly, as researchers have examined children's early lexicon (the first 50–75 words), two different types of vocabularies have emerged (e.g., Nelson, 1973), possibly indicating two different language learning strategies. One group of children has been described as **referential**, or analytical, and the other as **expressive**, or gestalt (Nelson et al., 1993; Plunkett, 1993; Thal & Bates, 1990). The vocabulary of referential children is dominated by common nouns (object labels) and is used primarily for labeling the environment. The referential child primarily connects a string of phonemes, that is, a word, to an object or concept in the environment by labeling it (Bates et al., 1994). In contrast, an expressive child focuses more on interaction and has a vocabulary that consists of more proper names, action-type words, and social-communication words such as *go bye bye*, *thank you*, and *stop it* (Nelson, 1973; Hampson, 1989). The expressive children seemed to use language primarily for social interaction or instrumental functions (Bates et al., 1994).

The Learning Process

Nelson (1974) made several observations about the acquisition of first words or first vocabularies. First, she noted that, initially, a small set of words is learned early. These words tend to be dominated by categories such as people, animals, and food. As previously noted, early words seem to have some relevance in the child's environment, especially in the area of basic needs, and are often associated with movement (Reed, 1986). Although children follow a general pattern of development, there is a great deal of variation in the rate of learning (Bates et al., 1994). In general, the first 50 words tend to emerge slowly, followed by a spurt in vocabulary development.

Second, Nelson noted that children will make up words if they do not have a word to describe something. Children enjoy playing with language and will create new words to fill in gaps in their vocabularies. They may use attributes in this process and also interchange classes of words, such as using nouns to create new verbs (Clark, 1981). For example, in an attempt to let her mother know she had a stomach ache, a young 2-year-old said, *Body Boo Boo.* Using an attribute of shape, another child described a pumpkin-shaped house as *pumpkin house* (Kit-Fong Au, 1990).

Finally, Nelson noted that acquired words are often generalized by children. In the early productive language of young children, two processes occur, **overextension** and **underextension**. These processes aid children in the hypothesis testing of the mechanics and meaning of language. They occur most frequently between the ages of 1 and 2½. If these processes continue beyond this age period, they may be indicative of a language delay.

Overextension is the overgeneralization of meaning and occurs when the range of meaning for a particular word is much greater than it is for the adult's referent for that word. Lindfors (1987) described this process as the child *making-the-most-of-what-you've-got* strategy (p. 193).

For example, a young child may call his regular babysitter *MaMa.* Much to the parent's dismay, the child has overgeneralized the meaning of *MaMa* to all caregivers. The young child is only attempting to communicate his or her limited knowledge about the world with an even more limited lexicon. This is a process that continues for some time. For example, a 2-year-old discovers the Walt Disney Movie *Dumbo,* after which all elephants are called *dumbo.*

Young preschoolers tend to use certain features to produce these overextensions. The features most often used to categorize or determine sameness are perceptual features and, occasionally, functional features (Clark, 1973; Nelson, 1974). The perceptual features most often identified in this overextension process are shape, movement, size, sound, texture, and taste. Table 8–2 contains examples from Clark (1973).

Overextension may be the result of a comprehension error or a performance error (Naigles & Gelman, 1995). A comprehension error could occur if the child does not have adequate semantic representation. In contrast, a performance error in overextension could be the result of

TABLE 8–2. Examples of overextension.

Category	Word	First Referent	Overextension Examples	Language
SHAPE	*mooi*	moon	→cakes →round marks on book →round postmarks →letter O	English
	buti	ball	→toy →radish →stone spheres at park entrances	Georgian
	tick-tick	watch	→clocks→gas meter →firehose on spool →bathroom scales with round dial	English
SIZE	*fly*	fly	→specks of dirt →dust →all small insects →his own toes→bread crumbs →small toad	English
	bebe	baby	→other babies →all small statues →figures in small prints and pictures	French
MOVEMENT	*bird*	sparrows	→cows→dogs→cats →any animal moving	English
SOUND	*fafer* (chemin de fer)	sound of train	→steaming coffee pot →anything that hissed or made a noise	French
TEXTURE	*va*	white plush dog	→muffler→cat →father's fur coat	Russian
TASTE	*cola*	chocolate	→sugar→tarts →grapes, figs, peaches	French

Source: From "Some aspects of the conceptual basis for first language acquisition" by E.V. Clark, 1974, p. 112. In R. L. Schiefelbusch & L. L. Lloyd (Eds.), *Language perspectives: Acquisition, retardation, and intervention*. Baltimore: University Park Press. Copyright 1974 by University Park Press/Pro-Ed. Adapted with permission.

limited vocabulary (i.e., the child knows there is a difference but does not have the adequate vocabulary to express it) or a retrieval problem (the child is unable to retrieve the correct vocabulary term).

The other process that occurs is **underextension.** This occurs when the range of meaning for a particular word is more limited than the adult's meaning of that word. For example, the child learns *kitty* for his pet but then only uses *kitty* for his cat and not other cats with which he may come in contact.

SEMANTIC DEVELOPMENT AT THE TWO-WORD TO SENTENCE LEVEL

After a rather slow start for the first 50 words, typically, vocabulary development will then increase at a rapid rate (Reznick & Goldfield, 1992) as indicated in Figure 8–2. Vocabulary development continues at this rapid pace throughout the preschool years. Assessment of vocabulary development continues to be a discriminating task into adolescence (Prather, 1984). Prather found vocabulary test scores to be significantly higher for 12th graders than for 5th graders. In contrast, tests (or subtests) focus-

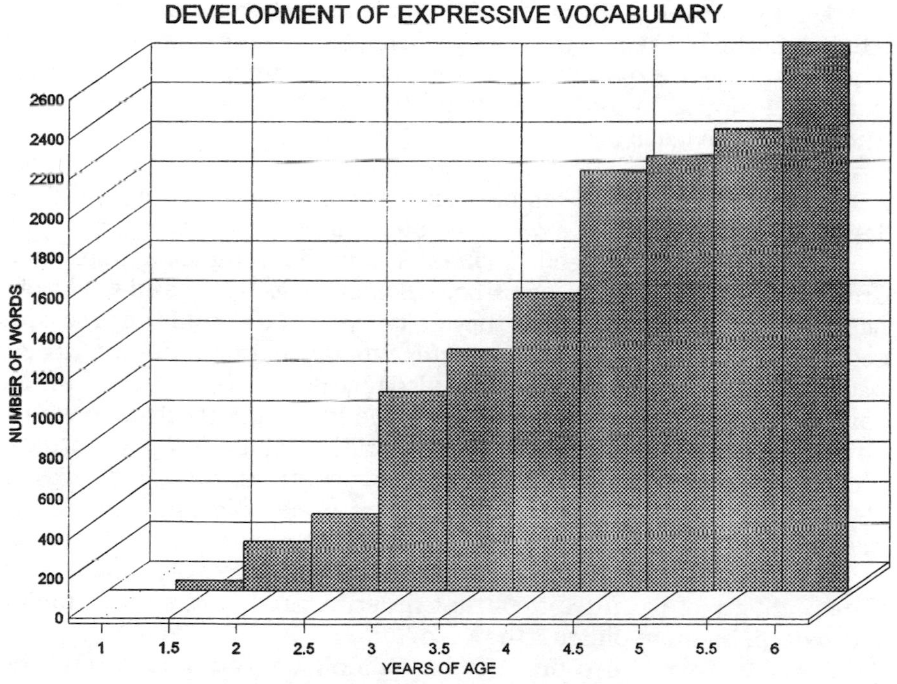

Figure 8–2. Average number of vocabulary words used by children at specific ages of development. (Adapted from *Language development: An introduction*, 3rd ed., by R. E. Owens, 1992. New York: Merrill.)

ing on syntax and morphology showed less noticeable increases. This implies that the size and scope of a typical student's vocabulary will continue to grow at a noticeable level throughout adolescence.

As the child becomes older, Wiig, Freedman, and Secord (1992) noted that the old principle of *world knowledge* translating into *word knowledge* does not hold. Instead, in the middle and secondary school years, vocabulary understanding will aid in the understanding of the world and in the development of efficient strategies for problem solving. Some vocabulary terms prove particularly difficult for children, and more so for many children with disabilities. Specifically, these vocabulary terms are known as shifters, relationals, and kinship terms. A **shifter** is a word that changes its referent depending on who the speaker is and where and when he or she is speaking (Reich, 1986). The problem is that these words lack a one-to-one correspondence with a referent. For example, pronouns (e.g., *I, me, my, mine, you, yours*) will shift referents depending on who the speaker is. *I* refers to the speaker and obviously the speaker changes. *I* becomes *you* when you are talking about me. This concept is very difficult for young children and generally is not mastered until after the age of 5. Interestingly, caregivers, when speaking to young children in child-directed speech (CDS), tend to avoid using pronouns; possibly recognizing the level of difficulty, they attempt to make language easier to understand. In learning pronoun shifters it is common to first witness some redundancy, as in *Mary me going*. It is also developmental to initially use *me* as the first person pronoun and later replace it with *I*.

The use of the shifters, *this/that* and *here/there*, depends on the location of the referent to the speaker. *This book* is the exact same book when it is moved across the room and becomes *that book*. *Come/go* will indicate a motion (although an opposite motion) from one location to another but usage is dependent on the direction.

Relationals are vocabulary terms that express a relationship between two or more objects or events and depend on context (Reich, 1986). Examples include *more/less, big/little*, and *before/after*.

As previously discussed in Chapter 6 under complex syntax, children will find temporals, such as *before, after, until, since*, and *while*, difficult and will use word order if they do not yet understand the time concept. Locational terms, such as *inside/outside, in, on, under, at, above, below, top, in front of*, and *behind* are also relationals. These terms, which can be quite complex, are commonly found in directions given to young children in school. Terms that depend on the relationship of physical attributes include, among many others, *more/less, hard/soft, big/little*, and *thick/thin*. The positive terms are usually learned before the negative and both may be interpreted first as the positive attribute, for example, *more* before *less* and *big* before *little*. Complexity depends on the specificity of the attributes that must be analyzed, so that *wide/narrow* will be more difficult than *big/little*.

Kinship terms also prove to be difficult for young children. The level of difficulty will depend on the complexity of the relationship, so that acquisition of *mother, father, sister*, and *brother* will precede *son, daughter, grandfather*, and *grandmother*. *Aunt, uncle, niece*, and *nephew* are learned even later (Reich, 1986).

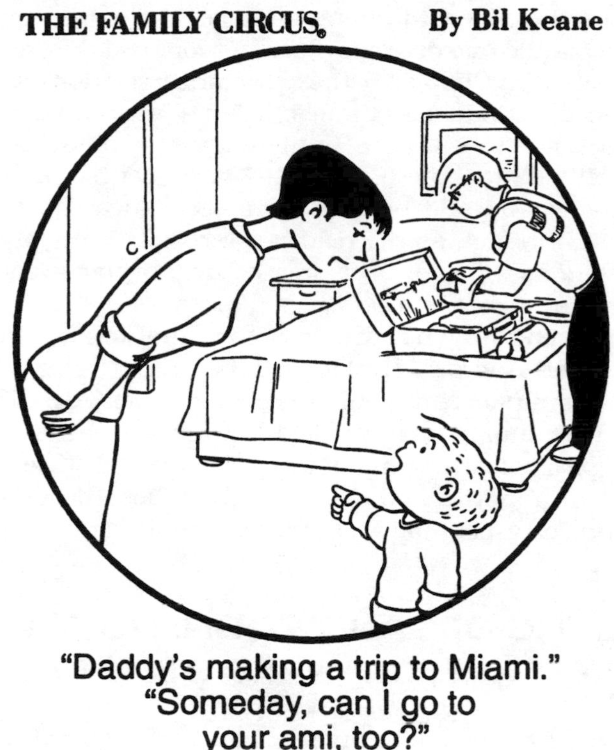

"Daddy's making a trip to Miami."
"Someday, can I go to your ami, too?"

Although previous research has indicated that children in preschool and early elementary school have difficulty learning homonyms (Peters & Zaidel, 1980), more recently, Backsheider and Gelman (1995) discovered that children as young as 3 years (and possibly younger) know some homonyms. This means that young children realize that labels can be misleading and that a single label can represent different categories. The fact that homonyms exist complicates the encoding of meaning, sometimes referred to as **semantic mapping**. Each time a new word is learned, the child must map that word into previous knowledge (Backsheider & Gelman, 1995); unfortunately there are a number of possible mappings (Quine, 1960), contributing to the possibility of error.

Semantic Relations

At around 18 months of age, children begin to combine words into multiword utterances. These utterances expand the usefulness and define the relationship between semantic categories (McLean, Bailey, & Wolery, 1996). Chapter 6 included the semantic relations expressed in early language. Bloom and Lahey (1978) discussed the importance of the interrelationship of syntactic and semantic roles once the child moves beyond the one-word utterance stage. The same word may play a different semantic role depending on the word order (syntax). As previously discussed in Chapter 6, these semantic relations are dominated by certain combinations or rules: agent + action, action + object, agent + object, action + locative, entity + locative, possessor + possession, and entity + attribute (Brown, 1973). Of course, these meaning relationships expand and become more sophisticated as the child's MLU increases. In fact, as the reader will recall, many of these early semantic relations will later be expressed by morphological or syntactic markers. For example, *Daddy shoe* (possessor + possession) will later be expressed by the use of a possessive marker: *Daddy's shoe.*

Yonovitz and Andrews (1995) described an informal assessment instrument to evaluate early semantic content categories. Their checklist offers a nice summary and provides examples of these categories, which are typically learned and used by the age of 5. (See Figure 8–3.) Appendix E in Yonovitz and Andrews describes the developmental sequence and corresponding ages for these relations.

SEMANTIC ORGANIZATION: MULTIWORD, SENTENCE, CONVERSATION LEVEL

At this point, the individual has reached a level of semantic sophistication that allows the comprehension of language by processing pragmatic, syntactic, morphological, and lexical information simultaneously. This allows the understanding of multiple and complex ideas, events, theories, and so forth. Conversely, this level of semantic sophistication allows the individual to competently translate complicated events and abstract ideas into language through accurate structure and appropriate use. In addition, these language abilities will affect the encoding of experience to memory and the retrievability of that experience at a later date (Lindfors, 1987).

Figurative Language

School-age children develop figurative language skills which allow for creativity. Hakes (1982) reports that the linguistic creativity of younger children results from their not knowing enough not to be creative. Preschool children invent many creative terms because of a lack of vocabulary. For example, Gardner and Winner (1979) related the description of a bald man by a preschooler as having *a barefoot head.* Owens (1992) recalled his daughter's description of the Lincoln Memorial with its many columns as *Lincoln's crib.* Early use of figurative language is based on physical resemblance or similarities of use or function (Owens, 1992).

Owens (1992) described the development of figurative language. Metaphors become less frequent after age 6 as the child's basic vocabulary increases, requiring less of a need to create new words. And per-

Language Content Probe: Checklist

DATE:____________________

NAME:____________________________________ AGE:____________________

\+ - EXISTENCE Reference to objects or persons in the environment (e.g., "car", "That a dog.")

\+ - RECURRENCE Reference to the reappearance (e.g. "dog again") or another instance ("another dog", "more cars") of an object or event.

\+ - NONEXISTENCE-DISAPPEARANCE Reference to disappearance (e.g., "dog all gone") or nonexistence of an expected objec t (e.g., "no cars") or an expected action (e.g., "no open")

\+ - REJECTION Opposition to an action or event (e.g., "no take car", "girl not drive") or an object (e.g., "car too little"

\+ - DENIAL Negation of the identity, state or event expressed in the preceding utterance, (e.g., "That's not a dog."

\+ - ATTRIBUTION Reference to properties of objects regarding inherent state or features that distinguish it from others in its class (e.g., "the metal car", "the red one")

\+ - POSSESSION Indication that an object is associated with particular person, permanently or temporarily (e.g., "girl's car", "his chair")

\+ - LOCATIVE ACTION Reference to movement resulting in change of location of a person or object (e.g., "Daddy go bed", "(You) put him there", "(You) sit down")

\+ - ACTION Reference to movement of persons or objects, not to change location (e.g., "girl eat", "dog jumping")

\+ - LOCATIVE STATE Reference to static spatial location (e.g., "daddy on chair")

\+ - QUANTITY Designation of more than one person or object through use of number words (e.g., "two chairs"), plural inflection (e.g., "dogs gone"), or quantitative adjectives (e.g., "many", "some", "all")

INTERNAL STATE References to subjective response to situations or events:

\+ - ATTITUDE/EMOTION Likes/dislikes, felt needs, feelings (e.g., "like", "sad", "I need a hug", "I'm hungry")

\+ - VOLITION/INTENTION Wants, intentions (e.g., "I want to . . . ", "He's going to . . . "); need statements that are more a preference than a felt necessity (e.g., "I don't need any help!")

\+ - OBLIGATION Rules, agreement, demands (e.g., "should", "have to", "supposed to", "gotta")

\+ - POSSIBILITY Proposed or suggested activities, event, or states of affairs (e.g., "would", "could", "maybe", "what if", "let's pretend")

\+ - EXTERNAL STATE References to weather, climate, natural or environmental conditions ("cold", "windy", "dark")

\+ - ATTRIBUTIVE STATE Reference to the condition or properties of a person, place or thing (e.g., "broken", "too small", "the one that's red"

\+ - POSSESSIVE STATE Reference to a temporary or permanent state of ownership (e.g., "it's mine", "that car isn't hers")

\+ - DATIVE Reference to the recipient of an action or object, with or without a preposition (e.g., "give it to me", "she gave him the basket")

\+ - ADDITIVE Chaining of references to two or more objects, events, or states without a temporal or causal relationship between them (e.g., "I can pick apples, and I can be the best picker")

\+ - TEMPORAL Reference to a time aspect of an event, use of tense to mark a time relationship, coding of a sequence or simultaneous occurrence of events ("not right now", "she told me", "first", "before")

\+ - CAUSAL Reference to a means-end or cause-effect relationship ("I need apples, so I can make apple pie", "He put on his coat because it was cold.")

\+ - ADVERSATIVE Reference to contrasting characteristics of person, place, thing, or event ("The ones at the top are big, but the ones at the bottom are little.")

\+ - EPISTEMIC References to intellectual events (e.g., "know", "think", "wonder", "remember")

\+ - SPECIFICATION Identification of a particular person, place or thing ("the basket that she had given him", "the big, juicy apples")

\+ - COMMUNICATION Utterances containing a verb that codes a communicative act and a complement that indicates what is to be communicated ("she told me to get the apples", "tell her where you are")

Figure 8–3. Checklist for early language content (From "A play and story telling probe for assessing," by L. Yonovitz and K. Andrews, 1995. *Journal of Childhood Communication Disorders, 16*, p. 15. Copyright 1995 Council of Exceptional Children, Division for Children's Communicative Development. Reprinted with permission.)

THE FAMILY CIRCUS
By Bil Keane
CHILD'S MIND
I THINK WE SHOULD STRIKE WHILE THE IRON IS HOT!
UNFAIR!
THE LINE'S BUSY.
LOOK, I CAN SEE THE HANDWRITING ON THE WALL.

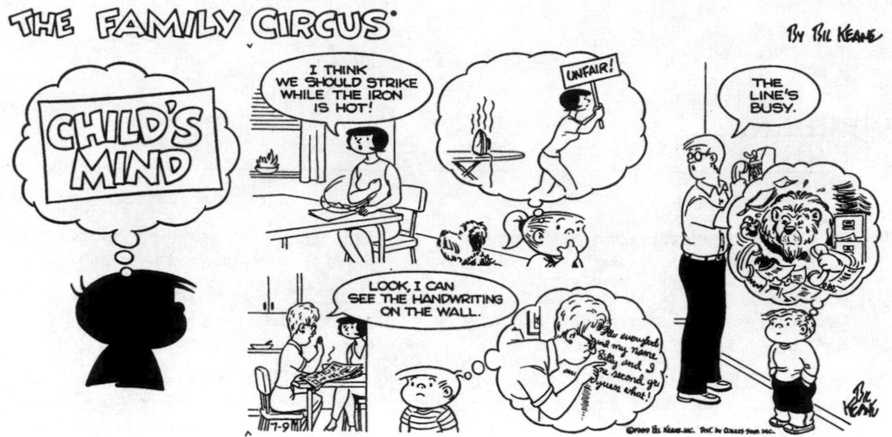

haps parents begin to correct or discourage such language creativity as it has also been suggested that school leaves little room at this time for creativity (Gardner & Winner, 1979). The decline in spontaneous production may also be evidence of the elementary school child's focus on the real and the literal. Usually the quantity of metaphors increases in creative writing in later elementary school.

Whereas spontaneous production of figures of speech declines with age, comprehension increases. The 8- to 9-year-old begins to appreciate psychological states such as *feeling blue* and *being a cold person*, although misinterpretation may still occur.

However, proverbs, such as *don't put the cart before the horse*, are very difficult for young school-age children and may be interpreted literally. The ability to understand proverbs and idioms develops slowly throughout childhood, adolescence, and adulthood (Nippold, 1985). Figurative expressions are easier for adolescents to comprehend in context than in isolation, and interpretation may depend on how transparent they are. Thus, *hold your tongue* would be easier than *kick the bucket*.

✓ SUMMARY CHECKLIST

☐ **Definition of Semantics**

Semantics is the study of the meaning system of language.

☐ **Semantic Development at the Word Level**

Referential Meaning

Semantic Feature Hypothesis

Synonyms

Antonyms

Selection Restrictions

Functional Core Hypothesis

Schemes

Prototypic Complex Hypothesis

Prototype

Early Expressive Vocabulary

Substantive Words

Relational Words

Reflexive

Attribution

Action (Protoverbs)

Location

Possessive

Lexicon Types

Referential

Expressive

Learning Process

Overextension

Underextension

☐ **Semantic Development at the Two-Word to Sentence Level**

Shifters

Relationals

Kinship Terms

Semantic Mapping

Semantic Relations

☐ **Semantic Organization: Multiword, Sentence, Conversation**

Figurative Language

CHAPTER

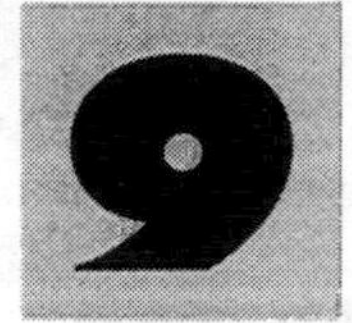

SEMANTICS: ANALYSIS AND INTERVENTION

ANALYSIS

Semantics involves the meaning of single words, of combinations and relations of words, and the meaning expressed through the development of sentences and discourse. Thus, semantic difficulties are evaluated by the explicitness of meaning at the word level, the sentence level, and through conversation. The evaluation of semantic proficiency becomes more difficult to delineate beyond the word level because of the interdependence of other language component skills (e.g., syntax) and the dependence on memory.

Problems in Vocabulary Development

Historically, vocabulary is the area of semantics that has received the most attention. The evaluation of vocabulary knowledge (size and depth) is a common component of cognitive assessments and comprehensive language evaluations. In fact, in a survey of assessment procedures used by SLPs in Illinois (Beck, 1996) and in California (Wilson, Blackmon, Hall, & Elcholtz, 1991), language assessment included receptive and expressive vocabulary tests across age groups. Beck (1996) found that the *Expressive One-Word Picture Vocabulary Test* (EOWPVT) (Gardner, 1990) was listed highest in order of use for assessing expressive language skills in the age groups 3-5 years (preschool), 6-11 years (elementary school), and 12-18 years (secondary school). Likewise, the *Peabody Picture Vocabulary Test—Revised* (PPVT) (Dunn & Dunn,

1981) was the highest ranked assessment instrument for evaluating receptive language skills in all three age groups.

Toddlers with language delays or disorders may be first identified by delays in reaching developmental age milestones. Most children say their first word around 12 months and evidence a vocabulary spurt after the first 50 words are acquired. Thus, vocabulary may be evaluated by a comparison to age norms. (See Chapter 8, Figure 8–2.) The overall size of a student's vocabulary is a better diagnostic indicator of overall semantic abilities or overall language abilities with younger children than with older children.

Many students with disabilities will have difficulties in vocabulary development. For example, it is typical for children with hearing impairments to have a reduction in the overall number of words that they both understand and use. Very commonly, a 2–3 year lag will be demonstrated. Likewise, children with mental handicaps (i.e., mental retardation) consistently show smaller and poorer vocabularies when compared to their normally developing peers. And although all children will show a gap between receptive vocabulary and expressive vocabulary, this gap appears to be much larger with the child who has mental retardation.

Vocabulary can also be evaluated by breadth. In other words, whether the child is using a variety of words across word classes such as nouns, adjectives, and so forth. Preschoolers with a language delay may have a reduction in overall vocabulary words, or they may not. They may not have a reduction in the number of words that they use but may have whole classes of words that they have difficulty comprehending or fail to use.

Students with learning disabilities tend to know more nouns, mainly concrete nouns (Reed, 1986). Because this is very similar to early development, they may not always be distinguished from normally developing children in the preschool years (Reed, 1986), especially because most vocabulary tests focus more on nouns and the meanings of a word in isolation. In other words, the current vocabulary or semantic tests that are available (e.g., the PPVT) may not reveal the semantic difficulties of many of these children.

Specific terms or vocabulary that represent spatial or temporal concepts pose particular problems. Spatial terms such as *over, under, in,* and *out* and temporal terms such as *first, last, before,* and *after* are all very difficult. This may be because they are somewhat more abstract and occur later in normal development. They are normally acquired around age 6 but are acquired much later in students with learning disabilities.

Vocabulary development should be evaluated with both informal procedures such as a language sample and formal instruments. Vocabulary problems may be indicated by generic labeling, extended use of overgeneralizatons, word errors, neologisms, restricted meaning, and word retrieval problems.

Generic Labeling

One indicator of poor vocabulary is the use of **generic labeling**. Generic labeling is the use of a vague or generic term such as "stuff" or "thing" in place of a more explicit vocabulary word. Examples include:

The child says:	*I need some more stuff* instead of *I need some more Playdoh.*
The student says:	*I need the thingamajig to fix this thing.*

These examples highlight the vagueness that occurs in communication when generic labels are used, allowing for the possibility of miscommunication. However, in many cases, context clues would probably provide the necessary information to accurately interpret the message. Generic labeling may be the result of an inadequate lexicon or may be an indicator of word finding difficulties, which will be discussed later.

Overgeneralization

Another problem in the area of vocabulary is the use of overextensions or **overgeneralizations** beyond what would be considered the normal period of development. In the process of language learning, children do overgeneralize word use, especially at the toddler and preschool level. However, in a relatively short period of time, the child will narrow the meanings of words to their adult representations. If the meanings of words do not systematically narrow and become more specific, that is, if overgeneralized use continues, a problem may be indicated. Preschoolers with language disorders may continue to use overgeneralizations for a much longer period of time than the typically developing preschooler. In other words, the child does not refine the meaning of vocabulary terms.

In older students, deficiencies in the process of refining meaning can result in misconceptions of meaning (Wiig et al., 1992), or what Lindfors (1987) described as "shades of meaning." Wiig et al. offered the example of a student's understanding of the word *punctual*. The student defined *punctual* as "how many manners you have." The authors went on to relate that the student was very well mannered, however he was always late.

Semantic Word Errors

A **semantic word error** is the selection of an inappropriate or inadequate word. This may be due to a misunderstanding of the meaning of the semantic relations or the functional attributes of words (Smiley, 1991b). Examples include:

Qualitative adjectives: How *tall* is this pencil?

Quantitative adjectives:	The teacher told us not to put too *many* stuff in our boxes.
Prepositions:	I come back *on* ten o'clock.
Time and Space:	Don't worry you can buy some *yesterday*.

Word errors, as well as other semantic errors, are based on the child's personal life experiences, the cognitive coding of those experiences, and the efficiency of that coding. An example may best illustrate this.

One day when I was working on vocabulary and categorization with a group of prekindergarten students, we went out under the chickie hut to act out animal movements, sounds, and so forth. The next week, Kristy, one of the students, kept asking me to take her to the Pizza Hut. After several attempts to explain we could not go to Pizza Hut for lunch and much insistence on Kristy's part, I allowed her to drag me outside for clarification. There she directed me to the chickie hut. Only then did I realize that Kristy had coded the new vocabulary and new experience (i.e., the chickie hut) with the only hut she knew, the Pizza Hut.

Children with semantic difficulties are often described as being "way off base" or as being "out in left field." However, if investigated, a teacher may find a connection, albeit an odd one. Consider Paul, who, during a language screening test, responded to the question "what flies?" with the answer "air conditioners." His teacher had reported that Paul, a kindergartner, often responded to story comprehension questions with bizarre answers. However, when I pursued the "air conditioner" response, I learned that Paul had been car shopping over the weekend with his dad. At one of the car dealers, there was a window air conditioner with streamers attached that blew when the air conditioner was on; thus, the flying air conditioner. Throughout the rest of the year the teacher and I were able to pursue Paul's unusual answers and find the connection. We would then design interventions to help recode his experiences in more appropriate representations.

Neologisms

One of the unique processes in the development of language is the creation of new words known as **neologisms**. This may be the child's best effort with a limited lexicon to make sense of the world through words. Children do a wonderful job of using what they have in order to express meaning (Lindfors, 1987). If the situation proves to need a yet unknown vocabulary word, they will create one. Some of these are truly remarkable in their descriptiveness, as can be seen in the following examples.

They may use new combinations: I had a *cokasoda.*

They may play with suffixes: Where are the *nofiction* books.

They may use phonological cues: I want to go to the *pomcuter.*

My daughter, Molly, at age 2, called helicopters *happycopters* and at age 4 said *Elvis's glue* for Elmer's glue. In these last two instances, the new words appear to be formed through a process of using some phonological clues (/h/ for helicopters; *El* for Elmer's) and then using the vocabulary with which she was familiar. However, in the case of the *happycopters*, there seems to be some attempt at expressing interaction with the item. It seems appropriate; when most children see helicopters, there is an element of fascination and happiness, and they therefore enjoy it. *Happycopter* would appear to be an appropriate guess, given the limited vocabulary/language knowledge of the child and her reaction to helicopters.

The *Elvis's glue*, again, appears to be based on a phonological cue plus life experience. Molly did not know anyone or anything by the name of "Elmer." However, there was a bird in her preschool class named "Elvis." Molly used what she knew from her own limited life experiences.

In many ways, this exchange illustrates how much the child does know about language. First, she demonstrates phonological awareness. Second, she illustrates her knowledge about word classes; she substitutes a noun, and more specifically, a proper noun (i.e., *Elvis* for *Elmer*). In addition, the retrieval of *Elvis* may not be based solely on phonological awareness. The child was engaged in building a bird feeder at the time of the utterance. This may be an additional factor in her retrieval of *Elvis* (the bird's name). The activity probably activated the cognitive representations she had related to birds. Thus, there was easy access to the name *Elvis* due to personal experience.

Some neologisms may be based on function. For example, a *pull-on* for a boot or a *smoke machine* for the vaporizer (child, age 3). In Florida, where there are lizards that have sacks under their neck that inflate and deflate, Meridith, age 4, said "the lizard is blowing a bag."

Although the use of neologisms is evidenced in typical development (i.e., toddler/preschool years), it may indicate a semantic difficulty if evidenced in later years. If the neologism is replacing a vocabulary term the child has previously learned and had experience with, then the neologism may indicate deficiencies in labeling, memory, or word retrieval. However, the use of a neologism instead of the use of generic labeling may indicate a higher level of language usage and greater language problem-solving skills.

Narrow Concrete Meanings

The difficulty with narrow or concrete meanings can be demonstrated with multiple meaning words such as *trunk*, as in the *elephant's trunk*, the *car trunk*, the *tree trunk*. It is very difficult for the student to expand from whatever meaning is initially learned to understand that a single word can have more than one meaning depending on its use and context. For example, one day school was closed due to the threat of a hurricane. A previously scheduled teacher work-day was designated as a hurricane make-up day. Tina, a 5th-grade student with language learning disabilities, read the notice on the bulletin board that Friday was hurricane make-up day. Tina was thrilled that she was going to be able to wear lipstick, blush, mascara, eyeliner, and so forth! In another example, the same student appeared to have a crush on another student in the class. Whenever she would move about the room, she would constantly stare at David. She was told by her teacher "not to look at David when she was moving about the room." Tina interpreted that statement literally. When she went to sharpen her pencil, she closed her eyes completely and ran into the wall! And then there's Johnathan, a 13-year-old with moderate mental retardation, who asked his teacher, who was telling about her trip to the mouth of the Mississipi River, "What does it eat? What do you feed it?"

The difficulty with narrow or concrete meanings is often exhibited with idioms. A mentor (Barbara Ehren) described middle school students with learning disabilities at an assembly. The principal was trying to encourage them to start their new semester fresh. He said something similar to "please leave your baggage behind you, start fresh, and move on to the next term." When the auditorium was vacated, the students with learning disabilities had left their backpacks, books, and other paraphernalia behind them. And how about the students with learning disabilities who stood up with their books when told by the teacher that they "were going to go around the room reading."

Word Retrieval

Another area often mentioned in the literature is **word retrieval** problems. A word retrieval deficit is the inability to retrieve an appropriate word or label when needed. The student knows the particular term or item (i.e., it is stored in long-term memory), but he or she has difficulty retrieving the word from memory. This may be evidenced by indefinite

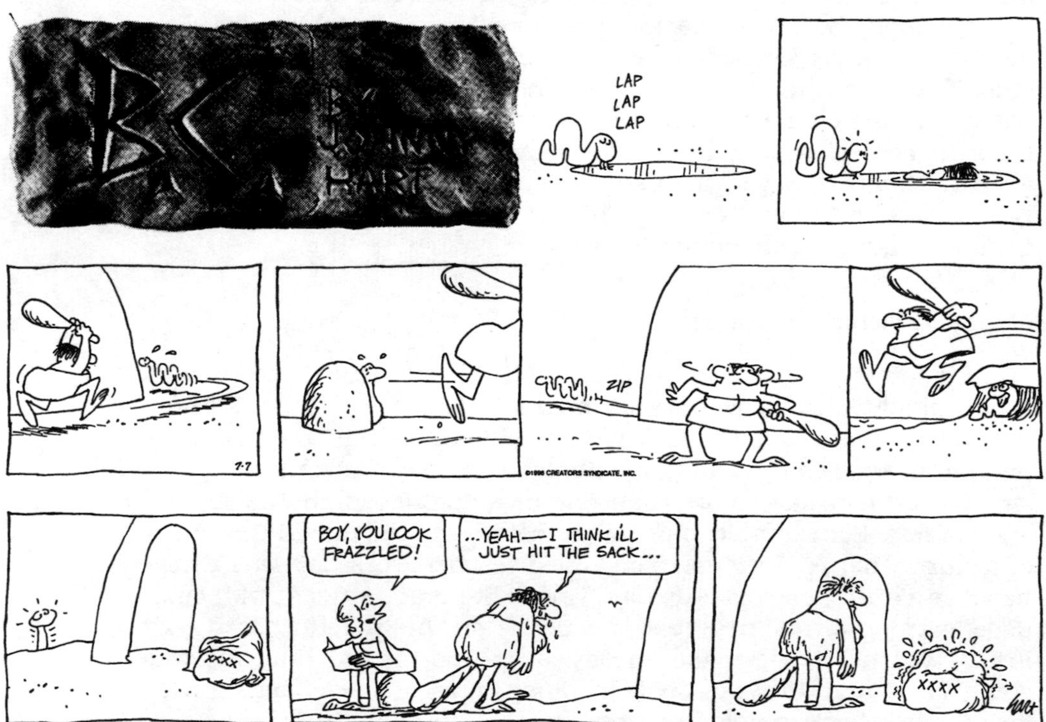

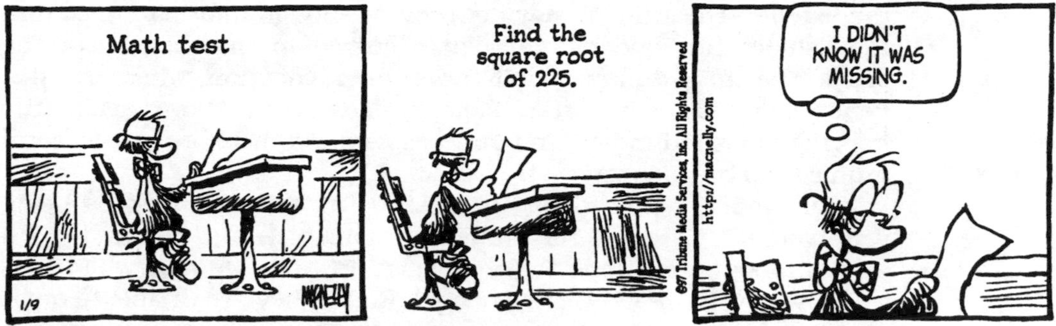

fillers, "I seen um, um things, like a guy who spit fire"; by questions, "um um what dya call it?"; may include signs and/or statements of frustration, "I don't know what they are, I don't remember"; as mentioned earlier, generic labeling, "stuff"; descriptions, "They're all squared up" for plaid; or even made-up words (i.e., use neologisms).

Students with learning disabilities often have expressive language problems. They may have difficulty with word retrieval. As a result they may use semantic word substitutions and choose a less specific word (Bos & Vaughn, 1988), use indefinite words such as "stuff" or "thing," use excessive fillers, use gestures/pointing, or have difficulty retelling stories, especially in sequencing (Merritt & Liles, 1987). This is illustrated by JJ, an 18-year-old student with learning disabilities, when trying to figure out the name of a shoe he wanted to use in a story he was writing:

> What's name of that shoe, you know with lightning bolt looking thing on side and . . . uh . . . they is sometimes blue and black and white and . . . uh . . . that other bluey color . . . you know what that shoe is called?

Echolalia

Echolalia is the restatement of a speaker's previously uttered words, phrases, paragraphs, or such, and may occur immediately after the speaker emits them or much later (**delayed echolalia**). The utterance usually lacks prosodic features that would characterize it as meaningful and is quite frequently more grammatically complex than the echolalic speaker's comprehension (Lucas, 1980). It is therefore critical that an assessment of the child's language include the level of spontaneous language as well as the limited echolalic level.

Organization and Formulation

Last, Smiley (1991b) discussed difficulties in conveying information. Students may have a difficult time formulating or organizing stories or directions in logical sequences that provide enough information for comprehension to occur. These problems may involve sequencing, redundancy, or organizing the main idea with supporting information.

Students with semantic organizational difficulties who may not be able to sequence their ideas in the correct order cause confusion for the listener. The student may not provide enough information so that the listener can understand what occurred in that activity or the event. The student may exhibit **verbal perseveration**, where the student tells the same important facts or ideas over and over again. The information is redundant and unnecessary and therefore causes communication breakdown.

Interestingly, sometimes these students are described as being very "verbal." These are the students who come up to you and go on and on about something that happened in their life, but when they walk away you are left there saying, "Huh?" They are unable to organize their verbalizations to make a point or main idea, or to present things in an orderly fashion. They may have a very good vocabulary. They may also have a command of the syntax and morphology. However, in organizing everything to convey information, they have a great deal of difficulty. Unfortunately, these students are often overlooked in terms of having a language problem. However, it will probably be evidenced in reading activities, such as finding a main idea or answering comprehension questions.

Confusion may also show up in phrases, especially with idioms. Examples include:

> He's like a loose bolt.
>
> Don't let the cat in the bag.
>
> Take your hand off or I'm going to break every finger of your bone.

INTERVENTION

Vocabulary

The expansion of word knowledge is a priority with students in special education. Larger vocabularies will enhance language abilities in the other component areas, aid word retrieval, and enhance learning across content areas. Decisions regarding the enhancement of vocabulary must include what to teach (target vocabulary) and how to teach.

Target Vocabulary

Targets for vocabulary teaching should be based on the student's needs, the student's environments, and age appropriateness. An ecological evaluation of the environments in which the student interacts will provide relevant target vocabulary that could enhance the quality and quantity of interactions. This must include at least the **home** and **school environments**. The target vocabulary based on an evaluation of the home environment would involve the many routines and relationships that occur in a family's life. Communication with the family about those routines is a necessity. For students who are very young or very limited in language abilities, the understanding and production of vocabulary related to basic needs would be a priority, for example, toileting and eating needs. An evaluation of the school environment would reveal appropriate target vocabulary related to academics, social interactions, and the language of teaching and learning. Instruction should always include the teaching of new vocabulary from all content areas. For instance, it is quite common to introduce new vocabulary for reading lessons. However, this must also be done for math, science, social studies, and other subjects.

It is also important to teach vocabulary that will promote positive social interactions, that is, vocabulary that is commonly used in interactions with both peers and adults. For example, in a recent study by Marvin and Hunt-Berg (1996), a preference for certain semantic themes was found in the pretend play of preschoolers. They demonstrated a preference for playing themselves and cartoon characters (e.g., Superman). They also demonstrated a preference for content that included food, people's actions/locations, toys, animals, buildings, places, and people's traits or conditions. Thus, teaching the vocabulary and routine scripts related to these themes would be appropriate for this age group. Marvin and Hunt-Berg suggested this will increase the socialization of young children with disabilities and their peers. This may be an appropriate practice for older children as well. In other words, it may be beneficial to teach vocabulary common in peer interactions as well as the vocabulary of academic areas.

In addition, the vocabulary related to teaching and learning, which is all too often assumed to be understood, needs to be targeted. The vocabulary involved in teaching and learning is the language of directions, the language of rules, the language of problem solving, as well as metalinguistic or metacognitive skills. Every day, teachers give directions for academic tasks and expectations of behavior. Every day, students face additional written directions in workbooks and worksheets. Every day, a student, in order to be successful in school, must first understand oral and written directions and, second, comply with those directions. Appendix B provides a list of vocabulary heard (oral) and seen (written) in directions given in classrooms (K–middle school). A review of this list highlights both the qualitative and quantitative vocabulary knowledge required in education.

Difficulties characteristic of certain disabilities also must be considered. For example, children with mental retardation tend to primarily use nouns. Thus, a teacher may want to focus on other parts of speech, such as verbs (Reed, 1986).

Procedures for Teaching

Using real objects and demonstrating real actions in familiar contexts facilitates vocabulary development. New vocabulary should be presented numerous times in a variety of contexts. The vocabulary should be described and contrasted with previously learned and used vocabulary. As mentioned earlier, students tend to categorize items through perceptual features. However, Kit-Fong Au (1990) noted that children could benefit from linguistic contrast. For example, the teacher or clinician can overcome the preference for shape by describing the material the object is made of. "It's not paper, it's cloth." Giving examples and nonexamples is recommended as good teaching strategy in all learning; vocabulary is no exception. In addition, the use of visual imagery and cloze procedures are also reported in the literature as facilitating vocabulary development.

Practice and reinforcement can occur through a variety of tasks. Comprehension checks in the form of rapid naming and categorization tasks will reinforce initial learning and maintenance of vocabulary by strengthening the semantic representation and network of the "word." Multiple elicitations of new vocabulary are important (Reed, 1986).

The teaching of language structure or content (along with use) can be greatly enhanced if placed within an activity that is familiar and comfortable for the child. Further enhancement can occur if the activity or task is predictable and if the child can easily retrieve a relevant cognitive representation of the information (Montgomery, 1996). In other words, the comprehension of language and language teaching occurs best in an educational and task environment with which the child is already familiar. This allows the child to pick out the "new" information. Children also seem to build on learning. As they go back to the same environment or the same task, they pull out more information each time. This gives credence to the use of repetition in teaching and may also explain why young children want the same story read over and over again and why they will watch the same video repeatedly.

Later Vocabulary/Concept Development

In the early years of development, vocabulary learning occurs in spoken contexts. However, after the fourth grade, vocabulary is learned primarily through written contexts. Likewise, classroom activities are more experientially based in the early grades and less contextually supported by middle and high school years (Wiig et al., 1992). In a program designed for a self-contained special education class (adolescents with learning disabilities and behavior disorders who were also speakers of English as a second language), Wiig et al. recommended a holistic and thematic approach to the acquisition of new vocabulary and concepts. The following approaches and procedures were implemented:

1. Collaboration
2. Student centeredness
3. Guided questioning and scaffolding
4. Semantic word webbing and comparisons
5. Problem solving strategy for strategy training

Although the greatest gains were seen with the students with learning disabilities, the procedures advocated are theoretically sound and reflect current trends in special education.

Collaboration

Collaboration among various personnel such as SLPs, special educators, and general educators can aid in the integration of vocabulary and concepts across disciplines. This approach is now being demonstrated in a variety of inclusionary models.

Coteaching and collaborative teaching models such as general education/special education teacher teams as well as speech-language pathologist/general education teacher teams are now viewed favorably within the educational community at large. In fact, in a study by Bland and Prelock (1995), students served in a collaborative model (teacher and SLP designing and implementing intervention in the classroom) were rated higher in the intelligibility and completeness of their oral language than students from a traditional pull-out model. These students ranged in age from 6 years 2 months to 9 years 9 months. Likewise, Wilcox, Kouri, and Caswell (1991) found that preschool children receiving speech/language services in the classroom, as opposed to a pull-out speech/language model, spontaneously used targeted vocabulary more frequently. Obviously, collaboration can help in the identification of appropriate vocabulary and concepts, as well as in the identification of appropriate teaching strategies (including preteaching) and evaluation.

Student Centeredness

The philosophy of **student centeredness** emphasizes the teacher's knowledge of the student. It is extremely important for the teacher to know what the student knows (content knowledge) and what the student can do (skill and abilities within a content area). Learning occurs in this "spacc" between where the student can perform a task independently and where the student requires assistance or guidance. Vygotsky (1934/1986) referred to this as the **zone of proximal development**. (See Berk & Winsler, 1995, for a review of Vygotsky's theories and perspectives.) Various academic areas refer to aspects of this in their curriculum, for example, reading often describes this as "Instructional Level" (Bormouth, 1968). In teaching, we must recognize individual instructional skill/knowledge levels so that learning for the student is secure, frustration is limited, and positive outcomes are produced: successful task completion, a sense of accomplishment, and self-confidence. However, student centeredness must expand beyond skill level. Teachers must also consider motivation, incentives for learning, development of rapport, and so forth. This is the student's **learning comfort zone** (LCZ). The LCZ is dependent on the zone of proximal development, the relationship between the teacher and learner, the students' expectations of their abilities, and other environmental factors, both internal and external to the student. A teacher must be teaching in the LCZ for learning to take place. However, it is important to remember that the LCZ is not static but dynamic.

How does this relate to vocabulary and concept learning? For instance, for science class students to understand the concept of *vol-*

ume, the students must first have an understanding of *space* and *measurement*. More specifically, they must understand the three-dimensional aspects of space and the various units of measurement. A teacher's attempt to teach *volume* without this prior knowledge would be unproductive instruction. It is therefore extremely important for teachers to know the specific knowledge and abilities of their students. This is best done informally, through interactions over time. However, to learn specifics in a particular context area, some pretests (either formal or informal) can be completed and constant monitoring of performance will be needed.

Hence, in order to successfully teach new concepts and vocabulary, the teacher must first have an understanding of each student's present level of knowledge in the content area. Because students always seem to be at different levels of knowledge, some preteaching intervention or other modifications to instruction may be needed. Thus, student centeredness provides the basis for generating instructional goals, objectives, procedures, and evaluation.

Guided Questioning and Scaffolding

This principle recognizes the student as an active learner and changes the role of the teacher to a guide or facilitator. Questions and scaffolding are effective strategies for enhancing learning within the child's LCZ and in evaluating a student's LCZ changes and advancement. Scaffolding describes the changing nature of support a teacher offers in the course of instruction. As competence increases, the teacher's support and guidance decreases (Berk, 1996). The teacher aids in the building (scaffolding) and assimilation of new knowledge on the child's existing foundation of world knowledge. The teacher enhances, clarifies, and questions to facilitate better understanding of the new topic (Wiig et al., 1992).

Semantic Word Webbing

As previously discussed, semantic word webbing is the process of comparing new vocabulary and new concepts for similarities and differences with existing knowledge. This can be translated into visual representations. Generating a visual representation to indicate various relationships, such as designing a semantic map (Heimlich & Pittelman, 1986), may help cue students to the word's relationship to their world knowledge. This process may begin by brainstorming for related words. Once a list of related words is generated, using a semantic map to categorize those words may help in organizing information for encoding (Hoggan & Strong, 1994). Figure 9–1 provides an example of this process. It is important in this process to teach the relevant features of a concept and the features that distinguish it from other similar vocabulary (Bos & Vaughn, 1994).

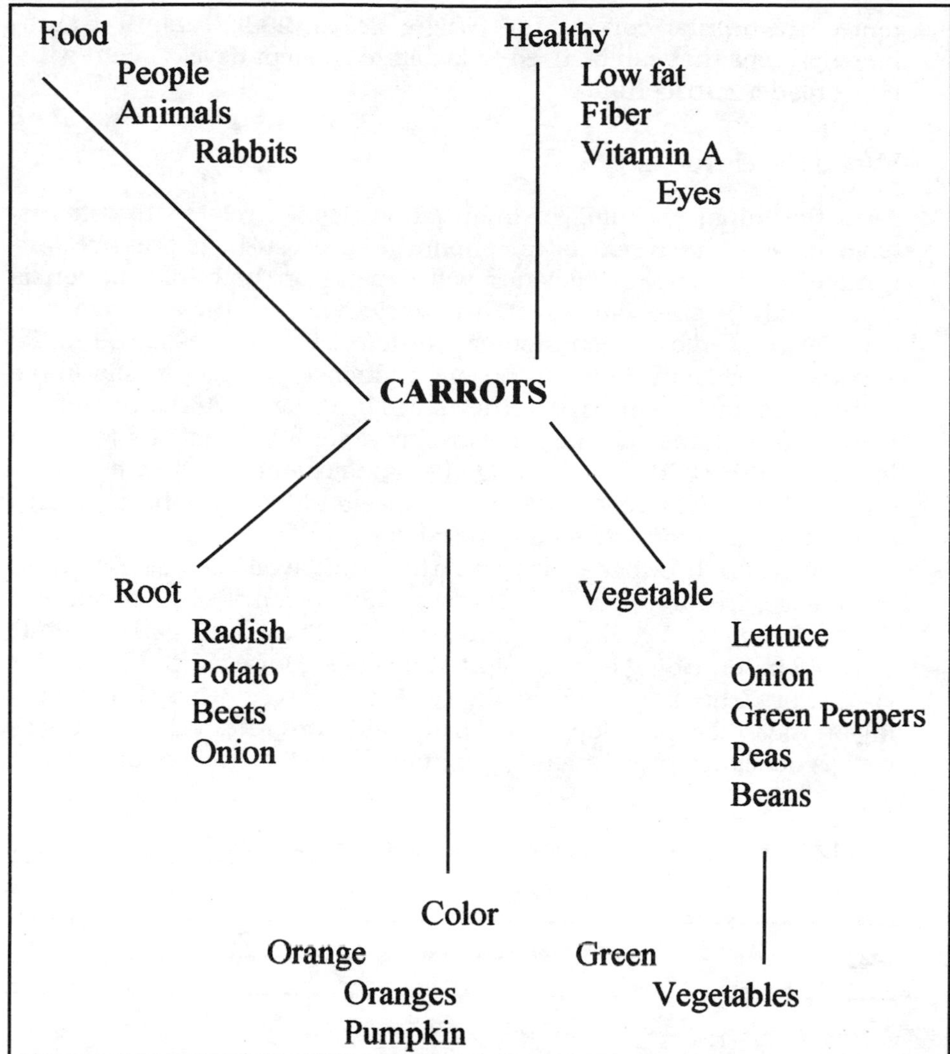

Figure 9–1. List of generated words and semantic word map for *carrots.* (From "The Magic of 'Once Upon a Time'" by K. C. Hoggan and C. J. Strong, 1994, p. 80. *Language, Speech, and Hearing Services in Schools,* 25. Copyright 1994 by The American Speech-Language-Hearing Association (ASHA). Reprinted with permission.)

Problem Solving

Finally, problem solving that utilizes a variety of skills and strategies is important for supporting the acquisition of a concept and its application across the curriculum and into the "real world." "The special educator may need to plan thematic units around vocabulary and concepts important for learning and living while staying within the content of the regular curriculum" (Wiig et al., p. 283). Table 9–1 summarizes steps that can be used to facilitate concept development within a broader curriculum.

Word Retrieval

After the initial encoding of information, issues related to retrieval emerge. **Word retrieval** is an important process in expressive language. Word retrieval efficiency will depend on how information is stored and the ease with which it is retrieved. Both the accuracy and complexity of information storage will affect this process. The initial experience with an item will heavily influence storage. If this initial storage is somehow in error, retrieval will be difficult. And if the refinement of this storage does not occur over several interactions (as often happens with children with language impairments), retrieval will remain difficult. As a result, timed activities and tests will be especially arduous (McGregor & Leonard, 1995).

Ease of retrieval depends on the cues available, overall word knowledge, frequency of item retrieval, and recency of item retrieval (Bjork & Bjork, 1992). Teachers in many instances can facilitate retrieval by providing and manipulating cues. However, the larger the vocabulary, the more efficient the retrieval process. Therefore, focusing on vocabulary development will also aid word retrieval problems as well as deficits in other areas of language behavior, such as narratives.

TABLE 9–1. Overview of planning steps for developing thematic lessons, units, and curricula.

Steps	*Activities/Considerations*
• Evaluate subject matter	Evaluate reasons (e.g., why it is/is not essential to teach) and relevance.
• Take a long-range view	Clarify importance and prioritize ideas and concepts to be taught.
• Identify vocabulary and concepts	Identify vocabulary associated with ideas and concepts; elaborate by referring to semantic category.
• Determine sequence, vocabulary, strategies, activities	Determine order for teaching related vocabulary/concepts; select teaching formats and strategies; design language-related activities.
• Design evaluation methods	Select/design evaluation methods that match what was taught and how (e.g., lab assignments, maps, portfolio).
• Teach, modify, enrich, generalize	Develop activities/lessons/units for opportunities to enrich, modify, broaden, transfer, generalize word meanings and concepts.

Source: From "Developing Words and Concepts in the Classroom—Thematic Approach," by E. Wiig, E. Freedman, and W. Secord, 1992, *Intervention in School and Clinic*, 27(5), pp. 278–285. Reprinted with permission.

These facts have resulted in two approaches to word retrieval problems, known as **elaboration strategy** intervention and **retrieval strategy** intervention. Elaboration approaches focus on increasing overall word knowledge, thus increasing the complexity of the semantic network. Techniques and strategies used to increase vocabulary knowledge discussed previously in this chapter are appropriate. For example, the use of themes is a recommended strategy for vocabulary development. In contrast, the use of random word lists would not be recommended (German, 1992). Teaching retrieval strategies could focus on the use of cues (e.g., phonological cues) to enhance word finding. Table 9–2 summarizes some strategies or techniques that might prove successful.

There is contradictory information when comparing the efficacy of these two approaches (German, 1992; McGregor & Leonard, 1995). In a review of efficacy studies of word finding intervention, German (1992) concluded that both the elaboration and retrieval strategies approaches may be beneficial for improving word finding, but there is insufficient evidence that this will translate into improved reading abilities.

Phrase/Sentence Level and Discourse

Idioms

The use of idioms by teachers (Lazar, Warr-Leeper, Nicholson & Johnson, 1989) and texts (Nippold, 1991) increases throughout the elementary grades. It may be necessary to directly teach the meaning of idioms to students. This can be done by presenting the idioms in a story context (Nippold, 1991), and, as in other reading activities, teaching the meanings through clues in the context of the story.

Comprehension of Classroom Discourse

To review/analyze comprehension in the classroom environment, it is important to attend to specific areas of concern (as has been just discussed) and also to take a more global perspective. The box on page 183 summarizes the processes or steps to classroom comprehension. These processes can be enhanced through the use of advance organizers. Advance organizers, such as prestory presentations, are an easy means of directing the student to attend to relevant detail and to anticipate what is to come. For example, in reading, the teacher or other support personnel can use prestory presentations to highlight important and possibly troublesome vocabulary and concepts (Hoggen & Strong, 1994). By reviewing the title and book cover, the student is given a lead into the story and an opportunity to discuss what he or she already knows about the subject. Small group brainstorming encourages the review of actual events experienced by the students that are related to the topic. This brings about a broader knowledge base in which to assimilate new information (Alverman, Smith, &

TABLE 9–2. Retrieval strategies and remedial techniques used in the remediation component of the Word Finding Intervention Program (WFIP).

Retrieval strategies		***Descriptions***
Attribute cuing	Phonemic cuing	The initial sound, vowel nucleus, digraph, or syllable is used to cue the target word.
	Semantic cuing	The category name or function is used to cue the target word.
	Graphemic cuing	The graphic schema is used to cue the target word.
	Imagery cuing	A revisualization of the referent is used to cue the target word.
	Gesture cuing	The motor schema of the target word action is used to cue the target word.
Associate cuing (story for book)		An intermediate word is used to cue the target word.
Semantic alternates	Synonym/category substitutions	Semantic components (synonym or category words) are substituted for the target word.
	Multiword substitutions	Semantic components (functions or descriptions) are substituted for the target word.
Reflective pausing		Constructive use of pausing is used to reduce inaccurate competitive responses.

Remedial techniques		***Descriptions***
Stabilization of phonological specifications	Rehearsal	Students practice saying or writing the target words five times alone and then in five different sentences.
	Rhythm + rehearsal	Each syllable is marked with a tap during the above rehearsal of the target word.
	Segmenting + rehearsal	A line is drawn between each syllable during the above rehearsal of the target word.
Rapid naming		Students rapidly say names of and phrases with target words until their response time is reduced.

Source: From "Word-Finding Intervention for Children and Adolescents," by D. German, 1992, *Topics in Language Disorders, 13*, p. 42. Copyright 1992 by Aspen Publishers, Inc. Reprinted with permission.

Attention	Attention or focus on task and relevant vocabulary, concepts, and ideas
Making Sense	The connection of new ideas and information into the student's current knowledge base
Knowing	Making this knowledge fluid
Using	Enhancing and expanding the understanding of this new application and use in new situations (i.e., generalization)

Readence, 1985). Summarizing the story in manageable chunks during and after the narrative reading aids student comprehension and highlights important events and activities. Students may also participate in summarizing by using the cloze procedure (Hoggin & Strong, 1994). In addition, extensions (elaboration) can be used to clarify meaning in stories (Hoggen & Strong, 1994) and expansions to enrich and raise the concept/vocabulary knowledge to a more complex and comprehensive level (Bos & Vaughn, 1994).

Lenz (1983) identified 10 steps in using an advance organizer (see Table 9–3). Many of these steps involve semantics. Vocabulary and concept development are highlighted in Steps 2, 6, 7, 9. The process of bridging information to an existing knowledge base is highlighted in Steps 5, 7, 8. In other words, if a teacher followed these steps, an organizational framework would be provided to learn the new information.

Narrative teaching strategies are frequently recommended in the reading literature for a variety of the previously mentioned processes. More recently these strategies have been recommended for students with language delays (see Hoggan & Strong, 1994). Table 9–4 lists the narrative teaching strategies cited in the literature. This table notes the story-presentation stage, the language focus (note that all address content), school level, and teaching context.

The repetition of stories and story enhancement activities help students understand more and more. On a higher level, discussion webs (Alverman, 1991) allow students to explore their own ideas and opposing ideas. Hoggan and Strong (1994) suggested initiating a discussion web in pairs. It may be helpful for enhancement activities to be a multimodality experience. Music may be an effective means for the facilitation of comprehension (Barclay & Walwer, 1992; Zoller, 1991). Townsend and Clarihew (1989) found a visual component improved learning. Likewise, Merrill and Jackson (1992) found that the inclusion of a picture illustrating a sentence would improve sentence recall

TABLE 9–3. Steps in using an advance organizer.

Step 1:	Inform students of advance organizers a. Announce advance organizer b. State benefits of advance organizer c. Suggest that students take notes on the advance organizer.
Step 2:	Identify topics of tasks a. Identify major topics or activities b. Identify subtopics or component activities
Step 3:	Provide an organizational framework a. Present an outline, list, or narrative of the lesson's content
Step 4:	Clarify action to be taken a. State teachers' actions b. State students' actions
Step 5:	Provide background information a. Relate topic to the course or previous lesson b. Relate topic to new information
Step 6:	State the concepts to be learned a. State specific concepts/ideas from the lesson b. State general concepts/ideas broader than the lesson's content
Step 7:	Clarify the concepts to be learned a. Clarify by examples or analogies b. Clarify by nonexamples c. Caution students of possible misunderstandings
Step 8:	Motivate student to learn a. Point out relevance to students b. Be specific, short-term, personalized, and believable
Step 9:	Introduce vocabulary a. Identify the new terms and define b. Repeat difficult terms and define
Step 10:	State the general outcome desired a. State objectives of instruction/learning b. Relate outcomes to test performance

Source: From "Promoting Active Learning Through Effective Instruction" by B. K. Lenz, 1983, *Pointer,* 27(2), p. 12. Copyright 1983 by Heldref Publications. Reprinted with permission.

abilities in subjects with mental retardation to the level demonstrated by subjects without mental retardation. Merrill and Jackson (1992) concluded that pictures assisted the subjects with mental retardation to use contextual information in their encoding of semantic representations of the sentence. In addition, such activities can give the student an opportunity to depict and clarify their understanding. Dramatic play

TABLE 9–4. Narrative teaching strategies by story-presentation stage, language-skill focus, grade/age level, and teaching context (listed alphabetically).

	Presentation Stage			***Language focus***			***Grade/age level***			***Teaching context***		
Strategy (Author, Year)	***Pre***	***During***	***Post***	***C***	***F***	***U***	***PG***	***LE***	***MS***	***LG***	***SG***	***Ind.***
Art activities (e.g., Berney & Barrera, 1990)			+	+	+	+	+	+	+	+	+	+
Directed reading/thinking (e.g., Nessel, 1989)	+	+	+	+		+	+	+	+	+	+	+
Discussion web (e.g., Alverman, 1991)			+	+		+	+	+	+	+	+	
Dramatic play (e.g., Putnam, 1991)			+	+	+	+	+	+			+	
Episode/story mapping (e.g., Davis & McPherson, 1989)		+	+	+		+	+	+	+	+	+	+
Extensions (e.g., Muma, 1971)		+		+			+	+	+	+	+	+
Flow charting (e.g., Geva, 1983)			+	+			+	+	+	+	+	+
Internal states (e.g., Dunning, 1992)			+	+			+	+	+	+	+	+
Journals (e.g., Staton et al., 1985; Wollman-Bonilla, 1989)			+	+	+	+		+	+	+	+	+
Music (e.g., Barclay & Walwer, 1992)	+		+	+	+	+	+	+	+	+	+	+
Preparatory sets (e.g., Alverman et al., 1985)	+			+			+	+	+	+	+	+
Question-answer relationship (e.g., Raphael, 1982)			+	+			+	+	+	+	+	+
Questioning (e.g., Panofsky, 1986)		+	+	+			+	+	+	+	+	+
Semantic word mapping (e.g., Hamayan, 1989)	+	+	+	+			+	+	+	+	+	+
Story generation (e.g., Trousdale, 1990)			+	+	+	+	+	+	+		+	+
Story-grammar cueing (e.g., Graves & Montague, 1991)			+	+	+	+		+	+	+	+	+
Story retelling (e.g., Peck, 1989)			+	+	+	+	+	+	+	+	+	+
Summarizing (e.g., Panofsky, 1986)	+	+	+	+			+	+	+	+	+	+
Think alouds (e.g., Davey, 1983)	+	+	+	+		+	+	+	+	+	+	+
Word substitutions (Beaumont, 1992)			+	+			+	+	+	+	+	+

Note: C = content; F = form; U = use; PG = primary grades; LE = late elementary grades; MS = middle/secondary grades; LC = large group; SC = small group; Ind. = individual.

Source: From "The Magic of 'Once Upon a Time,' by C. K. Hoggan and C. J. Strong, 1994, *Language Speech, and Hearing Services in Schools, 25*, p. 78. Copyright 1994 by American Speech-Language-Hearing Association. Reprinted with permission.

can be used for comprehension of stories (Pellegrini, 1984) or for routines such as restaurant visits.

Related Memory Skills

Memory abilities and skills will affect the comprehension and production of language (Cowan, 1996; Martin, 1993). If students are having difficulty with memory demanding tasks, it is very likely that those deficiencies will also affect the comprehension of language. Therefore, if memory skills can be strengthened, improved language comprehension may result.

Montgomery (1996) recommended a variety of strategies to improve short-term memory and working memory. He suggested the use of nursery rhymes for phonological memory abilities (as previously suggested in this text). Teaching verbal rehearsal strategies, as well as teaching why, when, and how to use them (Montgomery, 1996, p. 30), is important for initial learning and to "hold" information while encoding occurs. Another effective strategy is **chunking**. Chunking results in the dividing of linguistic material such as a sentence into manageable chunks. Paraphrasing strategies may be effective with language material that is larger than a sentence. Obviously, these strategies must be explicitly taught and practiced.

Parenté and Herrman (1996), in their research with adults with traumatic brain-injury, also recommendeded a variety of memory enhancing strategies, including training organization, training mediation, and training mental imagery. These may prove effective with students with language deficiencies. The purpose of organization training is to have the student identify semantic relations among items or information, for example, identifying categories. Mediation training directs the student to actively associate the new information to something "old" or familiar. This could be done by asking oneself questions (self-questioning) such as, "What does this look like? What does this remind me of?" or by mnemonics. **Mnemonics** are devices to aid memory and can be an effective mediation tool for both the memorization of lists and problem-solving strategies. Some of the most commonly used mnemonics include the "first letter" strategy. For example, HOMES can cue the student (through the cue of first letter) to remember the Great Lakes: **H**uron, **O**ntario, **M**ichigan, **E**rie, and **S**uperior.

The training of mental imagery is simply creating a visual cognitive image to include items to be remembered. Montgomery (1996) noted that this technique may not work well with low functioning persons and works best with concrete items.

✓ SUMMARY CHECKLIST

☐ **Analysis**

Vocabulary

Generic Labeling

Overgeneralization

Semantic Word Errors

Neologisms

Narrow Concrete Meanings

Word Retrieval

Echolalia

Organization and Formulation

Verbal Perseveration

☐ **Intervention**

Vocabulary

Target Vocabulary

Home Environment

School Environment

Teaching Procedures

Later Vocabulary/Concept Development

Collaboration

Student Centeredness

Zone of Proximal Development

Learning Comfort Zone

Guided Questioning and Scaffolding

Semantic Word Webbing

Problem Solving

Word Retrieval

Elaboration Strategy

Retrieval Strategy

Phrase/Sentence Level and Discourse

Idioms

Comprehension of Classroom Discourse

Related Memory Skills

Chunking

Mnemonics

CHAPTER

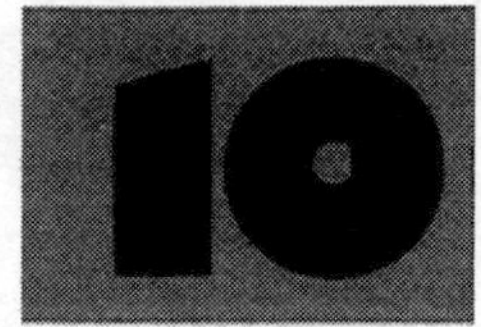

THE DEVELOPMENT OF PRAGMATICS

You are in a social situation such as dinner and your friend makes a comment. The comment is so inappropriate for the situation that it could easily be interpreted as an insult. You are sitting there saying to yourself, "I can't believe he just said that." You are totally embarrassed for your friend and yourself. He just can't seem to "read" situations very well.

This scenario demonstrates a problem of a pragmatic nature. Many students in special education seem unable to evaluate the social situation and determine the appropriateness of their verbal responses or their actions.

DEFINING PRAGMATICS

Pragmatics is a set of sociolinguistic rules related to language use in the communicative context. Pragmatics involves how language is used, rather than the way it is structured. Appropriate language, just like appropriate attire, changes from context to context. There is an unwritten rule not to wear shorts to a formal wedding reception and there are unwritten rules regarding language behavior depending on the context. What is socially and culturally acceptable in one situation may not be in another. For example, if I were speaking to a child and I wanted the window closed, I would probably say, "Close the window." If it were another adult, I would probably say, "Would you please close the window" or even, "It certainly is cold in here with that window open." This example demonstrates there must be pragmatic language rules that are affected by the age and/or relationship of the communication partners and that there are rules dictating the appropriate use of literal and implied meanings (Grice, 1975), as in the last example where the request to close the window was merely implied.

In this text, pragmatics is discussed as a separate, equally important, component of language. Some professionals in the fields of linguistics and speech and language view pragmatics as the umbrella that influences all the other components of language rather than as a single separate component. In other words, pragmatics is the whole and everything else is under it; the other components of language are ruled by the need to use language in context. Still others (e.g., Lucas, 1980) have suggested that phonology, syntax, and morphology interact with and are governed by semantics for a resulting pragmatic system. Although this textbook presents pragmatics in the more traditional approach as a separate component, it easily can be demonstrated that context and use influence choice of syntax and vocabulary. The decision to present pragmatics separately is governed by a desire for clarity and simplicity in presentation, not necessarily by theoretical viewpoint, and it is recommended throughout this text that intervention for individuals with language disorders, in any of the components of language, should take place in context, not in isolation.

ORGANIZATIONAL FRAMEWORK OF PRAGMATIC ABILITIES

There are many different aspects of pragmatics; an organizational framework for these aspects has been described by Roth and Spekman (1984). They included communicative intention, presupposition, and organization of discourse. Figure 10–1 illustrates the interrelationship of these areas and also delineates components of each.

Communicative Intention

Communicative intention is one's purpose or reason for speaking, that is, the act or force of illocution as discussed in Chapter 1. Communication is such an effective tool for humans, and it serves so many purposes; it is for this reason that we learn language in the first place. Depending on our intention, or illocutionary act, different language form and content will be used. The context in conjunction with those intentions will affect language production or the locutionary act.

There are numerous reasons for using language, including soliciting information, providing information, responding to requests, greeting others, and gaining attention. There are statements, assertions, denials, requests, commands, promises, apologies, thanks, condolences, warnings, and many other speech acts (Searle, 1976). In the earlier example, "Close the window" was a command and "Would you please close the window" was a request. These intents are closely related; others are not. Searle attempted to categorize illocutionary acts, or communicative intents; his classifications can be seen in Table 10–1.

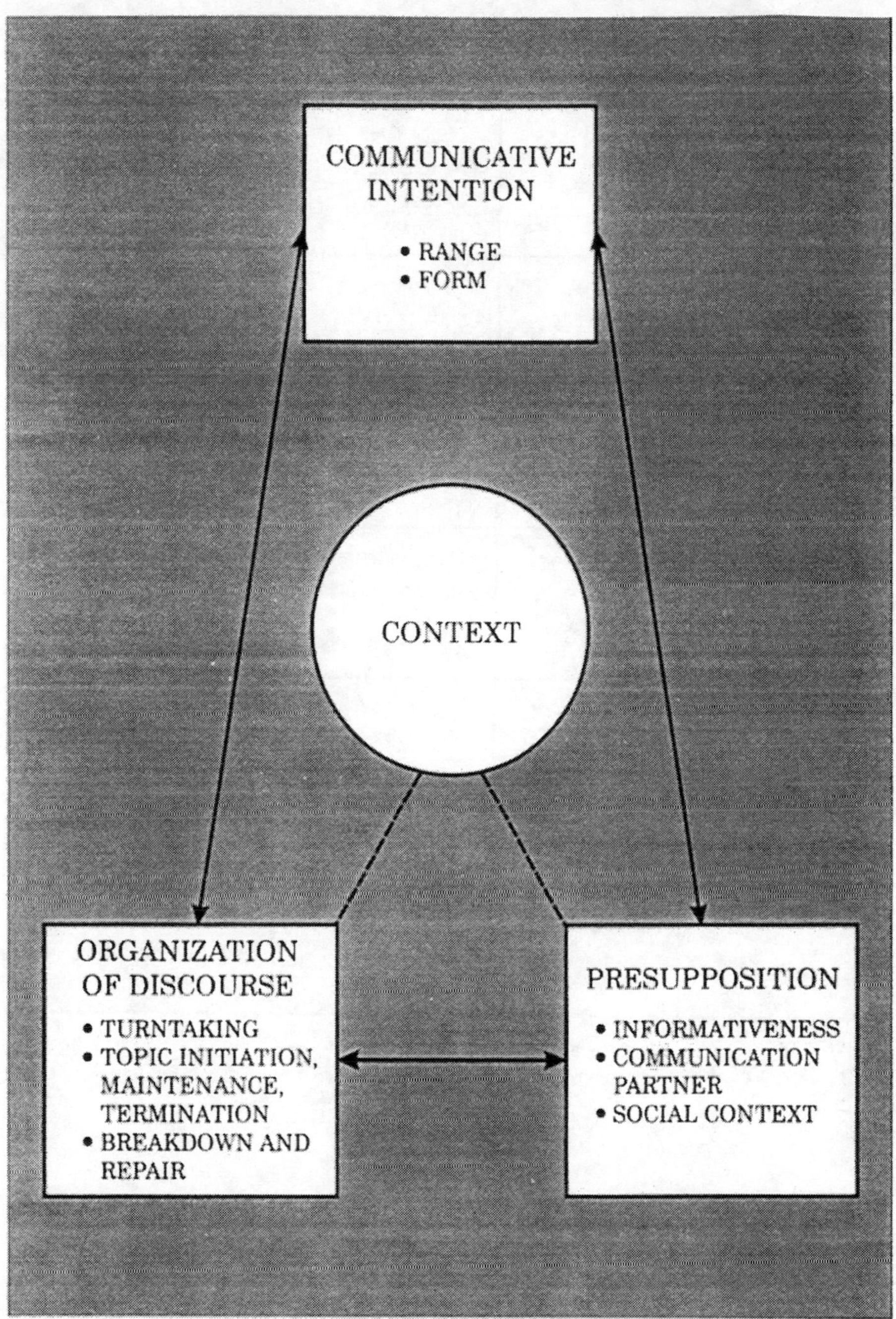

Figure 10–1. Organizational framework of pragmatic abilities. (From "An Intervention Framework for Learning Disabled Students with Communication Disorders," by N. J. Spekman and F. P. Roth, 1982, *Learning Disability Quarterly, 5*, p. 431. Copyright 1982 by *Learning Disability Quarterly*. Reprinted with permission.)

TABLE 10-1. Searle's classification of illocutionary acts.

Category	*Purpose*	*Example Statement*	*Examples of Acts Included*
Representative	Describe a state of affairs	*I have five more chapters to read.*	Stating, asserting, denying, confessing, admitting, notifying, concluding, predicting
Directive	Try to get someone to do something	*Underline the subject in each sentence.*	Requesting, ordering, forbidding, warning, advising, suggesting, insisting, recommending
Question	Get someone to provide information	*Where did Columbus land?*	Asking, inquiring
Commissive	Commit to doing something	*I will be there at about 6:00.*	Promising, vowing, volunteering, offering, guaranteeing, pledging, betting
Expressive	Express an emotional state	*I hate it when that happens.*	Apologizing, thanking, congratulating, condoling, welcoming, deploring, objecting
Declaration	Change the status of some entity	*You have been granted tenure.*	Appointing, naming, resigning, baptizing, surrendering, excommunicating, arresting

Source: From *Linguistics for Nonlinguists: A Primer with Exercises* (2nd ed., pp. 15–16), by F. Parker and K. Riley, 1994, Boston: Allyn and Bacon. Copyright 1994 by F. Parker and K. Riley. Adapted with permission.

Presupposition

Presupposition refers to the information that must be shared by the listener and the speaker in order for the message to be understood. If I came up to you on the street and I said, "Ed's going to be here next week," understanding the message would be a problem, because we do not share enough information for the message to have meaning. However, if I said, "I'm excited, because my brother Ed is coming into town next week and I will be able to show him the city," I would have provided enough information to be understood. (Provided it was appropriate for me to speak to you in the first place.)

Each time we speak, we evaluate and make assumptions about the knowledge a listener possesses. If those assumptions are accurate, then we will choose vocabulary and syntax that will provide the most efficient means of delivering our message. The message will be specific but not redundant. These choices will vary according to the listener's age, the formality of the social situation, and relationship to the speaker. For example, greeting a child will be very different from greeting a priest or senator and the greeting of a senator may be different at the Capitol than at a backyard barbecue.

Presupposition involves the ability to put yourself in someone else's shoes. Roth and Spekman (1984) described this as **role taking**. The speaker must be able to take the perspective of the listener. The speaker must determine what and how much information the listener needs to understand this message. The speaker must evaluate the knowledge and experiential base of the listener and must also consider cultural and linguistic influences.

Grice (1975) proposed four specific presuppositions that he called the Cooperative Principle in Conversation. These four simple maxims are the **Quantity Maxim**, **Quality Maxim**, **Relation Maxim**, and **Manner Maxim**, which are summarized in Table 10–2. Grice suggested that conversation is interpreted as if these maxims are being adhered to, but that the speaker may intentionally violate a maxim to convey another unstated implied message. Grice referred to this violation as **flouting**. An example of flouting the quantity maxim was illustrated in, "It certainly is cold in here with that window open." It is assumed that the listener will realize that there is a reason the speaker is making this statement and figure out that she would like the window closed, but perhaps does not want to directly impose her desires on the listener. The teacher who says to her student, "No one can hear you" is flouting the quantity maxim and is expecting her student to fill in the information omitted and realize that the teacher really means, "Speak up." The child in the room who does not fill in the missing information is likely to yell out, "I can hear her!" It is also possible that the speaker may unintentionally violate a maxim.

TABLE 10–2. Conversational maxims.

Maxim Name	***Rules of Conversation***
Maxim of Quantity	Contributions should be as informative as required, no less, no more
Maxim of Quality	Contributions should be truthful and based on sufficient evidence
Maxim of Relation	Contributions should be relevant to the subject
Maxim of Manner	Contributions should be expressed in reasonably clear fashion, not vague, ambiguous, or wordy

Source: Adapted from Logic and Conversation, by H. P. Grice, 1975. In P. Cole and J. L. Morgan (Eds.), *Syntax and Semantics 3: Speech Acts* (pp. 41–58). New York: Academic Press.

Organization of Discourse

Organization of discourse refers to the rules that must be mastered to effectively communicate in conversation or discourse. This includes skills related to **topic management**, such as **turn-taking**, as well as productive **repair** strategies.

Selection of a topic is important because it will influence the level of interest on the part of the listener and, as a result, influence the quantity and quality of social interaction that occurs. The **introduction** or **initiation** of a topic begins the social communication and must be presented in a manner acceptable to the listener and in a way that encourages participation. This is extremely important for positive peer interaction.

Topic **maintenance** refers to the ability to respond appropriately during a conversation in order to keep the conversation going. There must be some level of responsiveness on the part of the listener, or the conversation will not be maintained. The listener must demonstrate skills that acknowledge attention to the speaker and include making meaningful comments about the topic in an order that makes sense and increases understanding.

During a conversation, there will be times when the conversant changes topics. A **change** in topic requires a smooth transition, closure to the previous topic, and then the introduction of a new topic. Once again, appropriate selection, introduction, and maintenance of the new topic must be practiced.

Conversation is an exchange between two or more individuals with some level of responsiveness required of the parties involved. During conversation **turn-taking** is required. Turn-taking involves the ability to take the role of both listener and speaker and the knowledge of when to appropriately switch roles. A conversation partner listens to comments and then makes a statement regarding the topic, asks a question, and/or uses verbal and nonverbal modes to indicate listening and interest, such as a nod or verbal acknowledgments, such as "okay," "uh huh."

For all speakers, there are times when the intended message is not understood. The speaker must recognize this misunderstanding and then **repair** the communication breakdown. This can be accomplished through a variety of strategies, including revisions to the language form and content.

Nonverbal aspects such as eye contact and physical proximity that affect social communication will overlap these three aspects of pragmatics. Many intentions are revealed through nonverbal means. Listeners supply speakers with information regarding interest and comprehension through nonverbal means. And always remember these nonverbal aspects have a strong cultural base.

In summary, many language abilities fall within the area of pragmatics. Prutting and Kirchner's (1987) pragmatic protocol provides a comprehensive list of these abilities (see Table 10–3). However, to suggest that these abilities are "purely pragmatic" would be incorrect (Gerber, 1991). Many of these pragmatic abilities are dependent on seman-

TABLE 10–3. Pragmatic Protocol.

NAME:____________________ DATE:____________________

COMMUNICATIVE SETTING OBSERVED____________________ COMMUNICATIVE PARTNER'S RELATIONSHIP____________________

Communicative act	***Appropriate***	***Inappropriate***	***No opportunity to observe***	***Examples and comments***
Verbal aspects				
A. Speech acts				
1. Speech act pair analysis				
2. Variety of speech acts				
B. Topic				
3. Selection				
4. Introduction				
5. Maintenance				
6. Change				
C. Turn taking				
7. Initiation				
8. Response				
9. Repair/revision				
10. Pause time				
11. Interruption/overlap				
12. Feedback to speakers				
13. Adjacency				
14. Contingency				
15. Quantity/conciseness				
D. Lexical selection/use across speech acts				
16. Specificity/accuracy				
17. Cohesion				
E. Stylistic variations				
18. The varying of communicative style				
Paralinguistic aspects				
F. Intelligibility and prosodics				
19. Intelligibility				
20. Vocal intensity				
21. Vocal quality				
22. Prosody				
23. Fluency				

(continued)

TABLE 10–3. *(continued)*

Communicative act	Appropriate	Inappropriate	No opportunity to observe	Examples and comments
Nonverbal aspects				
G. Kenesics and proxemics				
24. Physical proximity				
25. Physical contacts				
26. Body posture				
27. Foot/leg and hand/arm movements				
28. Gestures				
29. Facial expression				
30. Eye gaze				

Source: From "A Clinical Appraisal of the Pragmatic Aspects of Language" by C. Prutting and D. Kirchner, 1987, *Journal of Speech and Hearing Disorders, 52*, p. 117. Copyright 1987 by the American Speech, Language, and Hearing Association. Reprinted with permission.

tic and syntactic flexibility, for example, the ability to revise statements when communication breakdown occurs.

PRAGMATIC DEVELOPMENT

As with other areas of language development, there is a gradual increase in pragmatic skills through infancy and toddlerhood. Then, during the preschool years with the advent of peer interaction, there is a rapid increase in pragmatic skill development. However, although other areas of language development are fairly well documented, the typical development of pragmatics is still being studied.

Communicative Intentions

Communicative intentions can be recognized in infancy. The infant can express intent through a variety of nonverbal means including cries, reaches, gazes, smiles, babbling and jargon, pointing, and pushing.

Parents respond to infants as if their early cooing and nonverbal movements have communicative intention. The child learns early that language is intricately tied to interaction with the most important persons in his or her life and that wants and needs can be achieved through the encouragement of such interaction. A range of intentions will be demonstrated at the one-word level. For example, the child may request information as in "Ball?" or may request the cessation of an activity as in "No!" or simply identify or label items in his or her environment such as "doggie." The range of intentions will continue to expand at the multiword stages as illustrated in Table 10–4.

Presupposition

Presupposition is the process of making adjustments to what we say and how we say it according to what we know about the listener. Re-

TABLE 10-4. Communicative intentions expressed at the multiword stage.

Intention	*Purposes of Utterances*	*Example*
Requesting information	Solicit information permission, confirmation, or repetition	*Where's Mary?* *Can I come?*
Requesting action	Solicit action or cessation of action	*Give me the doll.* *Stop it.* *Don't do that.*
Responding to requests	Supply solicited information or acknowledge preceding messages	*Okay.* *Mary is over there.* *No, you can't come.* *It's blue.*
Stating or commenting	State facts or rules, express beliefs, attitudes, or emotions, or describe environmental aspects	*This is a bird.* *You have to throw the dice, first.* *I dont like dogs.* *I'm happy today.* *My school is two blocks away.* *He can do it.*
Regulating conversational behavior	Monitor and regulate interpersonal contact	*Hey, Marvin!* *Yes, I see.* *Hi, Bye, Please.* *Here you are.* *Know what I did?*
Other performatives	Tease, warn, claim, exclaim, or convey humor	*You can't catch me.* *It's my turn.* *The dog said, "moo."*

Source: From "Assessing the Pragmatic Abilities of Children: Part 1. Organizational Framework and Assessment Parameters," by R. Roth and N. Spekman, 1984, *Journal of Speech and Hearing Disorders, 49*. p. 5. Copyright 1984 by ASHA. Reprinted with permission.

search indicates that young children (preschool age) will adjust their language to the age or developmental level of the listener. They will adjust their language when speaking to younger children, children with developmental delays, and children with language delay (Guralnick & Paul-Brown, 1980; Perner & Leekam, 1986; Shatz & Gelman, 1973). It is assumed that this ability to take the perspective of the listener is refined over time.

Organization of Discourse

Young children's conversation types can be classified in terms of the degree to which they are associated with normal socialized conversation (Reich, 1986). In early studies of young children's language, Piaget (1926, 1959) classified the language of young children into two groups based on functions, egocentric and socialized speech. In **egocentric speech**, the child talks, whether alone or in the presence of others, but only about himself with no apparent concern for who the audience is or whether anyone listens. **Socialized speech** shows a gradual increase in concern for the audience and communicating. Closer examination of these functions may provide clues to intervention for problems in discourse.

Monologues

Early "conversations" are characterized by the child's talking to him- or herself. There appears to be no interest in interacting with anyone else, but a great deal of pleasure in talking. The monologue still plays an important part in the language of 6- and 7-year-olds (Piaget, 1926, 1959). A simple monologue is illustrated in the language of Lev (age 5 years 11 months) as he sits down at his table alone.

> I want to do that drawing there . . . I want to draw something, I do. I shall need a big piece of paper to do that. (Piaget, 1926, 1959, p. 149)

Gallagher and Craig (1978) note that "monologues are a unique type of pragmatic speech act, a highly structured, semantically organized mechanism that permits action-based analysis of semantics, syntax, and conversation" (p. 116). Monologues are a mechanism for practicing language and all its components. In Gallagher and Craig's study of approximately 1,000 monologue utterances of children in Brown's Stages I, II, and III, 70% were declarative in sentence form. About 90% of declarative monologues were accounted for by four semantic categories, action (e.g., *He is jumping*), identity (e.g., *It doll*), attribute (e.g., *Baby cold*), and social (e.g., *Yeah, Okay*, and *Hi*), with action being the most frequent (40%). Several types of monologues will be described.

Self-Guidance Monologue. Children in this stage appear to use speech to help them focus attention on a task. The greater the difficulty of the task, the greater the amount of production of this type of monologue (e.g., Flavell, Beach, & Chinsky, 1966). Even as adults, we all remember times when we resort to this strategy in difficult tasks.

Affect Expressive Monologue. This describes periods when children sing, chat, repeat real and nonsense words, engage in verbal fantasy, and comment on their feelings (Klein, 1963, as cited in Reich, 1986). An example of this can be found in the language of Piaget's subject Pie (age 6 years 5 months) as he takes his arithmetic copy-book and turns the pages.

> 1, 2 . . . 3, 4, 5, 6, 7 . . . 8 . . . 8,8,8,8, and 8 . . . 9. Number 9, number 9, number 9 (singing) I want number 9 (p. 15).

Presleep Monologue. The most extensive studies of this language were those of Ruth Weir (1962), who placed a microphone under the crib of her son Anthony (age 28–30 months) and recorded his night-time monologues. A careful analysis of these monologues revealed four different types of sequences which are included, along with examples, in Table 10–5. In **build-ups**, Anthony uttered a word or phrase and then immediately repeated it in expanded form. **Breakdowns** involved the shortened version of a longer phrase immediately after its expression. **Completion** involved a second utterance that seemed to be the continuation of a thought after a complete sentence was uttered. Many of Anthony's longer sentences were **quotations** recognized as repetitions or close approximations of sentences he had heard earlier in the day. He was apparently thinking about the language he had heard that day. Three basic sentence

TABLE 10–5. Presleep monologues.

Monologue Type	*Example*
Build-up	Donkey. Fix the donkey.
Breakdown	Another big bottle Big bottle.
Completion	And put it Up there.
Quotation	Anthony wants to talk to Daddy.
Phonological Play	Bink. Let Bobo bink. Bink ben bink. Blue kink.
Grammatical Play	What color. What color blanket. What color mop. What color glass.

Source: Drawn from *Language in the Crib* by R. H. Weir, 1962. The Hague: Mouton.

types were distinguished: imperatives (e.g., *Move the yellow blanket*), declaratives (e.g., *Anthony want the blue one*), and interrogatives (e.g., *What color is BoBo*).

A great deal of play with sounds of words and the words themselves was found. Most of Anthony's presleep utterances seemed to be language play, including **phonological play** with alliterations, rhyming, and rhythm play, and **grammatical play** in the form of successive substitutions of words into sentence slots.

Collective Monologue. A more advanced type of conversation is the collective monologue where children talk about themselves without listening to each other (Piaget, 1926; 1959). At this point in development, children demonstrate turn-taking in the presence of other children; however, the content of utterances does not appear to be affected by the remarks of other participants in the conversation.

Pie (6-5): Where could we make another tunnel? Ah, here, Eun?

Eun (4-11): Look at my pretty frock. (Piaget, p. 58)

Associated Monologue. At this point, children are talking about the same topic, but other than the content there seems to be no evidence of communicative interaction. An example from Piaget (1926; 1959) occurs while children are drawing. Each is talking about his or her own picture with no attempt at cooperation, but at the same time they are talking about the same subject and listening to each other.

Lev (5-11): It begins with Goldylocks. I'm writing the story of the three bears. The daddy bear is dead. Only the daddy was too ill.

Gen (5-11): I used to live at Saleve. I lived in a little house and you had to take the funicular railway to go and buy things.

Geo (6-0): I can't do the bear.

Li (6-10): That's not Goldylocks.

Lev: I haven't got curls. (Piaget, p. 58)

Collaboration. Another step toward socialized speech reported by Piaget (1926, 1959) finds children's remarks affected by the previous remark made by another child, but not necessarily a direct response to it. In the following example, a memory is shared.

Arn (5-9): It's awfully funny at the circus when the wheels (of the tricycle) have come off.

Lev (5-11): Do you remember when the gymnastic man but who couldn't do gymnastics, fell down? (Piaget, p. 62)

Repetition. Some of children's repetitions, or imitations of the utterances of others, occur as simple monologues repeated just for the pleasure of using words (Piaget, 1926/1959). However, this event also occurs in the midst of conversation. Reich (1986) refers to this as *copycat talk* and suggests that it occurs when young children want to participate in a conversation, but have nothing to say.

Jac (7-2): Look, Ez, your pants are showing.

Pie (6-5): (From another part of the room.) My pants are showing, and my shirt, too. (This is not true.) (Piaget, p.12)

Socialized Speech

Piaget (1926; 1959) places the beginnings of socialization of thought somewhere between the ages of 7 and 8 years of age. A significant step toward completely socialized speech is evident in children's methods of quarreling and argument. Children are attending to others and responding to what is said. Examples of some of these common techniques suggested by Reich (1986) are illustrated in Table 10–6.

Topic Management Skills

One of the first skills that children learn is turn-taking. By 4 months of age, infants and caregivers will participate in **mutual gazing.** Mom looks at a toy and then the baby looks at the same toy. The quantity of this type of attentional interaction may affect early expressive language development (Dunham, Dunham, & Curwin, 1993). Early turn-taking skills are evidenced in both gaze and verbal interactions between infant and caregiver.

Current research, although still preliminary, suggests that young preschool children are able to produce utterances to maintain a topic.

Calvin and Hobbes **by Bill Watterson**

WHEN A PERSON PAUSES IN MID-SENTENCE TO CHOOSE A WORD, THAT'S THE BEST TIME TO JUMP IN AND CHANGE THE SUBJECT!
IT'S LIKE AN INTERCEPTION IN FOOTBALL! YOU GRAB THE OTHER GUY'S IDEA AND RUN THE OPPOSITE WAY WITH IT!

THE MORE SENTENCES YOU COMPLETE, THE HIGHER YOUR SCORE! THE IDEA IS TO BLOCK THE OTHER GUY'S THOUGHTS AND EXPRESS YOUR OWN! THAT'S HOW YOU WIN!

CONVERSATIONS AREN'T CONTESTS!
OK, A POINT FOR YOU, BUT I'M STILL AHEAD.

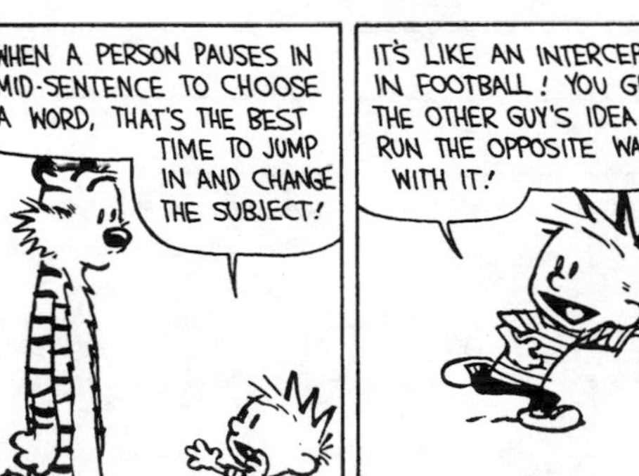

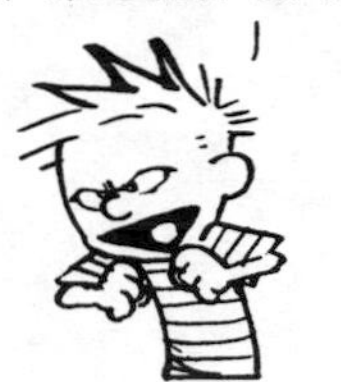

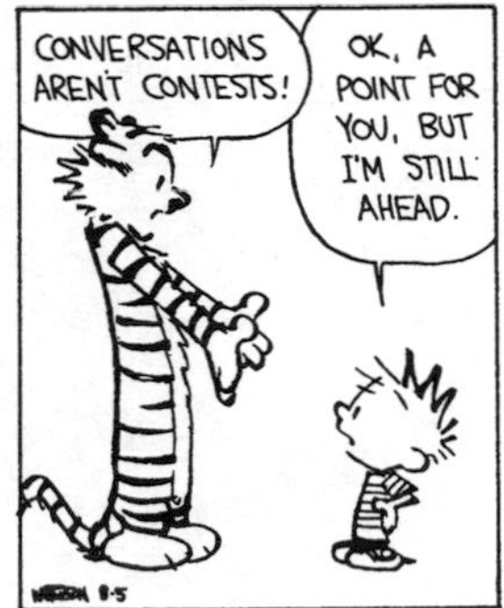

TABLE 10–6. Argument tactics.

Tactic	*Example*
Derogatory remark	I drew a better picture than you. You're stupid.
Possession assertion	That's mine. Gimme that truck.
Flat contradiction	Mia: My brother is bigger than yours. Sue: No, my brother is bigger. Mia: Oh yes, my brother's bigger. Sue: No he's not. Mia: Is too.
Content variation	Sean: I'll break your arm. JD: I'll tear yours off first. Sean: I'll punch your eyes out. JD: I'll rip your ear off.
Escalation	Jim: I can beat solitaire in two minutes. Suli: I can beat solitaire in one minute. Jim: Well, I beat solitaire and free cell in one minute with my eyes closed.
Giving a reason	Cause I said so.
Demand for proof	Who says so?
Stating disbelief	No way!
Ironic bribe	I'll give you a dollar if you can.
Threat	I'm going to tell the teacher on you.
Indifference	So what?
Nonword taunts	Nyeeh-nyeeh.

Source: Drawn from *Language Development*, by P.A. Reich, 1986.. Englewood Cliffs, NJ: Prentice-Hall.

Foster (1986) found that toddlers would produce an average of 3–4 utterances related to a specific topic. Interestingly, the number of utterances related to a topic would increase to 25–35 if the children were participating in a structured routine. This may have significance for intervention.

The development of topic management skills appears to be developmental (as one might expect). The ability to add significant information related to a topic increases with age (Brinton & Fujiki, 1984; Wanska & Bedrosian, 1985). Young children tend to introduce and change topics frequently. The tendency to introduce fewer topics in discourse and become more sophisticated with topic length and topic shifts increases in later childhood and adolescence (Brinton & Fujiki, 1984).

In conclusion, research on the typical development of pragmatics is still emerging. What we do know is that it appears to be developmental in nature and begins in infancy. Pragmatic performance may well be dependent on overall linguistic ability. As Prutting and Kirchner (1987) reported, children identified as having a language delay demonstrated more pragmatic deficits than children identified as normal and also children identified as having articulation disorders.

The knowledge that we do have regarding the development of pragmatic skills offers some groundwork for intervention practices. For instance, if the use of structured routines increases a child's abilities to contribute meaningful utterances to a topic, those routines may be a place to start intervention and practice.

✓ SUMMARY CHECKLIST

☐ **Definition of Pragmatics**

Pragmatics is a set of sociolinguistic rules related to language use in the communicative context.

☐ **Organizational Framework of Pragmatic Abilities**

Communicative Intention

Presupposition

Role Taking

Conversational Maxims

Quantity

Quality

Relation

Manner

Organization of Discourse

Topic Management

Topic Selection

Topic Initiation

Topic Maintenance

Change in Topic

Turn-taking

Repair

Nonverbal Aspects

☐ **Pragmatic Development**

Communicative Intentions

Nonverbal

One-word

Multi-word

Presupposition

Organization of Discourse

Monologues

Self-guidance

Affect Expressive

Presleep

Collective

Associated

Collaboration

Repetition

Socialized Speech

Topic Management Skills

CHAPTER

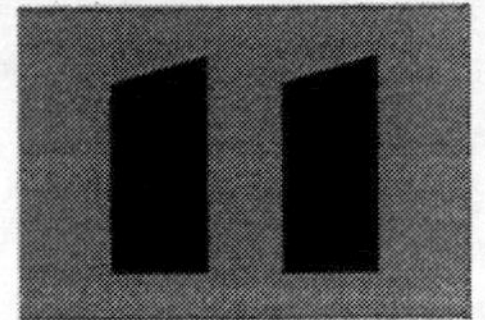

PRAGMATICS: ANALYSIS AND INTERVENTION

As described in Chapter 1, correlations have been found between a variety of disabilities and communication delays and disorders. Logically, the same students would be at risk for problems in the area of pragmatics as well. Current research supports this conclusion. McCord and Haynes (1988) found that 8- to 11-year-old students with learning disabilities differed from peers without learning disabilities in areas of topic maintenance, need for repetition, and failure to provide enough relevant information.

The DSM-IV criteria for students with attention deficit with hyperactivity disorder (ADHD) include difficulties in pragmatic skills such as turn-taking and topic management. Some students with mild/moderate retardation have difficulties with verbal aspects of pragmatics such as topic maintenance (Hunt, Alwell, Goetz, & Sailor, 1990) as well as nonverbal aspects such as touching (Bufkin & Altman, 1995).

Because pragmatic development is a part of social development, one might expect students with disabilities to be lacking in social competence. In fact, Bursuck (1989) reported that students with learning disabilities were rated significantly lower in social acceptance and perceived by peers and teachers as exhibiting fewer prosocial behaviors. Likewise, Westby and Cutler (1994) summarized a number of studies that indicated poor pragmatic skills in students with ADHD and the resulting social problems.

ANALYSIS

Communicative Intentions

A child has a problem in the area of communicative intentions if the range of intentions is limited and not age appropriate. For example, for a 4-year-old, it would be appropriate to look at a chart such as Table 10–3 in Chapter 10 and note the various intentions that are found at the multiword level. If the child is not demonstrating the full range of intentions noted, intervention may be appropriate.

Presupposition

One problem that exists in the area of presupposition is not providing sufficient information (i.e., a lack of specificity or accuracy) for a message to be understood. Consider the following example.

> My daughter Molly had acquired a fish tank. And as novice fish owners, there were numerous dead fish over the course of the first few months. One casualty was the "sucker fish." The sucker fish has a critical role in aquarium life; he eats all the algae on the glass of the aquarium.
>
> At the aquarium store, I explained that we needed to purchase a new sucker fish because our last one had died. The young sales clerk quickly responded: "What did the fish die of?" (Thinking to myself) . . . Darn, I forgot to do the autopsy.

The sales clerk had made the assumption that I was knowledgeable about fish and aquariums. For, you see, it is common knowledge that sucker fish often starve to death because the tank is not growing enough algae to sustain the fish. This is important information because it can be easily rectified by supplementing the fish's diet with algae treats. However, the clerk's assumption about my knowledge was erroneous and communication breakdown occurred. However, once explained, the additional information was a relief as I don't have time to play medical examiner for a bunch of dead fish.

It is always important to know who your audience is and add or delete information accordingly. Consider the following.

> For months, the Chair of our department discussed offering a "Sadie Hawkins Day" course in the summer. To clarify, Sadie Hawkins Day was a day when the girls asked the boys out instead of the traditional boy-ask-girl approach. So the Chair was suggesting that the school district choose the course it was in most need of rather than the traditional method whereby the department made the scheduling decision. Months after this discussion, one of our faculty members who was born and raised in India asked, "Who was Sadie Hawkins and what course did she choose?"

As can be seen from our discussion, some wrong assumptions had been made about our shared knowledge. Think about the student with a disability who tries to share information with the teacher or peer. Often, the listener will be found asking, "Who are you talking about?" "What are you talking about now?" "What's the situation?" This is because students with disabilities often don't supply enough information. The listener must then ask additional questions and piece together contextual information in order to understand the message. Many of the students assume the listener has the same knowledge that the speaker does. For example, the 9-year-old who calls the gym where his mom works out and asks, "Is my mom there?" Many students in special education have a very difficult time taking another's point of view, so they will have problems with the quality and quantity of information they give. Smiley (1991b) provided the following example of Jason, an 8-year-old with a learning disability, telling someone who has not seen it, what the movie *Look Who's Talking* was about.

> It's this baby which can talk, and the best part when I I like when he stucked his pretzel into a car when it was getting towed and the towed truck start up. An when he turned the tow truck turned and it was funny. And Mike he he he was um it was his father and going like that and he caught the baby. An and see we married each other and the baby goes maybe I should tell em my diaper's wet and he goes nah.

Jason obviously omitted a great deal of information that someone who has not seen this movie would need. Jason failed to consider his audience.

In contrast, if too much information is supplied for the listener/speaker relationship, redundancy can occur. In the case where a great deal of information is shared, less specificity is required. For example, if Mary Lou and I had been going out to dinner every Wednesday for the last 8 weeks at the same restaurant, I wouldn't have to say to Mary Lou, "We need to meet at 8:00 at The Grill so we can have dinner." I might easily say "We're on for Wednesday."

Many students may not be able to make the appropriate language adjustments according to age and social status. A student who says to a peer, "Get the hell out of my face" may not be perceived as friendly, but making this statement to a principal may have serious consequences.

The amount of information that is explicitly given will depend on the listener and the relationship of that listener to the speaker. If students are not being understood, it may be for reasons related to presupposition.

Organization of Discourse

Topic Related Problems

Topic management skills encompass topic choice, initiation, maintenance, and change. These skills will be dependent on semantic and syntactic proficiency. And, as with all the components of language, problems in one component area may well be the result of, or compounded by, deficiencies in other component areas.

There are appropriate and inappropriate times to discuss a topic. Certain topics should not be spoken about with certain people. Some students with disabilities appear to have difficulty learning these social subtleties. They may select topics that have nothing to do with what else is going on. Their teachers may be heard saying, "Arnold, this is not the time to be talking or discussing that issue. You need to deal with it later." Topic choice will influence both peer and adult interaction.

Topic Initiation. If a group of students are participating in an outdoor activity and the student with a disability wants to enter the group, he has to have the appropriate language and topic with which to do that. Unfortunately, the student, rather than saying, "Hi, what are you doing? Can I play too?" will more likely take the ball and bop one of the students on the head. What happens next? The students start screaming "Get away from us!" Students with disabilities inevitably end up with a lot of negative feedback because of the way they initiate contact with groups. They then end up with negative feelings about themselves and a vicious cycle has begun.

Students with disabilities may not initiate topics and social activities appropriately because of poor verbal skills. It may be difficult for them to form a sentence and find vocabulary. However, many students have sufficient language, but seem to not know how to use it. Rather than using language to get peers' attention, they will use inappropriate means to get it. Several studies have shown that children with disabilities initiate conversations much less frequently than their peers. Preschool children with speech and language impairments were more likely to initiate interaction with adults than with peers, and when interaction was initiated with peers, they were more likely to be ignored (Rice & Hadley, 1991; Rice, Sell, & Hadley, 1991). Likewise, students with mental retardation tend to take passive roles in all interactions, including language. This passivity may be a function of **learned helplessness**. Students who have mental handicaps often do a lot more responding than initiating. These, of course, are the children who need this interaction most in order to practice and enhance their conversational skills.

Conversely, students with disabilities may not be as responsive to conversational initiations as typically developing peers (for examples of students with learning disabilities, see Feagans & Short, 1986; for students with autism, see Newman, Buffington, & Hemmes, 1996). Rice, Sell, and Hadley (1991) and Rice and Hadley (1991) noted through observation that preschool children with speech and language impairments were less likely to respond to initiations by both peers and adults.

Topic Maintenance and Topic Change. Mentis (1994) discussed topic maintenance in terms of **local cohesion** and **global cohesion**. Local cohesion involves a relationship of one sentence to the previous one. Global cohesion is the relationship of the sentences to the topic. Mentis illustrated this with the examples in the box on the next page. The first example is locally coherent but not globally coherent. The sentences relate to one another, but there is no main idea. In this case, all of the sentences are linked to each other but not to a topic. The topic at the

EXAMPLE 1
Yesterday we looked at a house we wanted to buy. It had a wonderful garden with lots of fruit trees. I love fruit. I go to Farmer's market every Saturday morning to get the best fruit available. Sally also goes to Farmer's market. She's an old friend. We went to college together. Our reunion was last month. It was in California. The weather there is really lovely at this time of year.

EXAMPLE 2
Yesterday we looked at a house we wanted to buy. The renovations will cost a lot. The estate agent will let us know on Monday. It had a very modern kitchen. We'll never go to that bank again for a mortgage. Our son will love the garden.

Source: From "Topic Management in Discourse: Assessment and Intervention" by M. Mentis, 1994, *Topics in Language Disorders, 14*, 29–54.

beginning was about buying a house. In contrast, in the second example, all of the sentences are linked to the topic, but the speaker does not link one sentence to another.

The following example occurs in conversation and illustrates an abrupt change in topic by a listener. Note the lack of transition. Students are in the cafeteria line making comments:

S1 What are you having?

S2 A hot dog . . . I don't like that. (Points to the spinach)

S3 (Student with disabilities) (In line listening)

S1 I'm going to have ice cream.

S3 (Student with disabilities) It's raining.

It appears the last comment has nothing to do with the conversation already in progress. This example demonstrates a knowledge of turn-taking and a real desire to speak but little knowledge of the rules of topic maintenance. These rules must be mastered to participate successfully in a conversation. Unfortunately, lack of mastery may result in negative social interaction.

The example in the next box is of a 9-year-old student with a learning disability speaking with his teacher, Ms. Heather Benforado. This child does not maintain his own topics. It is possible that he misunderstood Ms. B.'s question about other parts he liked, but even if that were the case, he did not pick up on her confusion and the need to repair any breakdown. This difficulty in repair will be discussed later in the chapter.

What movies have you seen?	
	um: Aladdin and the king and the forty thieves/ um:
(S pauses)	
	Star Wars/ and um * Indiana Jones/
Wow/ Those sound like great movies/ Can you tell me what happened in the Indiana Jones movie?	
	I liked in the part when when * when the spikes was going down * and * and there was * and there___/ Indiana Jones/ and there was another kid with it s/c with him/ and there was___/ when they was coming they had s/c they saw bugs/ skulls/ and people was dead in it/
Ooh/ It sounds scary/	
	it was/ it was that was my favorite part/
(H laughing) It was!	
	mm-hmm/
Did you have any other parts you liked a lot?	
	okay/ um I liked the part when:* Aladdin's * Aladdin father was the king of thieves/
So this is the Aladdin movie now/	
	mm-hmm/ and Star Wars/ I liked it when the when they went the that the place got blowed up
What place?	
	um a __the: when the: when when the guys who was in the space ship blow up one giant ball and explode real hard/

Topics can be maintained through different strategies. One may use a repetition strategy or an enhancement strategy. The **repetition strategy** involves the repetition of the previous utterance in whole or part. It maintains the topic but contributes little to the propositional development of the topic. An enhancement strategy would elaborate, extend, and develop the topic by providing novel information. As many researchers have found, students with language delays are more likely to use repetition strategy or stereotypic responses (*okay, uh huh*), strategies that do not develop the topic but do maintain it. In summary, difficulties in these areas will be evidenced in the inability to begin a conversation, to enter an existing conversation, and to maintain the conversation.

Other Conversational Skills

Other problems related to conversation/discourse exist. Some areas suggested by Lucas (1980) and illustrated by Smiley (1991b) are presented next.

Topic Closure Difficulties. These problems involve rephrasing, rewording, or reiterating, because the speaker does not know when to quit.

> Todd, 11: When I came out of the store when it was stolen somebody must have put it in a truck because we were only in there for about two minutes and there was nobody in the sight when we went in there and I don't see how somebody can ride that fast cause there was nobody in sight . . .

Off-Target Responding. This is a response that is not the one that is expected in the context. The student is unaware of being off target and may not know the rules of conversation or may find the information too complex to respond to, so changes the topic.

> Edward, 8 (after raising his hand in response to teacher's asking if anyone has to go to the bathroom): Mrs. K., if I study I can pass my spelling test.

Tangentiality. In this response, the student hears the topic, associates it with something else, and goes on to that topic. It is sometimes difficult to recognize the association.

> Catherine, 8, when asked why she was late for school: My mom has a new car. (It turns out that she was late because she missed the bus and so her mom, who has a new car, brought her to school.)

Topic Identification Problems. These are evidenced by responses that are related to the previous question or statement, but not to the main topic. In this case, the student listens and is attempting to respond appropriately, but cannot determine the correct referent. This student will try again and may appear frustrated, unlike the off-target responder.

Bobby, 8th grade, in response to "Why is it important to ask questions about something before buying it?": How much will it cost?

Turn-Taking

Individuals who have difficulty with turn-taking are often perceived as rude, because they do not follow discourse rules related to turn-taking. For instance, they may interrupt the speaker or monopolize the conversation. This inability to follow rules of turn-taking may show up in other areas as well; for example, it may carry over into sports and games. It should also be noted that the rules of turn-taking are culture specific and teachers or clinicians should be sure to first determine whether they are correcting a problem in this skill or teaching another set of rules.

For effective conversational turn-taking to occur, the communication partners must attend and respond to one another. As previously mentioned, certain populations of students with disabilities do not respond to verbal initiations by others as frequently as typically developing students do. If a child is in a peer group situation and the child does not respond to peer initiations, the other children will decrease their initiations and may eventually leave the child alone. This, obviously, has social ramifications and will reduce the opportunities the child has to use, practice, and refine his or her language skills.

Likewise, Fujiki and Brinton (1994) described a situation where a preschooler with a language impairment is frequently nonresponsive to the mother's initiations. As a result, the mother-child interaction is less rewarding for the parent and may result in reduced initiations. Again, the child has fewer opportunities to refine all language skills, including pragmatic ones.

Repair and Revisions

As speakers, many students with disabilities will not repair or revise their language when needed (i.e., misunderstanding has occurred). This may result from two problems. One, they do not always recognize that a repair is needed, because they don't pick up on cues that the listener does not understand them. They may continue on and on with their message, never reading the confused look on the listener's face that is saying, "What are you talking about?" Most people don't need to have someone say "What?" or "I don't understand" to realize that the listener is not comprehending the message. Skilled teachers can often look out over the class and tell by facial expressions whether students are understanding the material or not. However, some students such as those with learning disabilities have been found to identify fewer emotions through facial expressions than normally achieving peers. However, they do show developmental increases and do better with interpreting gestures than facial expressions and posture (Nabuzoka & Smith, 1995).

Listeners may be less subtle and say, "What?" "Say that again," or "I don't understand." Once misunderstanding is recognized, it is time to rephrase the sentence or reemphasize the point. Unfortunately, the students with disabilities often repeat the message in exactly the same way. If initial misunderstanding is due to problems with presupposition, for example, the speaker is not giving the listener enough information in the first place, a restatement of the original statement will not increase the likelihood of understanding.

Conversely, as a listener, it may also be difficult for students with disabilities to let the speaker know when they do not understand a message, for example, in the case of students with learning disabilities (Donahue, 1984). And as Donahue (1997) stated, children are expected to spend significantly more time in the classroom listening (and understanding) than speaking, reading, and writing. One reason they may be having difficulties is that they do not always realize they do not understand (Kotsonis & Patterson, 1980). Sometimes students don't understand enough in some class situations/content areas to even know where to begin to ask. A base of knowledge of the content is needed in order to know what to ask. It is also possible that they simply do not know how to ask for clarification. However, Donahue (1984) found that teaching students with learning disabilities to ask questions did not improve their use of questions in situations where clarification was necessary. In other words, an improvement in the ability to ask questions did not translate in knowing when to use questions as a strategy for clarification. All too often, these students will just "go with the flow." In many cases, they may catch pieces of information but not the whole picture.

Another possible reason that students with disabilities do not ask for clarification is past history. This is especially true in the upper elementary and later grades. These students have received so much negative feedback for asking questions and letting people know they don't understand that they quit trying. Consider the following example.

> The teacher says "Does everybody understand what to do?"
>
> T: (After no response) Okay, go ahead and get started.
>
> Five minutes later, she notices Shannon sitting there with not a word on the paper. But the student has not let the teacher know that she does not have a clue to what's going on. The student feels it's just safer not to say anything.

Or does this sound like a familiar scenario?

> S: Raises hand and states he doesn't understand.
>
> T: What do you mean you don't understand? I **just** explained it. We did this yesterday.

Donahue (1997) proposed a different, however interesting, reason for such an occurrence. She suggested that these scenarios occur because of student beliefs. Students with learning disabilities may have erroneous beliefs about listening and the listener's role. Based on Grice's (1975) maxims, students believe that the speaker (i.e., the teacher) is informative, truthful, relevant, and clear (see Chapter 10 for a review of Grice's maxims). Therefore, if misunderstanding occurs, it must be the fault of the listener, not the speaker. In a summary of research in this area, Donahue noted students with learning disabilities were more likely to state that listener confusion was the fault of the listener. In other words, these students perceive all misunderstanding as their fault and attempt to hide their lack of comprehension in a variety of ways.

Nonverbal Aspects

Nonverbal aspects of language including proxemics, body posture, foot/leg and hand/arm movements (think about hyperactive students) also need to be considered. The student who is always shifting and tapping proves to be a difficult communication partner. Again, this behavior inhibits social interactions with peers. Inappropriate touching may also break down communication if the listener is uncomfortable with it. These will obviously affect interactions with adults, but will even more profoundly affect interactions with peers.

INTERVENTION

Perspective

It is important to note that the study of pragmatics or the study of language from a pragmatic perspective has had a dramatic effect on the understanding of specific language problems and their treatment. The study and understanding of children with autism has broadened and changed through pragmatic approaches (Geller, 1991). If one takes a pragmatic perspective of language intervention, then deficits in all component areas will need to be analyzed functionally and will need intervention both specifically and pragmatically. For example, as Prutting and Kirchner (1987) noted, word retrieval difficulties are treated as a semantic deficit. If, however, the child is using generic terms such as *thing* or *stuff*, communication will lack the pragmatic aspect of specificity. Therefore, intervention from a pragmatic perspective needs to include semantic strengthening, that is, naming, word knowledge, and semantic mapping, as well as pragmatic strengthening, such as strategies to correct communication breakdown (Gerber, 1991).

There is an overwhelming call for language intervention to target "real language" in "natural contexts." Goals are centered on the development of targets through natural discourse using natural linguistic responses instead of contrived situations with unnatural language. In other words, natural conversation should be the context for intervention in all component areas and language targets should be taught in the way they would naturally occur in conversation. Historically, in an attempt to emphasize and isolate a language target, SLPs encouraged unnatural discourse. Consider the following interaction, in which the clinician is attempting to have the child produce the present progressive form of the verb.

Clinician: Shows a picture of a boy riding his bike.
Asks, "What's the boy doing?"

Student: "Riding the bike"

Clinician: "Use a complete sentence."

Student: "The boy is riding the bike."

The student's first response is the natural way to answer such a question. However, with the clinician's interest in practicing the "is + ing" form, the student is required to respond in an unnatural way.

General Strategies

Environmental Arrangement

One of the best strategies to promote pragmatic language development is to create an environment that encourages verbal interaction. We are always amazed when college students have assignments to observe in special education classrooms in order to collect samples of language, and they return with two utterances. They report, "I was there for 3 hours, the teacher gave directions, and after that no one spoke." If students are to learn pragmatic skills, they **must** have an opportunity to use them. The classroom must be designed to encourage verbal participation. This is best done through engaging students with exciting materials and activities. The current focus on hands-on learning lends itself to facilitating language practice. Put a frog in a student's lap and you will generate a whole lot more language than if you slap a coloring page on the desk.

The use of script knowledge for familiar routines appears to provide a comfortable environment for practice of communication skills. If script knowledge and the use of familiar routines such as "preparing meals" can significantly increase the number of meaningful contributions a student will make on a topic (Foster, 1986; Schober-Peterson & Johnson, 1989) in typical development, then it may provide a facilitative environment for those delayed in pragmatic aspects. The use of scripts and the role playing of familiar events provides rehearsal for various roles and topic management skills (Fey, Catts, & Larrivee, 1995). Incorporating those types of routines (or variations of them) in the classroom will offer a supportive environment for conversation practice.

Teacher manipulation of the environment to encourage conversation at the preschool level can be done by providing toys or activities that encourage cooperation or by assigning specific roles in, for example, the housekeeping center (Fey, Catts, & Larrivee, 1995) or, for older students, the use of cooperative learning. If there are certain students who invoke particular concern in the area of pragmatics, the teacher or clinician should design activities that promote their targeted interests and talents (Fey, Catts, & Larrivee, 1995). Recognize the role language plays with the rest of the academic curriculum and treat it integratively, rather than separately. Englert and Mariage (1996) discussed how the integration of reading, writing, and discourse skills can be facilitated. They used a format called "Sharing Chair" in which a student, after writing in a journal, shares his or her writing with the group. The other students ask questions and make comments regarding the topic. This social interaction provides practice in presupposition as well as the organization of discourse. In turn, this process promotes the development of writing skills as well. The authors emphasized the need for scaffolding in this process. The teacher may need to initially provide models and/or prompts such as question words (*what, where*, etc.)

Observation

Teachers must be very good observers of social interaction. Teachers should be able to identify everyday situations in which students have difficulty. Intervention can occur immediately (i.e., during the difficulty) or be incorporated in a role-playing activity at a later time. Many times students with disabilities act the way they do because they have not thought of any other way of handling the situation. The behavior may have been an effective strategy in an earlier situation. They continue to use it even when it is not effective, because it is the only one they have. Therefore, we need to teach them alternatives.

Specific Strategies

More specific strategies and/or structured activities may be useful to teach specific skills. The difficulty with these approaches has traditionally been in the area of generalization. If the ultimate goal is positive social interactions, then we must teach flexibility and response options to a variety of situations.

There are many good social skills curricula available, such as *ASSET* (Hazel, Schumacher, Sherman, & Sheldon-Wildgen, 1981), *ACCEPTS* (Walker, McConnell, Holmes, Todis, Walker, & Golden, 1983), and *Skillstreaming the Elementary School Child* (McGinnis & Goldstein, 1984) or *Skillstreaming the Adolescent* (Goldstein, Sprafkin, Gershaw, & Klein, 1980), that include, as would be necessary, verbal interactions. They often incorporate role playing as a practice activity for specific situations. Teachers may want to target situations that they anticipate to be difficult for their students. Again, the teacher must be alert to encouraging these skills in naturally occurring situations throughout the day or generalization will not occur.

Direct instruction can be employed as an effective intervention technique. Certain skills and certain populations will lend themselves better to direct instruction than others. The more severe the area of disability, the more important the role of direct instruction may become. Persons with moderate mental retardation are poorer at perspective-taking than persons with mild mental retardation and may require more structured intervention. Other examples have been provided by Newman, Buffington, and Hemmes (1996), who determined that appropriate conversations could be increased with autistic teens by teaching them to use self-reinforcement; and Clement-Heist, Siegel, and Gaylord-Ross (1992), who were able to improve work-related social skills through a structured training program. Four high school students with learning disabilities were trained on ordering job duties, conversation skills, and giving instructions.

Role-Taking

A speaker must be able to take the perspective of the listener if successful communication is to occur. Roth, Spekman, and Fye (1995) suggested brainstorming about the kinds and quantity of information a speaker needs about a topic, how a speaker can know if enough information was given, and how listeners can let the speaker know they need more information through signals of misunderstanding. These discussions would include how to determine appropriate vocabulary and style in relation to listener characteristics (age, social status, etc.).

Bunce (1991) suggested a variety of tasks/activities that may facilitate areas of giving and following directions and asking clarification questions (see the box on the next page). Bunce suggested teaching specific strategies while using these activities, including the use of redundant information and contrasting skills. She emphasized the need for the speaker and listener to discuss and analyze the information given after the activity to determine areas of confusion and possible solutions. It is also wise for the speaker/listener dyad to switch roles.

Donahue (1997) suggested teaching about listening and communication breakdowns in order to change beliefs about misunderstandings. Her study, as previously discussed, revealed that many students with learning disabilities believed that, if a communication breakdown occurred, it must be due to their poor listening skills. Donahue stated that these students must realize that speakers sometimes are not clear and do not provide sufficient information and, therefore, clarification must be requested.

Topic Management

Teachers can easily increase topic management through manipulation of the environment, as previously mentioned, or by more direct interventions such as teacher prompts or modeling in a peer group situation. For students who tend to prefer adult interaction, redirection of students who need help or information to a peer is called for.

Referential Communication Training Tasks

Description tasks	Speaker describes an object or picture, listener selects from several alternatives
Word-pair tasks	Speaker gives a clue, listener selects from a pair of words
Twenty Questions	Participants ask questions until they can guess the target
Magic box task	An object is hidden, and the speaker gives directions to find it
Drawing task	Speaker describes a design, the listener attempts to reproduce from the directions
Map or Maze task	Speaker gives directions to reach a destination
Barrier games	A barrier is placed between the speaker and the listener, the speaker gives directions for an activity such as drawing design, map, etc.

Source: From "Referential Communication Skills: Guidelines for Therapy" by B. Bunce, 1991, *Language Speech, and Hearing Services in Schools, 22,* 296–301.

Mentis (1991) identified several strategies that appear to encourage the development of topic management skills. These include question-answer sequences, use of repetition, and the use of script knowledge. These strategies have been documented as occurring naturally in typical development, thus they may have intervention significance on a slightly more structured and purposeful level. The question-answer strategy, initially used in mother-child dyads, is an appropriate technique for teacher-student dyads to facilitate topic management skills. This technique provides the opportunity to scaffold the learning process so that the student is given the amount of support necessary to be an effective conversation partner. This technique can easily be accomplished through individual and small group story reading (McNeil & Fowler, 1996).

It is also extremely important to encourage students to acknowledge that they don't understand and teach them appropriate ways of letting speakers know they don't comprehend. Remember that these students may have processing problems, and they may have difficulty with listening and short-term memory. Some students may learn a skill one day and not remember how to do it the next day. So, as teachers, what can we do to aid comprehension in the classroom? Some suggestions include:

1. Always review.
2. Provide frequent comprehension checks.
3. Devise systems that allow students to clarify through the teacher or a buddy.
4. Create an environment that allows students to feel comfortable in letting you know they don't understand. (Keep in mind that students with disabilities may take this to the limit if they discover they can get a lot of attention just by saying they don't understand. The teacher must impose some boundaries and encourage self-management techniques to prevent misunderstandings. However, the students must know that it's all right to ask questions and say they don't understand.)

As speakers, students with disabilities need to be taught to recognize confusion and to use effective repair strategies. They need to know how to repeat the same message with different emphasis or to revise the message in terms of form and vocabulary selection. They also need to be able to analyze the message in terms of specificity of information and cohesion.

Nonverbal Skills

Many nonverbal behaviors need to be addressed as well in intervention. Eye contact and physical proximity can have a great impact on communication. The student who does not provide eye contact or is inclined to touch the listener will distract the listener from the message. Appropriate pausing and interruptions may need to be taught and practiced, as well as how to give feedback to speakers (e.g., good listeners nod their heads and intermittently say "uh huh," "okay," and "yea").

Pragmatics and Social Skills

The separation of pragmatic skills from social skills or social competence may be nebulous (Prutting, 1982; Windsor, 1995). Social interactions are verbal and nonverbal participatory behaviors are dependent on cognitive, emotional, and adaptive development. What this implies is that pragmatic skills may not only be interwoven across language domains but across developmental domains as well (Gerber, 1991).

This, of course, has implications for intervention with children with language deficits. An understanding of the whole child (i.e., across developmental areas) is needed for a better understanding of relevant factors affecting language performance. There may be difficulties in the cognitive and social domains that are influencing language performance, and not the reverse. Or it may be the scaffolding or spiraling of these domains that ultimately affect one another. In other words, a deficit in any one area will have a rippling effect across domains. Assessment and intervention must be responsive to these effects.

However, our goal of positive social interactions is an important one. So, as teachers, we must employ whatever means are necessary to accomplish this objective. It is successful social interactions that will determine satisfying interpersonal relationships, successful employment, and community acceptance.

✓ SUMMARY CHECKLIST

☐ **Analysis**

Communicative Intentions

Presupposition

Organization of Discourse

Topic Related Problems

Topic Initiation

Learned Helplessness

Topic Maintenance and Topic Change

Local Cohesion

Global Cohesion

Repetition Strategy

Enhancement Strategy

Other Conversational Skills

Topic Closure Difficulties

Off-Target Responding

Tangentiality

Topic Identification Problems

Turn Taking

Repair and Revisions

Nonverbal Aspects

☐ **Intervention**

There is an overwhelming call for all language intervention to target real language in natural contexts.

General Strategies

Environmental Arrangement

Observation

Specific Strategies

Social Skills Curricula

Direct Instruction

Role-Taking

Topic Management

Nonverbal Skills

Pragmatics and Social Skills

CHAPTER

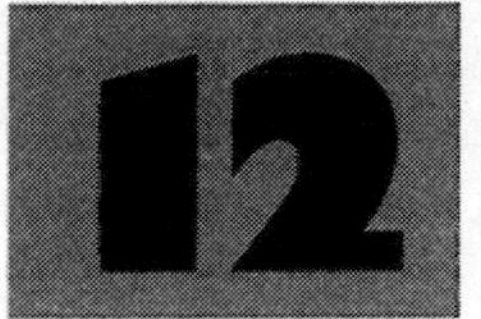

DIALECT DIFFERENCES

All languages have dialects that are rule-governed variations of the language. Everyone speaks in a dialect, not just those people down the road or across the country. A rule of thumb often used for defining a dialect is that, although dialects differ systematically from each other, speakers of different dialects of a language are mutually intelligible, that is, they can understand each other (e.g, Akmajian, et al., 1990; Fromkin & Rodman, 1988; Wardhaugh, 1977). Speakers of different languages are generally mutually unintelligible. A Texan and a New Yorker can understand each other, but a monolingual speaker of English and a monolingual speaker of French will have much difficulty communicating with each other.

Differences may arise from the influences of many factors other than region. Vocabulary differences may be noted among speakers in particular occupations. For example, the weather forecaster may be more likely to use the words *forecast*, *prognosis*, and *prediction*. The researcher using quantitative methods or the student studying research methodology may find the terms *significant*, *variables*, *correlation*, and *as a function of*, entering his or her everyday conversation. The special educator can be spotted in the grocery store telling her acting out child that his "behavior is inappropriate." In fact, the special educator may be picked out from the general educator as the one who speaks in so many letters (e.g., EH, LD, MR, IEP, ITP, IDEA) and numbers (e.g., 94–142, 99–457). Age may also influence one's language as in the use of *ice box* for a refrigerator or *spider* for frying pan or skillet.

The most significant differences in a language, however, are due to two factors, **regional** and **social** (see Figure 12–1). Dialectical diversity develops among people who are separated from each other geographically and socially. When enough differences give the language

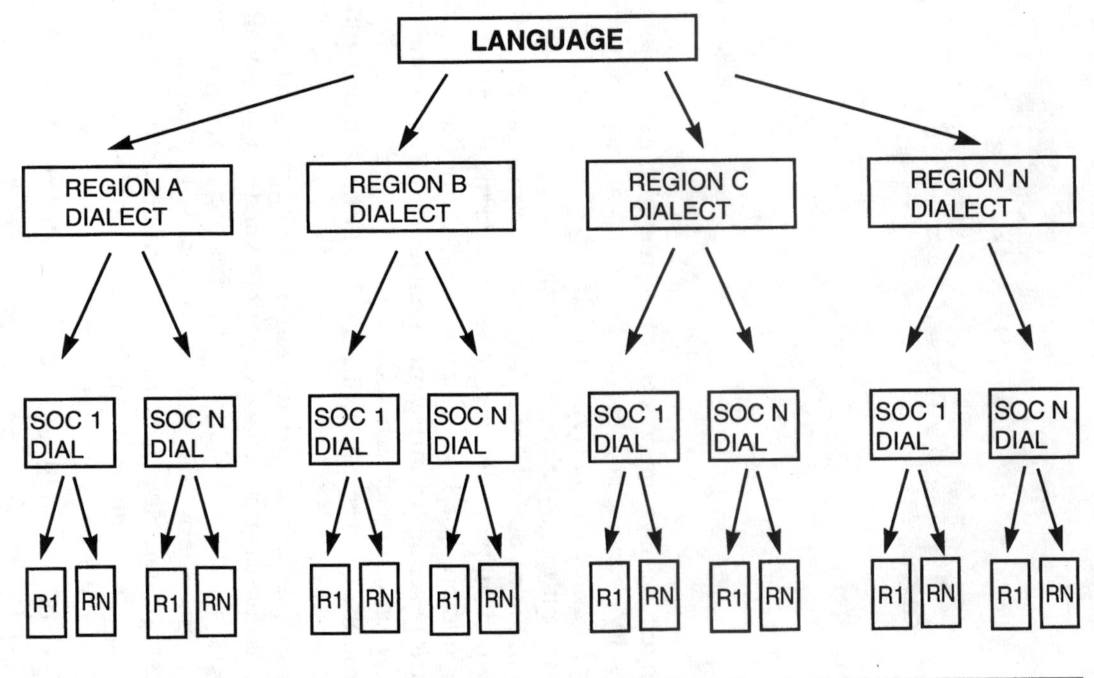

Figure 12–1. Factors influencing language variations.

spoken in a particular region its own "flavor," that version of the language is referred to as a regional dialect (Fromkin & Rodman, 1988). The region could be the city of Boston or the southern part of the United States (U.S.).

Historically, the origin of regional differences in the U.S. can be traced to settlement patterns and physical geography in North America during the 17th and 18th centuries. The east coast of the continent was colonized by settlers from different parts of England with great differences in dialect. The U.S. has traditionally been thought of as having three major dialect areas running horizontally from the East Coast to the Mississippi River: Northern, Midland, and Southern (Parker & Riley, 1994) as seen in Figure 12–2. The development of regional dialects was illustrated by Fromkin and Rodman (1988) by changes in pronunciation of words with /r/. As early as the 18th century, the British in southern England were already dropping their /r/s before consonants (lengthening the preceding vowel) and at the end of words, for example, /fa:m/ for *farm* and /fa:ðə/ for *father* and *farther*. By the end of the 18th century, this practice was a general rule among early settlers in New England and the southern Atlantic seaboard. This r-deletion rule was reinforced by close commercial ties maintained between New England and London, and Southerners' sending their children to England to be educated. The "r-less" dialects still spoken in Boston, New York, and Savannah maintain this characteristic.

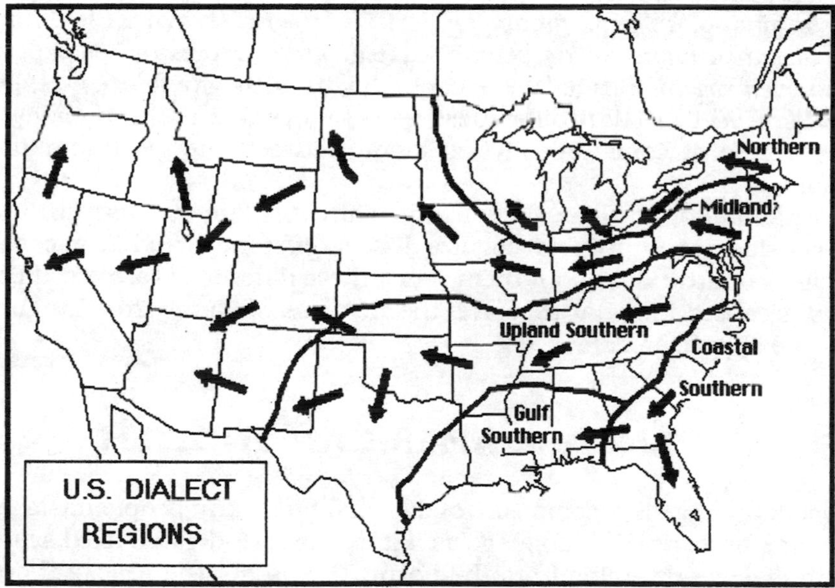

Figure 12–2. Map of United States dialect regions.

Later settlers came from northern England where the /r/ had been retained; as the frontier moved westward, so did the /r/.

As migration to the West took place, dialect patterns moved horizontally. For example, people from western New York who moved to Michigan, Wisconsin, northern Illinois, and northern Ohio took their western New York dialect with them (Shuy, 1967). As pioneers from all three dialect areas spread westward, the intermingling of their dialects "leveled" many of the differences (Fromkin & Rodman, 1988). Of course, other, later immigration patterns also enriched American English. The influence of German settlers on the vocabulary and syntax of certain parts of Pennsylvania has long been recognized; likewise, Polish terms can easily be found in Detroit, Hungarian in Cleveland, and Spanish in Los Angeles (Shuy, 1967). Still today, however, the most clearly defined differences in regional dialects are found on the East Coast.

Within a geographical region there will be similarities, but there will also be differences mostly related to socioeconomic status and ethnicity. In other words, there will be similarities in all speakers from Boston, but not all speakers will sound like the Kennedy family. Social dialects are subcategories of regional dialects, as indicated in Figure 12–1. Certain characteristics of English within a region have been found to be correlated with specific social variables. For example, working-class New Yorkers use postvocalic r-deletions more often than middle-class New Yorkers do (Parker & Riley, 1994). Within each social dialect, there also exist different styles, or **registers**, which are influenced by the situation in which the speaker finds him- or herself.

Regional and social dialects, as well as stylistic changes, may differ in phonology (e.g., *greasy* as /grizi/ or /grisi/), syntax (e.g., *may be able to* or *might could*), semantics (e.g., *green pepper* or *bell pepper*), and even pragmatics (e.g., eye contact with authority figure = respect or disrespect). Dialect differences tend to increase proportionately to the degree of communicative isolation between groups (Fromkin & Rodman, 1988).

In addition to these facts about dialects, there are also attitudes to consider. Most people recognize dialect differences and have certain feelings or attitudes about them. Once these differences are recognized and accepted for what they are, the richness of variety in a language can be appreciated.

STANDARD AMERICAN ENGLISH

Every language is a composite of dialects, but many people mistakenly think and speak of language as if it were a well-defined fixed system with dialects diverging from the norm. This is not the case, although a particular dialect may enjoy such prestige that it becomes equated with the language. This is the dialect taught in school, generally used by mass media newscasters, often used by political leaders, taught to non-native speakers, and used in most printed documents. It is viewed as more important and more used; therefore it is used more, and becomes more important, and so the cycle continues. This particular dialect becomes the dominant or prestige dialect and is thus the **standard dialect**. In other words, Standard American English (SAE) is the dialect that most Americans *almost* speak. Though standard dialects share some features from region to region, they also include regional differences (Lindfors, 1987).

SAE is not defined precisely, and it is constantly changing. Although throughout history language purists (prescriptivists) have attempted to keep language the same, it continues to change; however, this change does not mean corruption as the purists would have us believe and as many of us were taught. One need only survey speakers of English in the 1990s to realize that the subjective use of the pronoun for the noun complement in *It is I*, dominant in the 1950s, has been replaced by the objective case of the pronoun, as in *It is me*, for the majority of speakers. Lederer (1991) pointed out in his popular book, *Crazy English*, that ultimately language is a set of laws made by lawbreakers, and although using double negatives is frowned on by purists today, it wasn't in Chaucer's time, and may be accepted again in the future. Considering that *wide-width*, *broad-breadth*, and *long-length* are accepted today, *heighth* may one day make it as well.

Another difficulty faced by purists wishing to dictate the correct forms of words and syntax is that it is not always clear which is correct. A debate today has arisen over the plural of the *mouse* used with the computer. Are two of them *mice* or *mouses*? Or are we stuck with one *mouse*, two *pointing devices*?

Although SAE may have social functions or provide a common written form, it is in no linguistic way superior to other dialects, nor is

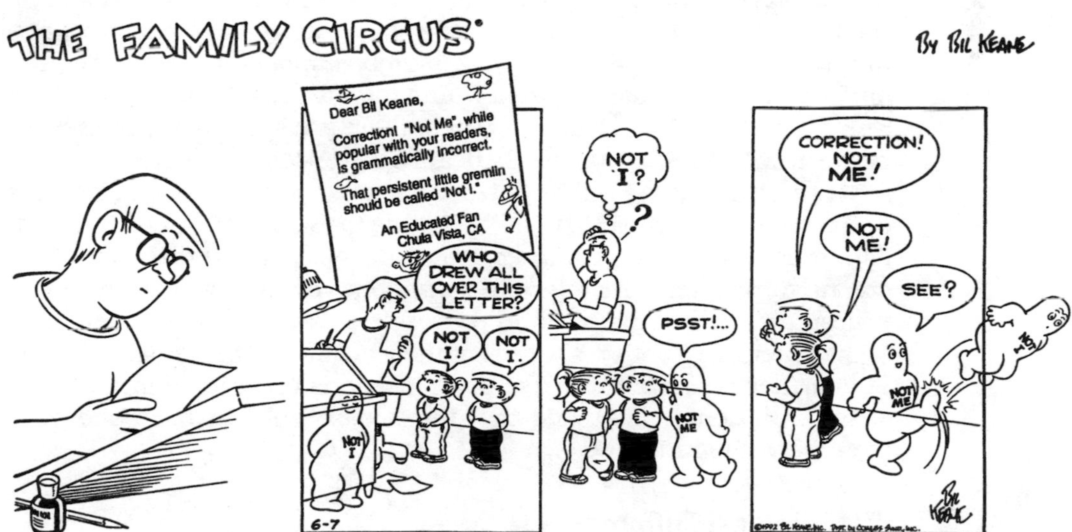

it more expressive, more complex, nor more regular than other dialects (Fromkin & Rodman, 1988). One dialect is not better than another; it is simply different. Any judgments of superiority are social judgments, not linguistic or scientific ones.

BLACK ENGLISH

Whereas most U.S. dialects are free from stigma, especially the many regional dialects, one dialect has been a victim of prejudicial ignorance. This dialect, or actually a collection of closely related dialects, has been variously referred to as *Black English, Black Vernacular, African American English,* and more recently, the much publicized and highly controversial *Ebonics,* from *ebony* and *phonics.* Not only is this the most publicized and stigmatizing dialect in schools today, it is also the dialect that has been most studied. For these reasons, this chapter focuses on it and uses the more traditional term Black English (BE). All of these terms have an easily misinterpreted or misleading component, that is, Black or African American. Although the dialect is spoken by a large section of non-middle-class blacks, it is not spoken by all blacks, or African Americans, nor is it spoken only by blacks. The distinguishing features of this dialect have persisted for social, educational, and economic reasons. Where social isolation exists, dialect differences have intensified; and, more recently, it has become a means of positive black identification (Fromkin & Rodman, 1988).

The characteristics and origins of BE have been studied and debated since the mid-1930s when anthropologist Melville Hereskovits traced black cultural traits, including some language elements, to West African origins (Wilson & Ferriss, 1989). In the 1960s, BE became the focus of national attention with the onset of the civil rights movement. Increasingly, evidence supports the influence of African languages on the early development of what is today's BE dialect. For example, certain words (*gumbo, tote, okra, jazz, mumbo-jumbo*) and the affirmative and negative expressions *uh-huh* and *unh-uh* reached BE and later SAE from Africa. Whatever its origins, there are systematic differences between BE and SAE, just as there are differences between British and American English. As will be noted, none of the distinguishing features of BE are unique to BE. Battle (1996) defined African American English, or BE, as "a rule-governed linguistic system and discourse variety used primarily in informal situations by many working class African Americans and by lower or working class people in many parts of the American South regardless of their racial or ethnic origin" (p. 22). She further noted that the use of BE depends on the age and context of the situation or task, and that the use of SAE has been shown to increase with grade level.

Phonological Differences

Battle (1996) pointed out that the pioneer sociolinguists Dillard (1972) and Fasold and Wolfram (1978), who identified the features that contrast BE and SAE, found that they occur primarily in the medial and final positions of words rather than in the initial position. Furthermore, most contrasts involve consonants.

R-Deletion

Just as British English and many other dialects of American English delete the /r/ after a vowel, BE is also characterized by an r-deletion rule. Thus, *guard* would be a homonym for *god, sore* for *saw*, and *fort* for *fought*. This r-deletion rule may be extended in some instances to the middle of words between vowels so that *Paris* becomes *Pass*.

L-Deletion

Some speakers may also have a deletion rule for the /l/ in similar instances. Thus, *school* is *schoo* and *help* is *hep*. The l-deletion rule exists in other dialects in consonant clusters such as *talk* (/tak/), *calm* (/kam/), and *palm* (/pam/). With both BE l- and r-deletion rules in operation, the speaker of BE may indicate, "I get hep from my teachə at schoo."

Consonant Cluster Simplification

This regular phonological rule in BE simplifies consonant clusters at the end of words, especially when one of the two consonants is alveolar (/t/, /d/, /s/, and /z/). For some speakers of BE, this means that *sand* rhymes with *man* and *bend* rhymes with *men*. A combination of the consonant cluster simplification rule and the l-deletion rule results in the statement, "I toe you so" for "I told you so."

It's important to remember that this refers to pronunciation and not spelling; *ball* and *bald* may be homonyms in BE, just as *know* and *no* are in SAE. One local teacher related the story of his high school student with mild mental retardation writing, "Mr. McGrath has a ball head." Realizing that the application of consonant cluster reduction and l-deletion rules result in *ball* and *bald* being pronounced the same, he explained that b-a-l-l was the spelling for the round object called a ball and that b-a-l-d was the spelling for the word meaning no hair on the head. The student returned to her writing and composed the following sentence, "Mr. McGrath has a ball head and a bald head." In reality, this was a very apt description of Mr. McGrath, who indeed has a rather round head. Mr. McGrath accepted this sentence as a very creative, correctly spelled construction.

The consonant cluster simplification rule may also result in the same pronunciation for past tense and present tense forms of some verbs; for example, *pass* and *passed* (/st/) would both be pronounced as *pass*. This should not be interpreted as the lack of a past tense marker. This rule may also affect the pronunciation of some plurals, so that *two fans* becomes *two fan*. Again, this is not the omission of a plural marker, but rather a difference in pronunciation. Also, consider what the plural of *test*, pronounced *tess* in BE, would be with the correct assumption that the morphophonemic rule for the plural marker is the same in BE and SAE.

/ɛ/ Before a Nasal

As in other dialects of American English, the /ɛ/, or "short e" sound, before a nasal consonant is not distinguished from the /ɪ/, or "short i" sound. Thus *pin* and *pen*, and *since*, *sense*, and *cents* are pronounced the same.

"TH" Sounds /θ/ and /ð/

Some interesting variations occur with these two sounds. The voiceless "th" /θ/ sound in the final position of a word or syllable may be pronounced as /f/, as in *Ruf* for *Ruth* and *birfday* for *birthday*. Seymour and Ralabate (1985) reported that while first- and second-grade students who speak BE use the final /θ/–/f/ contrast in both spontaneous conversations and structured picture labeling tasks, third and fourth graders use /f/ in spontaneous conversation, but use the final /θ/ in the structured task.

This /θ/–/f/ correspondence also exists in some British English dialects, where even *think* is regularly pronounced as *fink* in Cockney English (Fromkin & Rodman, 1988). At the beginning of words, /θ/ may be pronounced by some BE speakers as /t/, as in *tink* for *think*. This also exists in some Northern American dialects, as in "What dya tink you're doing?"

The voiced "th" sound /ð/ at the beginning of words may be pronounced as /d/ by some speakers of BE (and other dialects of American English), so that *this* is *dis*, *them* is *dem*, and *those* is *dose*. In the middle of a word, the voiced "th," /ð/, may be pronounced as /v/ as in *brovah* for *brother*.

Suprasegmentals

Some different stress patterns which are common to many Southern dialects may also be noted in BE. These include stress on the first syllable of *po-lice* and *ho-tel*, and stress on the last syllable of *ambu-lance*. Deletion of unstressed syllables at the beginning of words may also result in *'potent* for *important* and *'pose* for *suppose*.

These are only some of the phonological variations that may occur in the speech of the BE speaker. Not all of these will occur for all speakers of BE, and those that do occur may not occur in all situations. However, from the variations presented here, it is evident that it is quite possible, even probable, that the unaware teacher's accepted responses to questions on such forms as homonyms and rhyming words will not match those that the speaker of BE may give. It is very important for teachers to consider the student's pronunciation in judging correctness of responses, just as the pronunciation of *vase* should be considered for speakers of SAE in a phonics lesson on the "long a" sound.

It is also imperative that a phonological assessment of the speaker of BE take into account the contrasts between SAE and BE. Phoneme inventory differences between BE and SAE are not evident until after 5 years of age (Seymour & Seymour, 1981), because the features that contrast in the two dialects do not develop until after age 5. At that point, awareness of features where there is no contrast is necessary to correctly distinguish normal from disordered speech among children who speak BE (Battle, 1996). Results of a study by Cole and Taylor (1990) clearly indicated that a failure to take dialect differences into account substantially increases the likelihood of misdiagnosing normally speaking African-American children as having articulation disorders. If standardized tests are used, they recommended that scoring criteria modifications be made based on knowledge of items that may elicit the use of BE rules. This requires determination of the number of potentially biased items included on the instrument, considering both the frequency of biased items and the linguistic environment, or word position, in which the phoneme is presented. The data generated by their study suggest a higher error rate in the word-final position than in other positions. Cole and Taylor further suggested that articulation tests should not be used as the sole basis for judging a speech problem; many sources of assessment should be used, including naturalistic observations in keeping with the child's linguistic and cultural community.

Morphological and Syntactic Differences

Just as with phonological differences, differences in morphology and syntax are systematic and rule-governed. Although syntactic differences have been used to illustrate the "illogic" of BE, it is just these differences that point out the fact that BE is as complex and "logical" as SAE. In fact, Craig and Washington (1994, 1995) have demonstrated a positive relationship between low-income preschoolers' use of BE forms and linguistic complexity; that is, they found that the higher the percentage frequencies of BE use, the higher the percentage use of complex sentences. This was true for the variety of types of complex sentences, as well as frequency of use. Craig and Washington pointed out that these findings underscore the inappropriateness of viewing BE as a deficient form of SAE.

A familiarity with some of the major features of BE is necessary for a true assessment of a BE student's performance in morphology and syntax. The literature on children who speak BE suggests that the use of morphosyntactic features among school-age children is a function of the social situation and communicative intent (Battle, 1996). An assessment of morphology and syntax must also take this into consideration.

In examining the features of BE, it should be noted that in some cases of morphological and syntactic differences, the BE rules eliminate redundancy in SAE by marking once what SAE marks twice. In other cases, BE marks more than once what SAE marks only once. Other BE rules may not exist at all in SAE.

Present Progressive

Whereas SAE marks the present progressive twice, once with an auxiliary and once with the {ing} morpheme, BE marks it only once, with the use of the {ing} morpheme.

SAE: He *is* go*ing* home. BE: He go*ing* home.

The {ing} morpheme alone in BE indicates that the action is ongoing.

Present Perfect

In SAE, the perfective tense is marked with an auxiliary and with a past tense marker; BE requires only one of these markers.

SAE: I *have* liv*ed* here two years.

BE: I *have* live here two years. OR: I lived here two years.

An interesting variation of the present perfect tense formation can be noted in some speakers from New York who state, "I'*m living* here two years now." A driver in West Palm Beach was quoted in the *Palm Beach Post* in May, 1993, as saying, "I'*m driving* a car for about 70 years and I never had an accident." Then with a nudge from his wife: "Well, I had about four recently." Driving record aside, note the use of the present perfect tense.

Deletion of "to be"

Wherever SAE can use a contraction, BE can use deletion of the copula or auxiliary *to be*. Standard Russian also omits the copula in sentences of this type.

SAE: He is a friend/He's a friend. BE: He a friend.

SAE: He is tired/He's tired. BE: He tired.

SAE: He is going/He's going. BE: He going.

SAE: There he is. BE: There he is.

SAE: How nice you are. BE: How nice you are.

It should be noted that in instances where SAE does not allow a contraction, BE does not allow a deletion. Furthermore, an utterance with a pronominal phrase (*He* a boy) has a higher probability of deleting the copula than an utterance with a noun phrase (*John* is a boy) (Battle 1996).

Uninflected Form of "to be"

In BE, an uninflected form of *to be* is used to indicate habitual action. Whereas this distinction can be made syntactically in BE and in some other languages, such as Russian, it can be made in SAE only with the addition of more words.

BE: John be happy.	SAE: John is always happy.
BE: John happy.	SAE: John is happy now.
BE: Dr. Smiley be late.	SAE: Dr. Smiley is habitually late.
BE: Dr. Smiley late.	SAE: Dr. Smiley is late this time.
BE: Do you be joking?	SAE: Are you generally joking?
BE: You joking?	SAE: Are you joking now?

With this in mind, it would certainly seem preferable to be told, "You ugly" as opposed to "You be ugly."

Possessive

Another regular rule in BE deletes the possessive morpheme whenever possession is redundantly specified by word order.

SAE: That is John's hat.	BE: That John hat.
SAE: That is your hat.	BE: That you hat.
SAE: That hat is John's.	BE: That hat John's.
SAE: That hat is yours	BE: That hat yours.

It should be noted that when word order is eliminated as an indicator of possession, the relationship is marked the same in BE as it is in SAE.

Plural

When a quantifier is used with a noun, SAE also requires a plural marker. BE does not require that a plural morpheme be used if a quantifier precedes the noun.

SAE: He's got five dollars.	BE: He got five dollar.
SAE: Look at the hats.	BE: Look at the hats.

A systematic rule is applied to differing cases in BE.

Indefinite Article

Although the rules for the uses of the definite and the indefinite articles are the same in BE and SAE, some speakers of BE do not use *an* to precede words beginning with a vowel as required by SAE.

SAE: a ball, an elephant, an alarm

BE: a ball, a elephant, a alarm

Actually, as this rule is a morphophonemic requirement in SAE, this may be considered a phonological difference. The deletion of the article is not optional in BE or SAE and an utterance such as *Mary is girl* would indicate a disorder in speakers of both BE and SAE (Battle, 1996).

Subject-Verb Agreement

Whereas SAE adds a morpheme to the third person singular verb form in the present tense, BE regularizes the verb forms. Again, redundancy is marked in SAE as the subject already indicates the person and number. The need to mark person and number in only one place may show up in other constructions in BE as well.

SAE: She has a bike.	BE: She have a bike.
SAE: They were going.	BE: They was going.

As the BE speaker learns SAE, an overgeneralization may sometimes occur on the irregular SAE third person singular form of *says*, resulting in say + /z/ (/sez/) instead of the irregular form /sɛz/.

Double Negative

In BE, when the verb is negated, the indefinite pronouns *something*, *somebody*, and *some* become the negative indefinite pronouns *nothing*, *nobody*, and *none*. This rule is common in other languages (e.g., French and Spanish) and once existed for all dialects of English (Fromkin & Rodman, 1988). In SAE, if the forms *nothing*, *nobody*, and *none* are used, the verb is not negated.

SAE: He says something.	BE: He say something.
SAE: He doesn't say anything.	BE: He don't say nothing.
SAE: He says nothing.	BE: He say nothing.

The rules are essentially the same but differ in detail. BE also allows more than one negative marker in a sentence as in *I ain't got no pencil.* Russian, Spanish, French, and Hungarian do so also (Labov, 1969). For example, French marks the negative with *ne* before the verb and *pas* after the verb. Actually, SAE also uses a double negative form to indicate subtle differences in meaning. For example, compare *It's impossible that they will still make it* and *It's not impossible that they will still make it.* The second statement is not the same as *It's possible that they will still make it.* The betting woman would do well to place her money on the last guys.

Irregular Past

Some irregular verbs in SAE are marked by the null form (ø), resulting in no change in form. BE uses this rule also but extends it to other verbs as well, such as *come*, *see*, and *say*.

SAE: I put it there today and I put it there yesterday.

BE: I put it there today and I put it there yesterday.

SAE: I see it there now and I saw it there yesterday.

BE: I see it there now and I see it there yesterday.

This is the same rule in SAE and BE, but a larger class of words is affected in BE.

Pronoun Apposition

The use of the pronoun following the subject noun is common in BE as well as in many other languages, for example, French (*Jean il est* for *Jean is*).

SAE: David says, "Here I come."

BE: David, he say, "Here I come."

SAE also uses pronoun apposition but less frequently and in cases where the speaker wants to be sure to focus the attention of the listener on the topic or subject. *David said he's not coming, Sue said she couldn't be there, John said he has another appointment, but now* ***Mary, she*** *said she'd be glad to be there.*

Question Formation

SAE requires that an emphatic-*do* be present in a direct question, but not in the indirect question. BE does not require the emphatic-*do* in the direct question, but does use it in the indirect question.

Direct Questions	SAE:	What do you want?
	BE:	What you want?
	SAE:	Do you know what I'm saying?
	BE:	You know what I'm saying?
Indirect Questions	SAE:	Ask Albert if he knows how to play.
	BE:	Ask Albert do he know how to play.

Imperative

The direct imperative is formed the same in both SAE and BE, but the indirect is not. BE retains the form of the direct imperative in the indirect, whereas SAE requires a change in format.

Direct Imperative	SAE:	Don't do that!
	BE:	Don't do that!

Indirect Imperative SAE: I told you not to do that!

BE: I told you don't do that!

Relative Pronouns

SAE allows the relative conjunction to be deleted in the relative clause but requires that a relative pronoun be included. BE also allows the relative pronoun to be deleted.

SAE: That's the book (that) I like best.

BE: That the book I like best.

SAE: I went with my sister who lives down the street.

BE: I went with my sister live down the street.

Existential It

SAE makes use of what is termed an existential form of *there*; in the same instances that SAE uses the expletive *there*, BE uses *it*.

SAE: There's a party down the street.

BE: It's a party down the street.

The use of one is no less arbitrary than the use of the other.

There are other differences between the syntactic rules of SAE and BE, but the ones presented here should illustrate the fact that BE is a logical, rule-governed system of language. Labov (1969) stated that there is no reason to believe that any nonstandard dialect is in itself an obstacle to learning, but rather that the chief problem is ignorance on the part of all concerned. Through the abolition of this ignorance, an acceptance and respect for other dialects and the speakers of those dialects should evolve. No teacher wants his or her students to feel the way that Darlene unintentionally makes Celie feel in the excerpt from *The Color Purple* (Walker, 1982) found in the letter on the next page.

Semantic Differences

BE relies on and derives much of its semantic character from the use of nonliteral figurative devices such as metaphor, proverbs, sayings, folktales, signifying, marking, and sounding (Battle, 1996). BE-speaking children as young as 8–9 years display comprehension and usage of figurative language and metaphorical devices. This leads to a very rich language system that uses a great deal of narrative expression.

Vocabulary differences exist also. In fact, SAE has picked up many expressions from BE. In the 1940s, *cool* and *dig* originated as BE expressions; in the 1950s, *rap* and *right on* were adopted by SAE from BE. The number of terms adopted by SAE from BE has increased in the

Dear Nettie,

I am so happy. I got love, I got work, I got money, friends and time. And you alive and be home soon. With our children.

Jerene and Darlene come help me with the business. They twins. Never married. Love to sew. Plus, Darlene trying to teach me how to talk. She say *us* not so hot. A dead country giveaway. You say *us* where most folks say *we*, she say, and peoples think you dumb. Colored peoples think you a hick and white folks be amuse.

What I care? I ast. I'm happy.

But she say I feel more happier talking like she talk. Can't nothing make me happier than seeing you again, I think, but I don't say nothing. Every time I say something the way I say it, she correct me until I say it some other way. Pretty soon it feel like I can't think. My mind run up on a thought, git confuse, run back and sort of lay down.

You sure this worth it? I ast.

She say Yeah. Bring me a bunch of books. Whitefolks all over them, talking bout apples and dogs.

What I care bout dogs? I think.

Darlene keep trying. Think how much better Shug feel with you educated, she say. She won't be shame to take you anywhere.

Shug not shame no how, I say. But she don't believe this the truth. Sugar, she say one day when Shug home, don't you think it be nice if Celie could talk proper?

Shug say, She can talk in sign language for all I care. She make herself a nice cup of herb tea and start talking bout hot oiling her hair.

But I let Darlene worry on. Sometimes I think bout the apples and the dogs, sometimes I don't. Look like to me only a fool would want you to talk in a way that feel peculiar to your mind. But she sweet and she sew good and us need something to haggle over while us work.

I'm busy making pants for Sofia now. One leg be purple, one leg be red. I dream Sofia wearing these pants, one day she was jumping over the moon.

Amen,
Your sister, Celie

Source: From *The Color Purple* (pp. 190–191), by A. Walker, 1982, Boston: G. K. Hall.

last few decades. Of course, some terms remain unique to BE. In 1972, Robert Williams at Washington University in St. Louis developed a dialect- and culture-specific test, primarily for adolescents and adults, which contained many vocabulary items and informational facts taken from the "Black experience." The purpose was to provide an evaluation of BE speakers, as well as measure awareness and familiarity of "whites" to determine how much information they have about the Black experience and to examine changes in the extent "whites" are willing to engage themselves in the Black experience. Some of the vocabulary may now be outdated as language changes over time, for example, *process*, correct response *conk*, a hair-straightening process; other items remain and have even been incorporated into the mainstream vocabulary, for example, *shades* for sunglasses. Most important, the concept of increasing awareness and change is one that should always be considered for teachers, clinicians, and counselors who are working with students from diverse populations.

Pragmatic Differences

Table 12–1 includes some possible sources of miscommunication that Orlando Taylor suggests may exist between a Black English speaking group and members of other cultural groups (Cole, 1989). This is not meant to be an exhaustive list nor should it be assumed that all speakers of BE will demonstrate them all, but it contains many examples of potential differences of which teachers and SLPs should be aware.

A preference for narrative style is found in the speech of BE speakers. The stories of working-class African American children are usually personal, with less chronicity and few formulaic openings or closings (Battle, 1996). They include many judgment statements about the characters and their behaviors. The stories of African Americans are very expressive, with the inclusion of a variety of paralinguistic cues such as loudness, stress, intonation, exclamations, and repetitions to enhance the story or the characters. For example, Battle reported that **marking** is used in telling folktales or describing a scene. Narrators provide prosodic cues through the use of variation in rate, intonation, duration, pause, and kinesthetic cues through gestures and movements. The narrative includes a lot of imitation and quotes, and repetition of short segments leading to a succession of mini-climaxes and an ongoing, open-ended line. Listeners not accustomed to African American style may have difficulty identifying the topic and may ask poorly timed questions that interrupt the flow of the narrative and throw the speaker off balance. The result may be perceived as an expressive language disorder, when actually it is the child trying to deal with interruptions in narrative style.

A match between school-language discourse plays a role in ensuring success of both language acquisition and school performance (Langdon, 1996). Lindfors (1987) pointed out that there are some specific **home-school mismatches** that may affect the student who comes from a BE speaking family. Mainstream children are more often from backgrounds that prepare and prime them for reading and writing. On the other hand, most BE speaking cultures emphasize skillful verbal performance. A variety of verbal communication techniques exist, including rapping, signifying, and playing the dozens. The better one

TABLE 12-1. Some possible verbal and nonverbal sources of miscommunication between cultural groups.

Black Culture	***Mainstream Culture***
Preference for indirect eye contact during listening, direct eye contact during speaking as signs of attentiveness and respect.	Preference for direct eye contact during listening and indirect eye contact during speaking as signs of attention and respect.
Public behavior may be emotionally intense, dynamic, and demonstrative.	Public behavior is expected to be modest and emotionally restrained. Emotional displays are seen as irresponsible or in bad taste.
Clear distinction between "argument" and "fight." Verbal abuse is not necessarily a precursor to violence.	Heated arguments are viewed as suggesting that violence is imminent.
Use of direct question is sometimes seen as harassment (e.g., asking when something will be finished is seen as rushing that person to finish).	Use of direct questions for personal information is permissible.
Asking personal questions of someone one has met for the first time is seen as improper and intrusive.	Inquiring about jobs, family, and so forth of someone one has met for the first time is seen as friendly.
Interruption during conversation is usually tolerated. Access to the floor is granted to the person who is most assertive.	Rules of turn-taking in conversation dictate that one person has the floor at a time until all his points are made.
Silence denotes refutation of accusation. To state that you feel accused is regarded as an admission of guilt.	Silence denotes acceptance of an accusation. Guilt is verbally denied.

Source: From "E Pluribus Pluribus: Multicultural Imperatives for the 1990s and Beyond," by L. Cole, 1989, *Asha, 31*, p. 69. Copyright 1989 by ASHA. Adapted by permission of the American Speech-Language-Hearing Association.

is at mastering and using these skills in street interactions, the more respect one commands. When these verbally skilled children enter school, the mainstream emphasis on written language places them at a disadvantage. Typically, verbal skills are slighted rather than encouraged, respected, and developed in all children. For example, a language experience approach to reading where a child's oral language is written down and used as the basis for teaching reading skills could be an ideal approach for the child who has learned to greatly respect oral language.

Taylor (in Cole, 1989) described a difference in the use of **eye contact** in conversation. Lindfors (1987) pointed out another difference in the rules of eye contact. Many readers can remember, as these authors do, being firmly told by their fathers, "Look at me when I speak to you." In the mainstream, direct eye contact was considered respect for authority. Members of most BE speaking cultures, as well as other cultures and subcultures of the U.S., are taught just the opposite, that is, to make direct eye contact is to defy authority and show disrespect. In an ideal world, teachers and other adults from the mainstream would be aware of, accept, and respect different sets of rules for familiar devices of communication. However, as most settings are not ideal, it may benefit students to be taught to code-switch in nonverbal skills as well as verbal. A strategy for the use of a different set of rules for eye contact in particular settings, such as Ms. White's room down the hall or in a job interview, may be developed, taught, and practiced in the informed teacher's classroom. Figure 12–3 illustrates such a strategy devised by a South Florida teacher. Practice may need to begin with role-playing and result in prompts to remind the student to use the skill once it is mastered. Without such survival skills, students' appropriate use of a different set of rules may result in the misinterpretation of respectful as disrespectful, sneaky, deceitful, or "so guilty that he can't even look me in the eye."

Another difference in rules exists in the role of the member of an audience, that is, **passive versus participative** (Lindfors, 1980). Consider the mainstream classroom where the child is expected to sit quietly while listening and speak only when called on. Now compare this to the traditional Black church service where appreciation and understanding are shown through participation, as with responses of *oh yes*, *uh huh*, and *Amen* (which, of course, means *so be it!*). The students who choose to show appreciation to the uninformed mainstream teacher in the same way may find themselves labeled hyperactive, noisy, unruly, or undisciplined due to misinterpretation of their behavior, possibly leading to total cessation of participation. The ideal solution to this problem is to be sure all teachers are knowledgeable and respectful of the existence of other rules. What may be needed is to teach another set of rules to use in settings where misinterpretation may occur. The informed teacher will provide practice by structuring some lessons in which the rules of passive responses are used and others in which the participative rules are used and encouraged.

Two other characteristics of the BE speaker's background and behavior may lead to misinterpretation on the part of an uninformed mainstream teacher. Although the mainstream child has learned to consider adults as the main sources of information, BE speakers have often learned to rely on other children, particularly older siblings, as their source of information. Related to this are differences in the view of competition and cooperation. Mainstream schools typically emphasize doing your own work and being the best in the class, while most

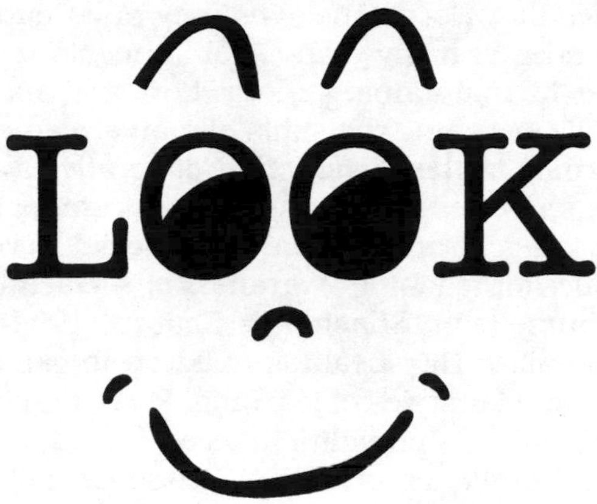

Lift my face toward
person talking

Open my eyes and look
at person's eyes

Open my ears and listen

Keep on looking and listening
until conversation is over

Figure 12-3. Learning strategy for eye contact. (Courtesy of Michele Barbieri, 1993.)

BE speaking children have learned that work is a time for cooperation in getting the job done. Once their home responsibilities have been fulfilled, individual prowess may be demonstrated in play. Of course, at mainstream schools, children are expected to play cooperatively. The students who look to other students as sources of information and cooperative partners in work are often misunderstood and labeled as "unruly cheaters." Once again, these children may be punished for not following a set of rules that violate the ones they have learned and operated successfully under for many years. Again, the informed teacher can make a difference in maintaining motivation and participation for these children, while enriching the skills of mainstreamers, by varying the format for learning in the classroom. Cooperative learning groups in which students share responsibility for task completion have been shown to foster academic, intellectual, and social development and provide opportunities for teaching awareness of social interactions and variations in discourse (e.g., Shachar & Sharan, 1994). Group work such as this would allow BE speaking children to capitalize on their strengths and use familiar styles of learning. Peer and cross-age tutoring also lend themselves to providing successful experiences for this group. All of these techniques benefit all students, not just the nonmainstream students, and should be a part of every classroom along with lessons where students are *taught* to "do their own work."

In the cooperative learning situation, varying amounts of responsibility may be assigned to different students through differing roles (e.g., the role of facilitator and the role of recorder). This, too, is an important consideration for children who have more than likely carried out responsibilities in their families that would surprise many mainstream teachers, who consider leading a line to lunch a major responsibility for the first grader and perhaps too great a responsibility for the kindergartner. In fact, the 5-year-old from the BE home, where an extended family may require many more responsibilities at an earlier age, may have helped care for a 2-year-old in the home, may have gone to the store down the block to buy bread and return with the change, or may have regular responsibilities for helping with dinner preparation. Appreciation for these capabilities may be shown at school through the assignment of greater responsibilities in the classroom and in learning. These first graders may well be ready to run errands to the principal's office and should make very good peer or cross-age tutors or facilitators in cooperative learning groups.

WRITTEN LANGUAGE

For some time, education has failed to meet the needs of many African Americans, and assignment to special education has led to labeling and poor treatment of some students (Obiakor, 1992). Reading is an area that has been of concern since the 1960s. The thinking of that time was that perhaps the reading problems evidenced by so many African Americans who were labeled "disadvantaged" were due to another home-school mismatch, that is, a mismatch between spoken dialect and the dialect of the readers in school. At that point, teaching the child in his or her own dialect was investigated at the Center for Applied Linguistics by researchers who developed materials in the "native dialect" (Baratz & Shuy, 1969). Of course, it quickly became apparent that this was a difficult, if not impossible, task as there was not a uniform BE dialect even in the Washington, D.C., area. Stewart (1969) suggested using a three-stage language experience approach in which reading materials are first written in the child's dialect as dictated (e.g., *Charles and David they out playin'*). At the second stage, the most important syntactic features of SAE are introduced (e.g., *Charles and Michael they are outside playing*). At the third stage, sentences are brought into full conformity with the SAE form.

In the 1960s, another group of reading researchers was investigating the use of the child's own dialect for reading with the belief that it was the divergence between spoken and written language that was interfering in the success of so many BE speakers' reading. In the 1970s, however, they retracted their position and declared that the problems readers were having were related to discrimination against their dialect on the part of teachers (Goodman & Buck, 1973). What they noted was that, when readers were beginning to show some true comprehension of reading materials, they read the material in their own dialect—they translated it, indicating a strength in comprehension. The teachers, however, insisted that those were not the words on the page and asked them to go back to the level of decoding and read every word as it was printed ("the right way"). Of course, the result is obvious, a loss of interest in reading, leading to reading failure.

More recently, Lindfors (1987) noted that many educators are now sufficiently sophisticated to avoid making explicit statements about children's use of "deficient language," but still advocate using drills and worksheets clearly aimed at substituting SAE for BE. Lindfors may have been a bit optimistic about the level of sophistication. A local newspaper recently interviewed four young black boys who reported that they didn't like school because their teachers often criticize them and other blacks for the way they speak in class. "Every time I say 'I ain't done,' she say, 'That's Swahili talk.' She say, 'Chickens get done, humans get finished.'" The teacher's response to the reporter was that she believes she is sensitive to her students, whom she described as "street kids." There is evidence in the literature that the teacher's negative reactions to children's use of dialect is what appears to adversely affect their academic performance (Garcia, Pearson, & Jiminez, 1990).

Approaches such as the language experience approach to reading or a writing process approach to writing could and should be successful, for by writing in the student's own dialect or accepting writing in the student's own dialect, legitimacy is expressed. At that point, it may be more effective to indicate "here's another way of saying that," leading to code-switching abilities and judgments of appropriate situations in which to use SAE. To be successful, however, the teacher will need to have true respect for and understanding of Black English as a rule-governed system. A knowledge of cultural differences can also aid success in the classroom as evidenced by Heath (1982), who found that by changing questioning styles to match those of the families of African American students in the Carolina Piedmont, students were more willing to participate.

✓ SUMMARY CHECKLIST

- ☐ **Regional Differences**
  Social Differences
  Registers
  Standard American English
    Dominant and Constantly Changing

- ☐ **Black English**
    Phonological Differences
    Morphological and Syntactic Differences
    Semantic Differences
    Pragmatic Differences
      Nonverbal
      Narrative Marking
      Home-School Mismatches
        Verbal versus Written Emphasis
        Rules of Eye Contact
        Passive versus Participative Role Taking
        Information Sources
        Competition and Cooperation

- ☐ **Written Language**
    Language Experience Approach to Reading
    Writing Process Approach to Writing

CHAPTER

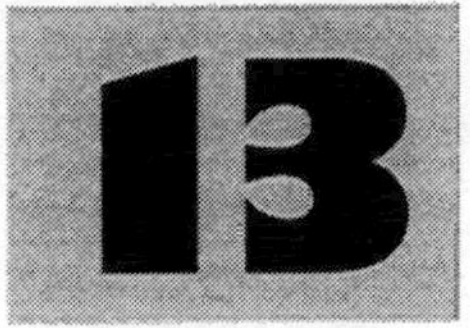

EMERGING ENGLISH LEARNERS

A bilingual person is proficient at speaking two languages and a multilingual person is proficient at speaking more than two languages. Four countries account for almost half of the world's population (China, India, the former USSR, and the USA) and extrapolating from estimates of bilingualism in these countries, Reich (1986) figured that between 45% and 50% of the world's population is bilingual. Unfortunately, his data also indicated that of the four largest countries, the USA has the lowest rate of bilingualism. Although the number of bilingual speakers in the USA is increasing, these data perhaps account for the often heard joke:

> What do you call a person who speaks two languages? . . . Bilingual.
>
> What do you call a person who speaks more than two languages? . . . Multilingual.
>
> What do you call a person who speaks only one language? . . . American.

Remaining this way, that is, monolingual, has too often appeared to be the goal of education in the U.S. as ever-increasing numbers of speakers of other languages enter our school systems. There is a subtle prejudice in the general American population against other languages and the non-English-speaking or bilingual child faces some danger in the schools, including educational placement (Owens, 1996). The teacher or clinician must be able to differentiate the child with limited language skills due to limited exposure to English from the child who has had exposure to English but still has difficulties.

Before discussing the issue of educating these children and some successful approaches used in bilingual special education classes, an understanding of how a second language is acquired is important. A second language can be acquired either naturally or through formal learning in schools, and natural bilingualism may occur simultaneously or sequentially (Reich, 1986).

SECOND LANGUAGE ACQUISITION

Natural Bilingualism

Natural bilingualism occurs in children when they hear two different languages in the home or when their family has moved to an area that speaks another language. The learning of two (or more) languages may occur simultaneously from birth or sequentially if a family moves after a child has established a first language. In an interesting review of case studies across time and languages, Reich (1986) drew a fairly consistent picture of natural bilingualism.

Simultaneous Bilingualism

For children learning two or more languages simultaneously, neither the rate nor the success of acquisition is affected by how closely related the languages are. The closely related languages of French and English are no less or more confusing to learn than the quite different languages of English and Japanese. Acquisition of a second language is smoothest when each person in contact with the child strictly uses one language. Children seem better able to place learned aspects of different languages in their appropriate "boxes." At age 2, children learning more than one language may appear to be delayed in language acquisition, but by age 4, children appear to have normal language development in both (or all) languages. The age most cited for language separation is from 3 to 5. Time of acquisition of specific rules is influenced by the complexity of the structure. For example, Slobin (1971a, 1973) reported that a child learning both Hungarian and Serbo-Croatian first used prepositions in Hungarian, which adds locative prepositions as suffixes to the noun that is the object of the preposition, before using them in Serbo-Croatian, which forms prepositions similarly to English, that is, preceding the object. Based on children's early strategies to attend to the end of words and sentences, this would be expected as suffixes are one of the most easily learned grammatical devices, whereas prepositions are more difficult.

In simultaneous language acquisition, **language interference,** or mixing of languages, occurs least in *phonology*, although children prefer easier phonemes in both languages and may evidence accents *at first*, then develop phonological accuracy at native speaker level. In 1965, Von Raffler-Engel (as cited in Reich, 1986) reported on children whose mothers spoke native French and whose fathers spoke French with an American accent. The children spoke French without an accent to their mothers but spoke French with an accent to their fathers.

In vocabulary (*semantics*), bilingual children may mix languages at first, but once they realize they are speaking two languages, they learn words from both simultaneously and may even ask for a name of an item learned in one language in the other language. *Syntax* is mixed for a longer time period or a single syntactic rule learned in one language is at first used in both languages. If syntactic structures are at the same level of complexity, they are acquired at the same time. As noted earlier in Slobin's example, if the level of complexity is different, the easier syntactic construction will appear first. The child becomes truly bilingual and can manage two language systems at about age 7 (Albert & Obler, 1978).

Sequential Bilingualism

Acquisition of a second language is generally referred to as sequential if it begins after the child's third birthday. Most bilingual children develop one language at home and a second with peers or in school (Owens, 1996). Reich reported from a review of case studies that, as with simultaneous acquisition, children are typically successful at sequential language acquisition. If thrown into a new language environment, a typical child under the age of 7 can successfully switch languages within a year. It is generally concluded that processes of learning the two languages are similar, even though analogy with the first language may be helpful. However, unless maintained in the home environment, the first language is apparently forgotten very quickly (3–6 months reported) due to lack of use, not the interference of a new language.

Processes of Second-Language Acquisition

Parker and Riley (1994) reported on how native speakers of one language (L1) later acquire another language (L2). Overall, speakers acquiring L2 go through a stage, or **interlanguage**, during which they construct a grammar different from that of both L1 and L2. The degree to which the L1 influences interlanguage is still subject to debate, but the influence of L1 on L2 acquisition cannot be ignored.

Language Transfer

Negative Transfer. Negative transfer, also known as interference, occurs when some property of L1 impedes L2 acquisition. For example, a native speaker of English while acquiring French may transfer English subject-verb-pronominal object word order to French, as in *Il veut les* (he wants them) for the correct French *Il les veut* (he them wants). Negative transfer is more apparent in phonology than syntax, thus the "foreign accent."

Positive Transfer. In positive transfer, some property of L1 promotes the acquisition of L2. For example, a native speaker of French while acquiring English may transfer French subject-verb-nominal object word order to English, as in *He wants the books.* Second-language learners must learn how to express meanings and interpret expressions of others, but they are perceptually and physically more mature and already possess abilities that they did not have when they learned L1 (Lindfors, 1987). For example, they know how to sort out, produce, and remember signals, and they know how language can be used by a speaker. Of course, the benefits of positive transfer require mastery of these aspects in the first language. The child who has a language delay or learning disorder may not have the necessary mastery, thus making his or her task of learning a second language that much more difficult.

Developmental Processes

Other factors that cannot be attributed to transfer also affect second-language acquisition and seem to account for the interlanguage grammar (Parker & Riley, 1994). It appears that the L2 learner goes through stages similar to those of speakers acquiring their native language. This can explain the production of structures such as *He not wrote the book* for an English negative even though this is not a pattern found in L1 or L2. The reader will recall from Chapter 6 that this is characteristic of a stage in the development of negatives in first-language acquisition. Other examples in English include consonant cluster simplification, use of Wh-words before interrogative reversal (Why I can't go?), and overgeneralization in semantics (*Daddy* for all men). It again appears that a second language is acquired much like a first language. This would suggest that a natural language sample with meaningful context and ample opportunity to practice language would best promote the successful acquisition of a second language. This is further supported by motivational processes that have been observed in children learning a L2.

Motivational Processes

Success in nonsimultaneous acquisition of a second language is most closely related to attitude, need, and identity with speakers of the L2. Fillmore (1976), in one of the most detailed early studies of second-language learners, identified three motivational stages that seemed to guide the learner's strategies for learning the L2. The first stage appeared to be focused on establishing social relationships with speakers of the second language. Interaction was the key and children depended heavily on fixed verbal formulas, such as "You know what?" "Guess what?" "Stupid," and "Shut up." Learners also relied on nonverbal communication and learning key words that would be useful for interactions. The purpose of the second stage was to communicate content, or messages, to L2 speakers and the L2 learners began creating more novel sentences and new combinations. More mixing of languages occurred here as the learner attempted to get his or her message across. The goal of the third and final stage was to be correct in speaking the L2. This stage was characterized by working on the finer points of form, incorporating grammatical devices and refinements that make language more "native-like." These stages would call for providing some cross-language interactions among children, but not necessarily to the exclusion of some instruction with other non-English-dominant speakers. This issue will be further considered later.

Characteristic Patterns and Challenges

Some specific patterns of acquisition and challenges beyond form need to be considered for each component of language. Parker and Riley (1994) noted that interlanguage phonology shows the strongest L1 transfer influence, whereas interlanguage morphology shows a strong developmental influence. Syntax evidences a complex interaction between transfer and developmental influences. Interlanguage semantics is strongly developmental with some negative transfer, but semantics is also influenced by developing cultural knowledge as no other component of interlanguage is. Cultural and social competence is also a very necessary part of L2 learning.

Phonology

Some accents may prevent learners of English as a second language from being fully accepted by members of the mainstream culture; some accents may be more widely accepted whereas others unfortunately may symbolize lower status (Cheng & Butler, 1989). Actually, speakers' accents are often the result of transfer from L1 to L2 in phonology, particularly if the L2 has phonemic distinctions that the L1 does not (Parker & Riley, 1994). For example, Japanese has no distinction between /l/ and /r/. Therefore, learning the English distinction is more difficult for Japanese speakers than vice versa. The Japanese speaker must learn a new distinction whereas the English speaker's distinction between /l/ and /r/ will go unnoticed by Japanese listeners (Parker & Riley, 1994). Some English speech sounds, such as /θ/ in *thin*, /ð/ in *then*, /z/ in *zip*, /š/ in *share*, /v/ in *vat*, /y/ in *you*, and the vowel sounds /ɪ/ in *ship*, /æ/ in *fat*, and /ʌ/ in *sun*, do not exist in Spanish, so these sounds are often distorted or replaced with another sound by Hispanic English speakers (Owens, 1996). Thus, interference may result in confusion with pronunciation and understanding of word pairs such as *thin-tin*, *then-den*, *zip-sip*, *chair-share*, and *vat-bat*. Words such as *pig* may become *peeg*, *fat* is *fet* and *sun* is *sahn*. Spanish has trill /r/ sounds that do not exist in English and thus will often be distorted or misunderstood by speakers of English learning Spanish. Short vowels in Arabic have very little significance, so when learning English, Arabic speakers tend to omit or confuse short vowel sounds, for example *bit* for *bet* (M. Wilson, 1996). In Arabic there is no distinction between /b/ and /p/, thus Arabic speakers randomly produce these sounds in American English, and they often drink *bebsi cola*; /v/ and /f/ are not distinguished in Arabic, so both are usually pronounced as /f/; /g/ and /k/ may be confused (Wilson, 1996).

English permits consonant clusters of up to three consonants such as in *street* or *splash*. A speaker whose native language does not permit such initial clusters may insert a vowel to break up the cluster in order to conform with the speaker's L1. Examples from Broselow (cited in Parker & Riley, 1994) include:

English Target	Egyptian Arabic	Iraqi Arabic
floor /flor/	/filor/	/iflor/
three /θri/	/θiri/	/iθri/

Both of these strategies result in forms that reflect an acceptable syllable structure in the L1. Hispanic English speakers use much the same strategy, for example, *espeak* for *speak* (Herrera, 1987), as do Hindu and Urdu speakers from India, for example, *ispeak* for *speak* (Shekar & Hegde, 1996).

Morphology and Syntax

Developmental processes play a major role in L2 acquisition among both adults and children learning English as an L2. For example, {PLU} is acquired before {POSS} and {PRES} similar to native speaker acquisition, that is, in the same order and according to morphological function not phonological form. Dulay and Burt (1983) found native speakers of Spanish used strategies that are not found in Spanish but do occur when children are acquiring English as a native language. For example, *He took her teeths off* and *I didn't weared any hat.*

Both transfer and developmental processes have been found to play a role in interlanguage syntax. For example, in English the verb *listen* requires a preposition, however, the equivalent French verb does not. Conversely, the English verb *obey* does not require a preposition, but the equivalent French verb does. Adjemian (1983) reported that English speakers commonly transfer English restrictions to French.

Interlanguage Form	English Use	Correct French
écouter à	listen to	écouter
obeir	obey	obeir a

This sheds light on the often heard native Spanish speaker asking someone to "Explain me what that means." Of course, there are some verbs that vary in a language depending on one's dialect. Just to make English more difficult to learn, some speakers say they *graduated from high school* whereas others (usually from New York) say they *graduated high school.*

Sometimes transfer and developmental processes interact. Anderson (1983) reported a study of a Spanish speaker learning English readily and acquiring the use of articles, which also exist in Spanish, whereas a Japanese speaker acquiring English omitted them, as Japanese does not have articles. This may be a function of both negative transfer and developmental processes.

Some structural contrasts between Spanish and English that may interfere with English as the L2 include adjective noun order (*cat, black*), postnoun possessive (*hat of my brother*), use of *no* before the verb for negation (*I no go*), use of longer forms of comparatives such as *more tall*, use of intonation rather than interrogative reversals (*Maria is going?*), and omission of the subject pronoun if previously identified (*My dog heard a noise outside. Is barking now.*)

Misplacement of English negatives may also occur in Arabic English, as negatives are formed in Arabic by placing a particle before the verb. Plurals are formed by internal vowel changes in Arabic (e.g., *walid* is *boy*, *awlad* is *boys*), so plural morphemes in English are often omitted at first. There are no copula, emphatic-do, modals, gerunds, or infinitive forms in Arabic, resulting in possible confusion in the formation of English verb tenses (M. Wilson, 1996).

Shekar and Hegde (1996) reported on some interferences that occur in the grammar of Indian speakers of English. For example, the absence of an article system in Indian languages results in structures such as *Office is closed* today for *The office is closed today.* Although stative verbs (e.g., *hear, touch, taste, smell, see, know, understand, have*) are not used in the progressive form in American English, Indian English speakers often use these verbs in the progressive, as in *I am smelling the flower.* Whereas the interrogative reversal required in American English Wh-questions may not be applied in Indian English, *What you would like to eat?*, it may be applied in the indirect question, *Tell me what are your duties?* Yes-no confusion may occur when an Indian English speaker gives a negative response where an American English speaker expects an affirmative: *You have no objection? Yes, I have no objection.* This is true for Arabic English speakers as well.

Semantics

Parker and Riley (1994) reported on some processes that occur when speakers are acquiring the vocabulary of English as a second language. One developmental strategy speakers may use is overgeneralization of superordinates such as *animal* for *dog.* Also, some speakers may rely heavily on the use of a few modifiers and generalize them to inappropriate contexts (e.g., *I have small money* for *I have little money*).

Another common developmental strategy is the inappropriate use of synonyms that may have similar meanings, but differ in selectional restrictions in words or categories with which they co-occur, in emotional associations of the word, and in level of formality. For example, *tall* and *long* are subsumed by one Arabic word, *tawil*; consequently, an Arabic speaker may produce a sentence in English such as *My father is a long thin man* (Parker & Riley, 1994). Related to descriptors is the fact that the Arabic language is rich with exaggeration and uses multiple adjectives. Eloquence is emphasized and admired; fluency and word usage are critical (Wilson, 1996).

It may also be the case that American English lacks words or markers that speakers of other languages commonly use. For example, speakers of Indian languages use markers of honor to show deference when they refer to their elders, teachers, and superiors. American English lacks such markers, so to circumvent this cultural dilemma, Indian English speakers tend to place a term such as *Sir* in front of names when addressing either teachers or elders (Shekar & Hegde, 1996). For example, a young woman who is married to one of the faculty members in our department is a Tamil speaker from India, as is her husband, and still, after 2 years of socializing together, sometimes refers to one of the authors as "Dr. Lydia" (I'm sure this is a mark of my profession and not my age).

Semantic problems may also arise with verbs that use particles, such as *run up*, *run down*, and *run out*. Nonnative speakers may prefer one-word equivalents (i.e., *incur*, *find*, and *expire*). Words that express reciprocal relations, such as *teach* and *learn*, may also cause difficulty. Confusion of words with similar sounds or spelling may occur. *People are unable to work and earn* ***efficient*** *[sufficient] money* (Parker & Riley, 1994). Another developmental strategy that may occur if vocabulary is lacking is the use of **circumlocutions**, or descriptions of objects rather than labels, for example, *a lady carrying a baby* for *pregnant*.

Many words have multiple meanings, and a large vocabulary may not be enough to comprehend all the different meanings of words or expressions (Cheng, 1996). For example, *He is in a critical state* may be interpreted as a place rather than a situation (Parker & Riley, 1994).

A common problem in semantics is difficulty with **idioms**, expressions that cannot be derived from their component words, for example *pull one's leg* for joke (Parker & Riley, 1994). Idioms can be particularly confusing for educated immigrants who are used to finding whatever they do not understand in the dictionary (Cheng, 1996). Other potential areas of confusion noted by Cheng involve humor, metaphors, and proverbs. Arabs make abundant use of proverbs, of which they have hundreds, and use metaphors and similes lavishly (Wilson, 1996).

Pragmatics

The process of acquiring cross-cultural communicative competence requires social and cultural knowledge beyond language form and content (Cheng, 1996; Rees & Gerber, 1992). Language use and function rather than language form alone have been the focus of language assessment and intervention for at least the past 15 years (Langdon, 1996). Children acquiring English as L2 may be knowledgeable about ways of appropriately communicating in their native language, but may need help in understanding and acquiring pragmatic skills in English (E. Garcia, 1994). Mastering a language means being able to say the right thing at the right time in the right manner (Cheng, 1996), and contrasts between languages also exist in pragmatic and nonlinguistic social arenas.

In an article by Cole (1989), Orlando Taylor noted several possible sources of miscommunication for different cultural groups learning English. These are presented in Tables 13–1, 13–2, and 13–3. These tables are to be viewed as general guidelines for consideration, for there are many tribal groups with very different lifestyles and cultures that are all designated Native American, just as there are many different cultural groups labeled Asian or Hispanic. Care must be taken not to stereotype ethnic groups and to be aware of individual differences (e.g., Keogh, Gallimore, & Weisner, 1997; Supple, 1996). These lists also represent only a sampling of potentially different behaviors for each of the groups. With this in mind, we may examine the tables from Taylor as useful information, using caution not to fall into the trap of stereotyping.

Taylor noted that eye contact is interpreted differently by many Hispanic and American English speakers, that is, direct eye contact signals attentiveness and respect to the American English speaker, but may indicate a challenge to authority by the Hispanic English speaker. Although most Americans let their gaze drift occasionally during conversation, Arabs constantly look each other in the eye (Wilson, 1996).

In Table 13–1, Taylor has noted that many Hispanic speakers precede business discussions with lengthy talk unrelated to the point of

TABLE 13–1. Pragmatic contrasts between Hispanic and Standard American English speakers.

Hispanic	***Standard American English***
Hissing to gain attention is acceptable.	Hissing is considered impolite and indicates contempt.
Touching is often observed between two people in conversation.	Touching is usually unacceptable and usually carries sexual overtone.
Avoidance of direct eye contact is sometimes a sign of attentiveness and respect; sustained direct eye contact may be interpreted as a challenge to authority.	Direct eye contact is a sign of attentiveness and respect.
Relative distance between two speakers in conversation is close.	Relative distance between two speakers in conversation is farther apart.
Official or business conversations are preceded by lengthy greetings, pleasantries, and other talk unrelated to the point of business.	Getting to the point quickly is valued.

Source: From "E Pluribus Pluribus: Multicultural Imperatives for the 1990s and Beyond," by L. Cole, 1989, *Asha, 31*. p.69. Copyright 1989 by ASHA. Adapted by permission of the American Speech-Language-Hearing Association.

TABLE 13–2. Pragmatic contrasts between Asian and Standard American English speakers.

Asian	*Standard American English*
Touching or hand-holding between members of the same sex is acceptable.	Touching or hand-holding between members of the same sex is considered as a sign of homosexuality.
Hand-holding/hugging/kissing between men and women in public looks ridiculous.	Hand-holding/hugging/kissing between men and women in public is acceptable.
A slap on the back is insulting.	A slap on the back denotes friendliness..
It is not customary to shake hands with persons of the opposite sex.	It is customary to shake hands with persons of the opposite sex.
Finger beckoning is only used by adults to call little children and not vice-versa.	Finger beckoning is often used to call people.

Source: From "E Pluribus Pluribus: Multicultural Imperatives for the 1990s and Beyond," by L. Cole, 1989, *Asha, 31*, p. 69. Copyright 1989 by ASHA. Adapted by permission of the American Speech-Language-Hearing Association..

TABLE 13–3. Pragmatic contrasts between Native Americans and Standard American English speakers.

Native American	*Standard American English*
Personal questions may be considered prying	Personal questions are acceptable particularly when establishing case history information.
Gushing over babies may endanger the child.	Gushing over babies shows admiration of the child.
A bowed head is a sign of respect.	Lack of eye contact is sign of shyness, guilt, or lying.
It is acceptable to ask the same question several times, if you doubt the truth of the person.	It is a sign of inattention if the same question is asked several times.

Source: From "E Pluribus Pluribus: Multicultural Imperatives for the 1990s and Beyond," by L. Cole, 1989, *Asha, 31*, p. 69. Copyright 1989 by ASHA. Adapted by permission of the American Speech-Language-Hearing Association.

business. Cheng (1996) reported that in Africa, it is also important to engage in lengthy greetings in social conversations before proceeding to other topics, no matter how urgent the topic may be. In Arabic, greetings are lengthy and formalized (Wilson, 1996), and there are at least 30 situations that call for predetermined expressions and required responses (Nydell, 1987).

In Table 13–2, Taylor has included nonverbal aspects of greetings that may differ culturally for Asians. Cheng (1996) added bowing in Japan, closing one's hands in Thailand, hugging and kissing in Spain and, in Africa, when greeting an older person, grasping his or her hand in both of the greeter's hands to show respect.

Gesturing also has different rules in operation in different cultures. For example, in East Africa when a vendor raises a fist when asked for the price, this means "five," and two fists hit together means "ten." One of the authors of this text experienced a difference in counting gestures in France when she received two beverages, thinking she was ordering one more by raising the index finger. She was unaware at the time that counting began with the thumb to indicate one and then the index finger to indicate two.

Rules of discourse are another area in which Cheng (1996) pointed out differences that can be significant in education. In Western discourse, an educated approach to writing a paper involves introducing a topic in a paper, developing it in the body of the paper, and then summarizing with conclusions. Asian verbal interaction, both spoken and written, is circular rather than linear, so that a paper may not have a topic sentence; thoughts or opinions may be presented in a circular manner without drawing conclusions. In fact, it may be considered condescending to draw conclusions for the reader. This is a difference that may require educators to explain more than just "this is the way it's done," for it's not done that way everywhere.

Concepts of time and space are different among cultures. How late a person may show up for an appointment without communicating disrespect varies. Rules for how closely one may stand to a conversational partner without being offensive also differ. Arabic, Hispanic, and Indian cultures all require less space between speakers during conversation than the American culture does. Germans, on the other hand, require greater personal space than Americans. Unawareness of differences may result in communication problems.

SHOE
by Jeff MacNelly

LATE AGAIN?
"LATE." THAT'S SUCH A NARROW-MINDED CONCEPT.
5/14
©97 Tribune Media Services, Inc.
All Rights Reserved
DO YOU KNOW THERE ARE SOME CULTURES THAT DON'T EVEN HAVE WORDS FOR "HOUR" OR "MINUTE"?
http://macnelly.com
DO THEY HAVE A WORD FOR "UNEMPLOYED"?
MACNELLY

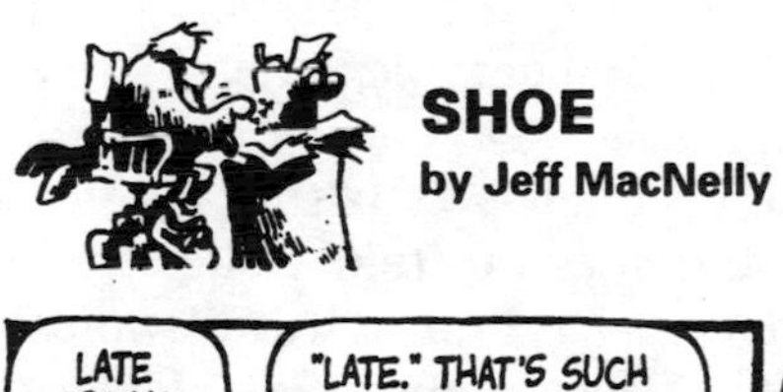

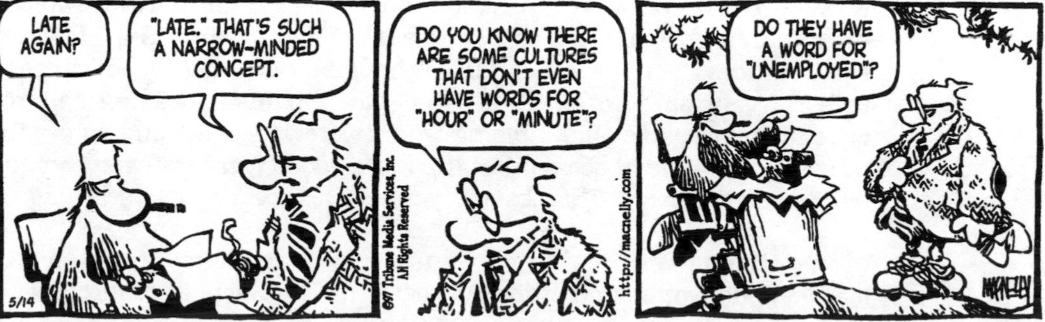

Wilson (1996) illustrated the importance of knowledge of other cultures in educational settings in her description of a contrast in the communication style of many Arab cultures and Americans. Whereas Americans generally place a high value on keeping promises, that is, "our word is as good as our bond," to Arabs, an oral promise has its own value as a response, and a request from a friend is never refused. A positive response is simply a declaration of intent and an expression of goodwill. In school, when a teacher or clinician asks parents to do something such as take their child to a physician or purchase particular school supplies, they are likely to agree to do so. However, it may not happen. Americans may judge this behavior as unreliable or dishonest, whereas the Arabic view is that the parents are behaving courteously. It would not be polite to refuse, so they say yes even though they may disagree with the request or be financially unable to follow through. "Yes" may mean "no" or "maybe" and should not be taken literally. Tactful inquiry may be necessary to determine agreement without putting the parents on the spot.

Cheng (1996) asserts that few individuals learning to speak other languages have the opportunity to learn the cultural aspects that are so essential to communication. Teachers and clinicians need to continuously pursue cultural/social information. A match between school-language discourse and home-language discourse plays a role in ensuring success of language acquisition and school performance (Langdon, 1996).

Nonlinguistic Influences

Forces other than linguistic factors may play a role in second-language acquisition.

Age. Although it is traditionally thought that acquiring a L2 is more difficult for an older learner than a younger one, this is not universally accepted (Parker & Riley, 1994). It is generally agreed, however, that phonology is the one area where adult learners lag behind, in that a nativelike accent is difficult to acquire if the L2 acquisition begins beyond the age of puberty. The issue of age is a complex one.

Personality Traits. Traits found to be correlated with success in L2 acquisition include extroversion and willingness to take risks. Extroversion has been found to be more advantageous in naturalistic settings than in formal learning settings (Parker & Riley, 1994). However, L. W. Filmore (1983) reported that, although most of her "good learners" in her 3-year study of 43 Cantonese- and Spanish-speaking children were highly sociable and outgoing, some were very quiet and somewhat uncommunicative. It seems that the latter "good learners" were very attentive and observant. This observer strategy also occurs in L1 learning.

Motivational Factors. As previously mentioned, factors such as the learner's motivation and attitude toward the L2 may play a role in learning. Motivation reflecting the language learner's desire to become part of the community or culture is seen as more important than motivation reflecting the learner's desire to learn the language for practical purposes, such as getting a job (Parker & Riley, 1994).

SECOND LANGUAGE ACQUISITION AND SCHOOL

There is no argument that the number of persons in the USA from nondominant cultural groups is increasing (Westby, 1995). The USA has struggled with the issue of how to best educate the children of these immigrants; yet, during the past decade, financial support for bilingual programs has dropped from 47% to only 8%, and it may decrease in the future (Langdon, 1996). Teachers with nonnative speakers of English in their classrooms do not know how to help them learn English or feel a part of the class nor do they understand the customs and values of the students any more than the students understand theirs (Freeman & Freeman, 1994).

The need to educate speakers with limited proficiency in English has become increasingly more important and the population more diverse. The debate on bilingual education has centered on the value of developing fluency in the English language but typically has not addressed aspects such as social and cultural values that are part of language (Bialystok & Hakuta, 1994).

Bilingual Education Programs

Programs that have been implemented in bilingual education include immersion, submersion, and transition.

Immersion

This program was first used to add French as a foundational language for English speakers in Canada. Students receive most of their elementary school instruction in their nonnative language by a bilingual teacher (Reich, 1986; Snow, 1990) who speaks only French to them. Successful implementation in Canada led to the incorrect assumption that it would also work for teaching English as a second language in the USA (Dicker, 1993).

Submersion

This term is a better description of early immersion programs in the U.S. Although all instruction occurred in English, there were several significant differences between the U.S. and Canadian programs, and research, as well as experience, have indicated that this has not been very successful and may actually have negative effects on children (Cummins, 1988; Reich, 1986).

Immersion in Canada was different in that all children were at the same level of L2 acquisition and the goal was the addition of the L2, not the replacement of the native language/culture. Programs in the U.S. include language minority students and the goal of most bilingual programs is a **language shift** to speak English, and English only. The teacher is often monolingual, not bilingual (Cummins, 1988). In the Canadian immersion programs, children are praised for a second language. In U.S. submersion programs, children are corrected and native language is often demeaned, and the program conveys the idea that the cultures and values of the language minority groups are inferior or do not matter at all. Furthermore, in Canada, English students learning French were exposed to English literacy in their homes; in the U.S., minority students learning English are not acquiring literacy in their native language (Dicker, 1993).

Transition

As an alternative, transitional bilingual education programs gradually move students into English language instruction and their native language is used in instruction throughout elementary school (Gersten & Woodward, 1995; Reich, 1986). The rationale is that the students need to know a language before reading it, otherwise they cannot understand what they are reading and they will fall behind in instruction. Moving students into English instruction too soon often results in "watered down" instruction to match the perceived competence of students (Gersten & Woodward, 1995).

Dicker (1993) described transitional bilingual education as reflecting an assimilationist approach to teaching minority language students in which the goal is still monolingualism in English, "weaning" students off their dependence on their native language. Although this approach attempts to take the students' needs into account, it may not show sensitivity to students' native languages and cultures. Dicker advocated a dual-language program, in which a classroom has an equal number of English-speaking and minority language students, and both languages are used for instruction. This would allow for L. W. Fillmore's stages of development described earlier in which social interaction with speakers of the L2 plays a great part in motivation to learn the L2.

Gersten and Woodward (1995) described a "sheltered English" immersion program that involves accelerating the introduction of English while maintaining the native language. This program stresses English language instruction presented in the context of content instruction and is sensitive to students' English proficiency. Ortiz (1997) noted that many of these children have such limited command of English that they cannot function effectively in classrooms taught entirely in English. There is extensive research to date on the benefits of instruction in children's first language for the first few years *as* they learn to speak, read, and write a second language (Bernhardt, 1991; Krashen, 1982; Krashen & Biber, 1988; Reich, 1986). This allows the development of cognitive academic level skills in their native language (Cummins, 1984) through providing experiences and activities that require them to perform at a higher cognitive level.

Unfortunately, the overwhelming evidence is that minority students experience limited academic success in public schools, and determination of the cause of school-related difficulties should begin with an examination of the educational programs provided to students (Ortiz, 1997). Students who are expected to learn English should receive the best instruction possible, in both special programs and in the general education classroom. Strategies that not only teach a second language, but also help maintain literacy and pride for the native language should be used (Freeman & Freeman, 1994). Although it is unrealistic to expect American teachers and SLPs to understand all the cultures and languages of the immigrants who have adopted the U.S. as their home, they can educate themselves in the linguistic and cultural differences of those they serve (Shekar & Hegde, 1996). Teachers should also encourage parents of minority language students to visit the classroom and share their culture and ideas (Milk, Mercado, & Sapiens, 1992).

If students are provided positive school and classroom contexts that accommodate individual differences or learning styles, most learning problems can be prevented; however, it is to be expected that, even with these accommodations, some students will have problems (Ortiz, 1997). At this point special education prereferral interventions should be implemented. If a teacher's adaptations or recommendations from consultants are ineffective, referral to special education may be warranted.

Specific Assessment Issues

For students with limited English proficiency (LEP), information about native language and English language proficiency is needed to determine whether they should be assessed in the native language (Ortiz, 1997). In addition, efforts should be made to obtain information from parents on whether the child's presenting problems are also evident in the home and community.

In assessing language proficiency, it is important to determine both basic interpersonal communication skills (BICS) and cognitive academic language proficiency (CALP) (Cummins, 1984) in L1 and L2. BICS are conversational abilities that LEP students may master quite easily. CALP entails the more complex, abstract language use related to problem solving, evaluating, and inferring. Students who are learning L2 generally acquire conversational skills in 1–2 years but may need 5–7 years to achieve academic language ability (Cummins, 1984). Students who have CALP proficiency in their first language will master critical literacy in a second language more easily and quickly than students who do not possess CALP in a first language (Westby, 1995). It is important to ensure that limited academic language proficiency is not misinterpreted as a learning disability (Ortiz, 1997). Westby suggested that diagnosing students who have had less than 5–7 years of learning school language as learning disabled or communication disordered is problematic.

Conversational ability should be assessed through observation of spontaneous language use and should focus on knowledge of discourse rules and language use (Ortiz, 1997). Storytelling activities can be used to assess expressive language and reveal information about a child's ability to organize information, sequence events, draw conclusions, and evaluate actions. Assessment of narrative competence reveals information about cognitive development. Informal, curriculum-based measures of literacy skills should also be administered in the native language and English (Ortiz & Garcia, 1990).

Assessment formats and procedures may be biased against non-mainstream children in many ways. Crago (1992) pointed out that the situation itself may have components that are unfamiliar to a child. For example, in some cultures, adults do not ask a child questions to which they already know the answer and in some cultures, children are not expected to be alone with adults. If the child is used to communicating mostly with peers, the testing situation may be very uncomfortable, resulting in incorrect conclusions.

Although language sampling as a method of assessment has been proposed as a solution to biases in standardized instruments, awareness of the cultural dimensions and socialization has significance for language sampling (Crago, 1992). The teacher or clinician needs to know the cultural situations, interactions, and interactants in a child's life in order to effectively structure the situation and the participants in the process. For example, if the teacher or clinician knows that Native American children talk more with peers than with adults, the procedure may be structured to include other children as communicative partners (Crago, 1992). Several cultures (e.g., Athabascan in Alberta, Canada and Hawaiian) expect audience participation in weaving a story, therefore the traditional expectation of a monlogue by the narrator would need to be adjusted to a more interactional format (Guitierrez-Clellen & Quinn, 1993).

Speech-language pathologists, psychologists, special educators, and classroom teachers need to be aware of the social context of the testing situation (Garcia, 1992). Guitierrez-Clellen and Quinn (1993) recommend using a dynamic assessment approach which identifies differences in narratives and gives children the opportunity to perform as expected when they understand the demands and rules of context.

Successful Teaching Approaches

Students from diverse linguistic backgrounds learn English best when teachers use clear instructions, provide feedback on students' progress, have a positive attitude toward the children and close contact with parents and families, and demonstrate a nonauthoritative interaction style (Langdon, 1996). Crago (1992) cautioned that, once children begin to learn a L2 in a nonbilingual school, they shift their use of L1 at home and parents increase their use of L2, often at the advice of the teacher or clinician (Cummins, 1989). Unfortunately, this results in a disruption of home patterns of communication and exposes children to a limited model of L2 at home as the parents are also L2 learners. The use of native language by parents should be encouraged, not discouraged (Cummins, 1984). Educators must remember that studies have documented that gains result from educating children in a culturally congruent manner (Crago, 1992). Students who use their native language effectively are likely to acquire and use English appropriately; students who evidence problems in their native language will experience problems in English as a second language (Krashen, 1992).

Communication in the classroom is enhanced through meaningful activities with opportunities for hands-on projects and small group interaction allowing verbal exchange and negotiation (Langdon, 1996). Willig, Swedo, and Ortiz (1987) found that children with disabilities, like their nondisabled peers, were more effectively engaged when they were provided instruction in their native language and lessons in English as a second language. Several interaction-oriented strategies that have been found to be successful in teaching literacy skills are described here.

Whole Language

Research on L2 acquisition suggests that whole language approaches are appropriate for LEP students who are being instructed in English, because this approach focuses first on developing communication skills in the very critical aspect of context before turning to the mechanics of oral and written communication (Ortiz, 1997). A literacy-rich environment is provided so that students experience reading and writing for purposes of communicating and learning. Lopez-Reyna (1996) described a bilingual special education class over a 2-year period as teachers and students made a transition from skills-based independent seatwork and worksheet activities to a whole language classroom with more personal student involvement in their reading and writing. The primary features of the approach were use of students' background experiences as a basis for each session, use of trade books and "big books" with predictable patterns, use of students' language of preference, and the use of student-selected writing topics. An adapted version of the experience-text-relationship (ETR) method (Au, 1979) was used. In the ETR approach, during the E-phase, the teacher and children discuss background experiences related to the story to be read. During the T-phase, students read segments of the story silently and then the teacher leads a group discussion. Finally, during the R-phase, the teacher helps the students draw relationships between their background experiences and text ideas (Westby, 1995).

Shared Literature

Ortiz (1997) described Shared Literature (Roser & Frith, 1988) as a program that has been successful in enhancing the reading and vocabulary skills of culturally and linguistically diverse students in general and special education classes. In the Shared Literature approach, award-winning children's literature is used for story reading in which ample opportunities are provided to discuss the stories read by the teacher. Activities such as writing, art, and drama are used to expand and refine language skills. This technique was used along with the Writing Workshop (Graves, 1983), both of which focus on meaningful context. B. Goldstein (1995) has provided a bibliography of children's literature, which can be used to initiate discussion on critical themes and issues for LEP Spanish speakers.

Writing Workshop

In Graves's Writing Workshop, children write every day, developing topics of their choice. The teacher conferences with students as they write, answering questions and evaluating skills. Lessons in mechanics are based on the teacher's and student's evaluation of the writing in progress. Students share and talk about their writing, which helps them develop both conversational and academic language skills. Students begin by expressing their thoughts and then move to proofreading and editing. As a result, students become better writers and enjoy writing more (Ortiz, 1997).

Talk Story

Garcia (1992) reported on the success of the Hawaiian Kamehameha Early Education Program (KEEP) (Au & Jordan, 1981) for increased reading comprehension. Hawaiian students in school engaged in a *talk story* similar to discourse patterns described by Boggs (1972, 1978) as common in the children's speech community. They responded very little to questions directed at them, but blurted out the answer when the question was directed to another student or to a group of students. Similar to the talk story common to the children's speech community, in KEEP, teachers initiate reading comprehension questions, then students respond by calling out their answers and building on each other's responses until the whole group has reacted. The talk story was combined with the ETR text discussion approach described previously. This approach is very different from the limited dialogue characterized by short statements and responses to known-answer questions that is typically used in this situation. In addition, this kind of restrained dialogue ensures all students share a common knowledge base and set of experiences (Lopez-Reyna, 1996).

Instructional Conversations

Instructional conversation (IC) is an approach that shows students how to interact with a text by engaging students in interactions that promote analysis, reflection, and critical thinking (Goldenberg, 1992–1993; Tharpe & Gallimore, 1988). ICs are instructional, but appear to be natural and spontaneous language interactions in which the teacher questions, prods, challenges, coaxes, or keeps quiet in order to point students toward a learning objective or goal (Goldenberg). The main components of the conversational elements include multiple interactive turns that build on and extend student contributions, promote complex language and expression through requests to expand what is said, and promote reasoning to support an argument. These structured, natural conversations revolve around a theme or idea selected by the teacher to serve as a starting point to focus the discussion. All instruction is thus contextualized and oral participation as well as student-to-student interaction is promoted during reading lessons, providing additional opportunities for language development. Through the use of instructional conversations, Echevarria (1995) found that Hispanic students with learning disabilities used higher levels of discourse when given the opportunity to do so. Echevarria and McDonough (1995) reported that the most significant adaptations of instructional conversations needed for special education were in theme selection and presentation, level of questioning, and behavior management.

Cooperative Learning

Cooperative learning, described in Chapter 12, holds much promise in fostering natural language use for LEP students and has been shown to provide positive benefits for bilingual special education students (Gersten, Brengelman, & Jimenez, 1994). Small cooperative groups allow students to interact with peers while doing school assignments.

Cognitive and Metacognitive Strategies

Cognitive and metacognitive strategies mentioned throughout this text help students learn how to learn and how to monitor and manage their own learning and are very important to success in school. These strategies depend on one's intraindividual use of language and are essential for students learning a second language. These may and should include strategies in problem solving, reflectivity, verbal rehearsal, verbal mediation, organization, self-instruction, self-monitoring, and self-evaluation.

KEY COMPONENTS OF SUCCESSFUL TEACHING

The main component in successful teaching approaches for bilingual education and bilingual special education is providing students with opportunities to participate in language practice at both the conversational level and the cognitive academic level. All too common are language-development curricula that rely on scripted teacher presentation and directed student responses. The institution of some of these more open approaches may result in what Echevarria and McDonough (1995) found when initiating instructional conversations. Teachers reported that initially students were "shocked to talk without raising their hands." The students had to be taught to participate spontaneously and formulate their own thoughts and expressions, because they were so unused to doing so. Along with encouraging oral participation and higher level cognitive language use, teachers, clinicians, and other professionals must value and appreciate students' native language and cultural heritage (Langdon, 1996) if we are to be successful in educating the emerging English learner. As Ramasamy (1996) noted, in reference to Navajo students, the task of education is to make teachng and learning compatible with the social structures in which students are most productive, engaged, and likely to learn.

✓ SUMMARY CHECKLIST

☐ **Second Language Acquisition**

Natural Bilingualism

Simultaneous Bilingualism

Language Interference

Sequential Bilingualism

Processes of Second-Language Acquisition

Interlanguage

Language Transfer

Negative Transfer

Positive Transfer

Developmental Processes

Motivational Processes

☐ **Characteristic Patterns and Challenges**

Phonology

Morphology and Syntax

Semantics

Pragmatics

Nonlinguistic Influences

Age

Personality Traits

Motivational Factors

☐ **Bilingual Education Programs**

Immersion

Submersion

Language Shift

Transition

☐ **Specific Assessment Issues**
- **Basic Interpersonal Communication Skills (BICS)**
- **Cognitive Academic Languge Proficiency (CALP)**
- **Format and Procedures**

☐ **Successful Teaching Approaches**
- **Whole Language**
- **Shared Literature**
- **Writing Workshop**
- **Talk Story**
- **Instructional Conversation**
- **Cooperative Learning**
- **Cognitive and Metacognitive Strategies**

APPENDIX

LANGUAGE SAMPLING

ELICITING A LANGUAGE SAMPLE

It is important for teachers or clinicians to elicit a sample of language, in naturalistic context, that is both spontaneous and representative of the highest level of language of which the student is capable. A teacher who has been listening to his or her students while working with them, perhaps even jotting down examples of the student's language that seem atypical, should have an idea of the level of language that is typical and representative of a student. To obtain a true representative sample of language, the teacher or clinician may need to guide and somewhat control the "spontaneous conversation." This conversation should be taped using a quality recorder to ensure clear playback. A counter will be helpful as some passages may have to be listened to many times to ensure exactness. The final sample should contain a minimum of 50 different utterances *representative* of the student's most complex language skills. An **utterance** is a complete thought that is divided from other utterances by sentence boundaries, pauses, and/or a drop in the voice (Owens, 1995). Fifty utterances are generally considered adequate for phonological and syntactic analysis; semantic and pragmatic analyses generally involve more than one observation (Lund & Duchan, 1993).

Some students are quite willing to talk a great deal with very little prodding or probing; others require much more encouragement and questioning. During this interaction, it is vital that the teacher show interest and enthusiasm. The following suggestions, adapted from Lee (1974) and Lund and Duchan (1988), should be helpful in eliciting a representative sample of language from a student:

1. **Use age-appropriate materials to stimulate conversation** or to change the topic if conversation seems to be lagging. Materials may include toys, puppets, picture cards, pictures of movie stars, rock stars or athletes, or advertisements for movies or Nintendo games. Materials are to be presented one at a time, as needed, and reading materials should be avoided for the result may be a sample of the student's reading abilities instead of speaking abilities.
2. **Elicit the highest level structures possible** as well as a variety of types of responses. The quality of the sample often depends on the quality of the questions asked. Questions requiring only one- or two-word responses will likely elicit just those responses. Questions should be open-ended and evaluative and include forms to elicit different, complex multiword responses. Examples: What will he do next? What did she say then? Why did they do that? How would you have acted?
3. **Do not talk more than is necessary** during the session and never interrupt the student. The student should be encouraged to take the lead and the teacher's comments should show interest and encourage higher level statements. The right topics alone can result in this. Topics that have been found to be especially successful include recent movies (Tell me what *Lion King* was about) and popular games (Tell me how to play *Myst*). Telling a story or giving directions will require organization of thoughts and sequencing, skills that are often difficult for students with language disorders. Avoid having a too familiar story told as it may be memorized.

TRANSCRIBING THE LANGUAGE SAMPLE

The tape should be transcribed as soon as possible after the recording so that recall may aid in the exactness of the transcription. Specific detail is extremely important. All fillers (*ums, uhs*) and interjections (*like, you know*) need to be included to allow for a complete analysis of language. The following conventions (adapted from Bloom and Lahey, 1978) may be used for transcribing:

1. **All comments by the student and to the student** are fully transcribed on paper divided by a hypothetical vertical line. Comments by the subject appear on the right side. Comments by other speakers appear on the left. This will be useful later when examining the context of what was said to the student prior to his or her response. A speaker is identified by an initial the first time he or she speaks—any changes in speaker need to be noted. Any **relevant situational context** that will be useful later in interpreting the student's response should be included in parentheses

(e.g., a description of the picture card that the student is explaining). **Differential use of verb tenses** aids in describing the situational context: present progressive for simultaneous action; simple present for actions or events that precede or follow.

(C makes a dragon noise)

then Adam eat the witch/
that's my story/

(C pointing to tape recorder)

now tape it/

2. The transcription moves down the page in a **chronological manner**. An action or event that occurs simultaneously with the subject utterance appears on the same line with that utterance. When an utterance precedes or follows an action or event, the utterance appears on the preceding or succeeding line. Utterances by a speaker that immediately succeed each other follow each other on the same line.

If you could buy a car,
what kind of car would you
buy?

I don't know/ the same
kind as my mom's/ kind
of like a station wagon
but it's not/

3. The **boundary (ending) of an utterance** is indicated with a slash (/). The boundary is determined by length of pause before the next comment and by its apparent terminal contour. The judgment is sometimes difficult to make. For older children and adults, the slash may be considered equivalent to a period, but it is important to make each judgment carefully and as objectively as possible. Sentences with conjoined or embedded clauses are considered single utterances.

Can you tell me the story of the
three little bears?

three little bears in the
house/ they left the house
and this girl Goldilocks
went into the house/

4. A **significant pause** within an utterance is indicated by an asterisk (*). The literature suggests that lengthy pauses are important clues to language production difficulties (Dollag-

han & Campbell, 1992). Based on data on adult conversations, Dollaghan and Campbell recommend a conservative estimate of a 2-second duration as the criterion for a significant silent pause.

just go in her closet/ look like * like* a store/

5. An **interrupted, unfinished utterance** is indicated with a line.

do you want some ________/

6. When a student **changes or corrects his or her own comment**, a self-correct symbol is used.

my mom s/c my dad likes the uh station wagon little bit/

7. When a word or portion of an utterance is totally unintelligible, it may be indicated by three dashes.

she says that she'll play with her for a little bit and then she'll go and play ---/

8. When a subject utterance seems to be a question because it has **rising intonation**, it should be followed by a rising arrow (↑)

(P shaking empty box) **no more in there↑/**

9. A colon is used to indicate that **a word is drawn out**.

no: it's it's like fur/

10. **Capitalization is not conventional**. Proper nouns and the pronoun I are capitalized; initial letter of subject utterance is not.

11. The symbol # is used to indicate that there is material on the tape that is **not transcribed**. It can **only appear on the left** side and usually represents conversations between adults or an interruption such as the PA system. The symbol is used only when the subject is not attending to the conversation or interruption. If the subject responds to it, it must be transcribed.

APPENDIX

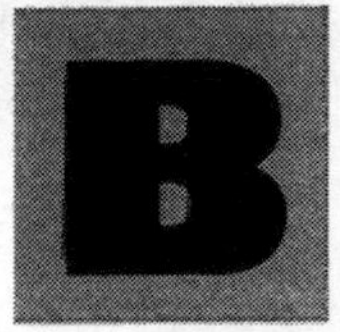

SCHOOL DIRECTION WORDS

Oral Directions: Primary (K–2)

After	Find	Raise
Behave	First	Ready
Bubble	Follow the directions	Repeat
Can	Give examples	Rhyme
Circle	Go	Show
Clear	Hold	Sing
Color	Imagine	Step
Come	Last	Stop
Copy	Line	Tell
Count	Listen	Then
Cut	Look	Think
Define	Next	Today
Discuss	Now	Trace
Do	Paste	Turn
Draw	Please	Walk
Enter	Point	Watch
Explain	Put an X on	Write

Written Directions: Primary (K–2)

Above
Add
Add the proper ending
Alphabetize
Answer Questions
Ask
Begin
Below
Bottom
Box
Bubble in
Categorize
Change
Choose
Circle
Classify
Color
Combine
Complete
Connect
Continue
Copy
Create
Cross-out
Cut
Describe
Draw
End
Enter
Fill
Fill-in-blank
Find
Finish
Follow
How
Label
Locate
Look
Loop
Make
Many
Margin
Matching (Draw a line to match)
Measure
Name
Page
Paste
Paste/Glue
Pick
Place
Point
Practice
Print
Put
Re-read
Read
Refer
Rewrite
Ring
Rule
See
Share
Sort
Start
Subtract
Tell
Think
Top
Trace
Trade
Turn
Underline
Underneath
Unscramble
Use
What
Where
Which
Write letter
Write word

Oral Directions: Intermediate (3–5)

After
Answer
Before
Begin
Build
Check
Circle
Clear
Close
Come
Continue
Correct
Count
Create
Decide
Define
Describe
Display
Do
Draw a line
During
Explain
Express
Feel
Fill in the word
Finally
Find
Finish
First
Flip
Focus
Follow
Go
Imitate
Include
Join
Know
Later
Learn
Leave
Listen
Look
Mark
Measure
Move
Name
Next
Notice
Now
Number
Only
Open
Outline
Pick
Place
Point
Practice
Prepare
Pronounce
Put
Raise
Re-read
Read
Remember
Reply
Report
Review
Revise
Say
Say the word
See
Select
Show
Sit
Solve
Soon
Speak
Spell
Stand
State
Stay
String
Study
Summarize
Take
Tell
Then
Think
Top
Total
Touch
Underline
Wait
Watch
What happened
When
Why did
Write

Written Directions: Intermediate (3–5)

Add
Analyze
Answer
Apply
Arrange
Browse
Change
Chart
Check
Choose
Circle
Color
Combine
Compare
Complete
Construct
Contrast
Copy
Count
Decide
Define
Describe
Divide
Double
Draw
Estimate
Examine
Exchange
Explain
Extend
Figure
Fill
Find
Finish
Form
Graph
Group
Include
Interpret
Join
Justify
List
Look
Make
Map
Match
Measure
Multiply
Note
Number
Observe
Omit
Order
Organize
Outline
Play
Point
Practice
Predict
Pretend
Proceed
Produce
Proofread
Read
Refer
Relate
Replace
Respond
Revise
Rewrite
Say
Separate
Shade
Show
Solve
Spell
Study
Subtract
Talk
Tell
Test
Total
Touch
Try
Underline
Unscramble
Use
Write

Oral Directions: Middle School (6–8)

Alphabetize	Generate	Proofread
Analyze	Highlight	Rank
Attach	Illustrate	Re-read
Best	Later	Recall
Better	Least	Refer
Beyond	Likely	Relationship
Bottom	Limit	Repeat
Center	List	Return
Check	Look	Revise
Choose	Margin	Rewrite
Continue	Mark	Share
Copy	Most	Solve
Correct	Next	Staple
Count	Note	Tent
Cover	Notice	Think
Data	Open	Top
Earlier	Order	Turn
Example	Pass up	Underline
Final	Practice	Unlikely
Focus	Pronounce	Vary

Written Directions: Middle School (6–8)

Align
Analysis
Apply
Attach
Balance
Circle
Classify
Compare
Connect
Construct
Continue
Contrast
Correlate
Count
Create
Delete
Describe
Develop
Diagram
Differentiate
Draw
Elaborate
Eliminate
Equate
Explain
Extend
Formulate
Graph
Height
Include
Indent
Interpret
Invert
Join
Length
Limit
Locate
Mark
Match
Measure
Order
Outline
Paraphrase
Range
Rearrange
Sequence
Simplify
Sketch
Solve
Summarize
Transfer
Underline
Width

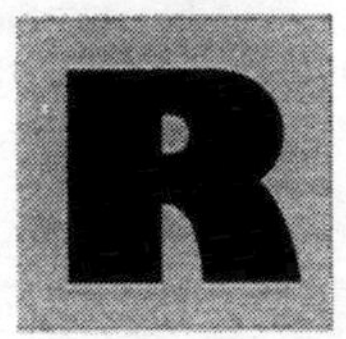

REFERENCES

Abrahamsen, E., & Rigrodsky, S. (1984). Comprehension of complex sentences in children at three levels of cognitive development. *Journal of Psycholinguistic Research, 13*, 333–350.

Adjemian, C. (1983). The transferability of lexical properties. In S. Gass & L. Selinker (Eds.), *Language transfer in language learning* (pp. 250–268). Rowley, MA: Newbury House.

Akmajian, A., Demers, R. A., Farmer, A. K., & Harnish, R. M. (1990). *Linguistics: An introduction to language and communication.* Cambridge, MA: MIT Press.

Albert, M. L., & Obler, L. K. (1978). *The bilingual brain: Neuropsychological and neurolinguistic aspects of bilingualism.* New York: Academic Press.

Alverman, D. (1991). The discussion web: A graphic aid for learning across the curriculum. *The Reading Teacher, 45*, 92–99.

Alverman, D. E., Smith, L. C., & Readence, J. (1985). Prior knowledge activation and the comprehension of compatible and incompatible text. *Reading Research Quarterly, 20*, 420–436.

American Speech-Hearing-Language Association. (1982). Definitions: Communicative disorders and variations. *Asha, 24*, 949–950.

Anderson, R. (1983). Transfer to somewhere. In S. Gass & L. Selinker (Eds.), *Language transfer in language learning* (pp. 177–201). Rowley, MA: Newbury House.

Apthorp, H. (1995). Phonetic coding and reading in college students with and without learning disabilities. *Journal of Learning Disabilities, 28*, 342–352.

Ardery, G. (1980). On coordination in child language. *Journal of Child Language, 7*, 305–320.

Atkinson-King, K. (1973). Children's acquisition of phonological stress contrasts. *UCLA Working Papers in Phonetics*, No. 25.

Au, K. H. (1979). Using the experience-text-relationship method with minority children. *Reading Teacher, 32*, 677–679.

Au, K. H., & Jordan, C. (1981). Teaching reading to Hawaiian children: Finding a culturally appropriate solution. In H Turega, G. Guthrie, & K. Au (Eds.), *Culture and the bilingual classroom: Studies in classroom ethnography* (pp. 139–152). Rowley, MA: Newbury House.

Austin, J. L. (1962). *How to do things with words.* New York: Oxford University Press.

Backscheider, A., & Gelman, S. (1995). Children's understanding of homonyms. *Journal of Child Language, 22*, 107–127.

Bain, B. A., Olswang, L. B., & Johnson, G. A. (1992). Language sampling for repeated measures wih language-impaired preschoolers: Comparison of two procedures. *Topics in Language Disorders, 12*(2), 13–27.

Baldie, B. M. (1976). The acquisition of the passive voice. *Journal of Child Language, 3*, 331–348.

Ball, E. W. (1997). Phonological awareness: Implications for whole language and emergent literacy programs. *Topics in Language Disorders, 17*(3), 14–26.

Ball, E. W., & Blachman, B. A. (1988). Phoneme segmentation training: Effect on reading readiness. *Annals of Dyslexia, 38*, 208–225.

Ball, E. W., & Blachman, B. A. (1991). Does phoneme awareness training in kindergarten make a difference in early word recognition and developmental spelling? *Reading Research Quarterly, 26*(1), 49–66.

Baratz, J. C., & Shuy, R. W. (Eds.). (1969). *Teaching black children to read.* Washington DC: Center for Applied Linguistics.

Barclay, D., & Walwer, L. (1992). Linking lyrics and literacy through song picture books. *Young Children, 14*, 76–85.

Bates, E., Marchman, V., Thal, D., Fenson, L., Dale, P., Reznick, J. S., Reilly, J., & Hartung, J. (1994). Developmental and stylistic variation in the composition of early vocabulary. *Journal of Child Language, 21*, 85–123.

Bates, E., & MacWhinney, B. (1987). Competition, variation, and language learning. In B. MacWhinney (Ed.), *Mechanisms of language acquisition* (pp. 157–194). Hillsdale, NJ: Lawrence Erlbaum.

Battle, D. E. (1996). Language learning and use by African American children. *Topics in Language Disorders, 16*(4), 22–37.

Beck, A. (1996). Language assessment methods for three age groups of children. *Journal of Children's Communication Development, 17*, 51–66.

Beers, J. W. (1974). *First and second grade children's developing orthographic concepts of tense and lax vowels* (Doctoral dissertation, University of Virginia, 1974). *Dissertation Abstracts International 35*(08), 4972. (University Microfilms, 1975 No. 75–4694)

Berk, L. (1994). *Infants and children: Prenatal through middle childhood.* Needham Heights, MA: Allyn & Bacon.

Berk, L. E. (1996). *Infants and children: Prenatal through middle childhood* (2nd ed.). Needham Heights, MA: Allyn & Bacon.

Berk, L. & Winsler, A. (1995). *Scaffolding children's learning: Vygotsky and early childhood education,* Washington, DC: National Association of Young Children.

Berko Gleason, J. (1971). The child's learning of English morphology. In B. A. Bar-Adon & W. F. Leopold (Eds.), *Child language: A book of readings* (pp. 153–167). Englewood Cliffs, NJ: Prentice-Hall. (Original work published 1958)

Berko Gleason, J. (1989). *The development of language* (2nd ed.). Columbus, OH: Merrill.

Berko Gleason, J. (1993). *The development of language* (3rd ed.). New York: Macmillan.

Bernhardt, E. (1991). *Reading development in a second language.* Norwood, NJ: Ablex.

Bernstein, D., & Tiegerman, E. (1993). *Language and communication disorders in children* (3rd ed.). New York: Merrill.

Bever, T. G. (1970). The cognitive basis for linguistic structures. In J. R. Hayes (Ed.), *Cognition and the development of language.* New York: John Wiley.

Bialystok, E., & Hakuta, K. (1994). *In other words: The science and psychology of second-language acquisition.* New York: Basic Books.

Bjork, R. A., & Bjork, E. L. (1992). A new theory of disuse and an old theory of stimulus fluctuation. In A. F. Healy, S. M. Kosslyn, & R. M. Shiffrin (Eds.), *From learning processes: Essays in honor of William K. Estes* (Vol. 2, pp. 35–67). Hillsdale, NJ: Lawrence Erlbaum.

Blachman, B. (1991). Early intervention for children's reading problems: Clinical applications of the research in phonological awareness. *Topics in Language Disorders, 12*(1), 51–65.

Blachman, B. (1994a). Early literacy acquisition: The role of phonological awareness. In G. Wallach & K. Butler (Eds.), *Language learning disabilities in school-age children and adolescents: Some principles and applications* (pp. 253–274). Needham Heights, MA: Allyn & Bacon.

Blachman, B. A. (1994b). What we have learned from longitudinal studies of phonological processing and reading, and some unanswered questions: A response to Torgesen, Wagner, and Rashotte. *Journal of Learning Disabilities, 27*(5), 287–291.

Bland, L. E., & Prelock, P. (1995). Effects of collaboration on language performance. *Journal of Children's Communication Development, 17*, 31–37.

Bloom, L. (1970). *Language development: Form and function of emerging grammars.* Cambridge: MIT Press.

Bloom, L. (1973). *One word at time: The use of single-word utterances before syntax.* The Hague: Mouton.

Bloom. L. (1988). What is language? In M. Lahey (Ed.), *Language disorders and language development.* New York: Merrill.

Bloom, L., & Lahey, M. (1978). *Language development and language disorders.* New York: John Wiley.

Bloom, L., Lahey, P., Hood, L., Lifter, K., & Fiess, K. (1980). Complex sentences: Acquisition of syntactic connectors and the semantic relations they encode. *Journal of Child Language, 7*, 235–262.

Boggs, S. T. (1972). The meaning of questions and narratives to Hawaiian children. In C. B. Cazden, V. P. John, & D. Hymes (Eds.), *Functions of language in the classroom* (pp. 299–327). New York: Teachers College Press.

Boggs, S. T. (1978). The development of verbal disputing in part-Hawaiian children. *Language in Society, 7*, 325–344.

Bornmouth, J. R. (Ed.). (1968). *Readability in 1968.* Urbana, IL: National Council of Teachers of English.

Bos C., & Vaughn, S. (1988). *Strategies for teaching students with learning and behavior problems.* Boston, MA: Allyn & Bacon.

Bos, C., & Vaughn, S. (1994). *Strategies for teaching students with learning and behavior problems* (3rd ed.). Boston, MA: Allyn & Bacon.

Bowerman, M. (1974). Discussion summary—Development of concepts underlying language. In R. Schiefelbusch & L. Lloyd (Eds.), *Language perspectives—Acquistion, retardation, and intervention* (pp. 191–209). Baltimore: University Park Press.

Bowerman, M. (1978). Systematizing semantic knowledge: Changes over time in the child's organization of word meaning. *Child Development, 49*, 977–987.

Bradley, L., & Bryant, P. (1978). Difficulties in auditory organization as a possible cause of reading backwardness. *Nature, 27*, 419–421.

Bradley, L., & Bryant, P. (1983). Categorizing sounds and learning to read: A causal connection. *Nature, 30*, 419–421.

Bradley, L., & Bryant, P. (1985). *Rhyme and reason in reading and spelling.* Ann Arbor, MI: University of Michigan Press.

Bradley, L., & Bryant, P. E. (1991). Phonological skills before and after leaning to read. In S. Brady & D. Shankweiler (Eds.), *Phonological processes in literacy* (pp. 47–54). Hillsdale, NJ: Lawrence Erlbaum.

Bridges, A. (1980). SVD comprehension strategies reconsidered: The evidence of individual patterns of response. *Journal of Child Language, 7*, 89–104.

Brinton, B., & Fujiki, M. (1984). Development of topic manipulation skills in discourse. *Journal of Speech and Hearing Research, 27*, 350–358.

Brown, A. L., & Palincsar, A. S. (1987). Reciprocal teaching of comprehension strategies: A natural history of one program for enhancing learning. In J. D. Day & J. G. Borkowski (Eds.), *Intelligence and exceptionality: New directions for theory, assessment, and instructional practices* (pp. 81–132). New York: Ablex.

Brown, R. (1970). The first sentences of child and chimpanzee. In R. Brown (Ed.), *Psycholinguistics: Selected papers* (pp. 208–231). New York: Free Press.

Brown, R. (1973). *A first language: The early stages.* Cambridge: Harvard University Press.

Brown, R., & Bellugi-Klima, U. (1971). Three processes in the child's acquisition of syntax. In B. A. Bar-Adon & W. F. Leopold (Eds.), *Child language: A book of readings* (pp. 307–318). Englewood Cliffs, NJ: Prentice-Hall. (Original work published 1964)

Brown, R., Cazden, C., & Bellugi-Klima, U. (1971). The child's grammar from I to III. In B. A. Bar-Adon & W. F. Leopold (Eds.), *Child language: A book of readings* (pp. 382–424). Englewood Cliffs, NJ: Prentice-Hall. (Original work published 1968)

Brown, R., & Fraser, C. (1963). The acquisition of syntax. In C. N. Cofer & B. S. Musgrave (Eds.), *Verbal behavior and learning* (pp. 158–197). New York: McGraw-Hill.

Bryson, B. (1990). *Mother tongue: English & how it got that way.* New York: Avon Books.

Bufkin, L., & Altman, R. (1995). A developmental study of nonverbal pragmatic communication in students with and without mild mental retardation. *Education and Training in Mental Retardation and Developmental Disabilities, 30*(3), 199–207.

Bunce, B. (1991). Referential communication skills: Guidelines for therapy. *Language Speech, and Hearing Services in Schools, 22*, 296–301.

Bursuck, W. (1989). A comparison of students with learning disabilities to low achieving and higher achieving students on three dimensions of social competence. *Journal of Learning Disabilities, 22*, 188–194.

Bybee, J., & Slobin, D. (1982). Rules and schemas in the development of the English past tense. *Language, 58*, 265–289.

Camarata, S., & Schwartz, R. (1985). Production of object words and action words: Evidence for a relationship between phonology and semantics. *Journal of Speech and Hearing Research, 28*, 323–330.

Cambon, J., & Sinclair, H. (1974). Relations between syntax and semantics: Are they "easy to see"? *British Journal of Psychology, 65*, 133–140.

Cantwell, D. P., & Baker, L. (1987). *Developmental speech and language disorders.* New York: Guilford Press.

Catts, H. W. (1996). Defining dyslexia as a developmental language disorder: An expanded view. *Topics in Languge Disorders, 16*(2), 14–29.

Chafe, W. (1970). *Meaning and the structure of language.* Chicago: University of Chicago Press.
Cheng, L. (1996). Beyond bilingualism: A quest for communicative competence. *Topics in Language Disorders, 16*(4), 9–21.
Cheng, L., & Butler, K. (1989). Code-switching: A natural phenomeonon vs. language deficiency. *World Englishes, 8,* 293–310.
Chomsky, C. S. (1969). *The acquisition of syntax in children from 5 to 10.* Cambridge, MA: MIT Press.
Chomsky, N. (1965). *Aspects of the theory of syntax.* Cambridge: MIT Press.
Clark, E. V. (1971). On the acquisition of before and after. *Journal of Verbal Learning and Verbal Behavior, 10,* 266–275.
Clark, E. V. (1973). What's in a word? On the child's acquisition of semantics in his first language. In T. E. Moore (Ed.), *Cognitive development and the acquisition of language* (pp. 65–110). New York: Academic Press.
Clark, E. V. (1974). Some aspects of the conceptual basis for first language acquisition. In R. L. Schiefelbusch & L. L. Lloyd (Eds.), *Language perspectives: Acquisition, retardation, and intervention* (pp. 105–128). Baltimore: University Park Press.
Clark, E. V. (1979). Building a vocabulary: Words for objects, actions, and relations. In P. Fletcher & M. Garman (Eds.), *Language acquisition.* Cambridge: Cambridge University Press.
Clark, E. V. (1981). Lexical innovations: How children learn to create new words. In W. Deutsch (Ed.), *The child's construction of language* (pp. 299–328). London: Academic Press.
Clark, E., Gelman, S., & Lane, N. (1985). Compound nouns and category structure in young children. *Child Development, 56,* 84–94.
Clark, H. H., & Clark, E. V. (1977). *Psychology and language: An introduction to psycholinguistics.* New York: Harcourt Brace Jovanovich.
Clarke-Klein, S. M. (1994). Expressive phonological deficiencies: Impact on spelling development. *Topics in Language Disorders, 14*(2), 40–55.
Clarke-Klein, S., & Hodson, B. W. (1995). A phonologically based analysis of misspellings by third graders with disordered-phonology histories. *Journal of Speech and Hearing Research, 38,* 839–849.
Clement-Heist, K., Siegel, S. & Gaylord-Ross,R. (1992). Simulated and *in situ* vocational social skills training for youths with learning disabilities. *Exceptional Children, 58,* 336–345.
Cole, L. (1989). E pluribus pluribus: Multicultural imperatives for the 1990s and beyond. *Asha, 31,* 65–70.
Cole, P. A., & Taylor, O. L. (1990). Performances of working class African American children on three tests of articulation. *Language, Speech, and Hearing Services in Schools, 21*(3), 171–176.
Cowan, N. (1996). Short-term memory, working memory and language processing. *Topics in Language Disorders, 17,* 1–18.
Crago, M. B. (1992). Ethnography and language socialization: A cross-cultural perspective. *Topics in Language Disorders, 12*(3), 28–39.
Craig, H. K., & Washington, J. A. (1994). The complex syntax skills of poor, urban, African-American preschoolers at school entry. *Language, Speech, and Hearing Services in Schools, 25*(3), 181–190.
Craig, H. K., & Washington, J. A. (1995). African-American English and linguistic complexity in preschool discourse: A second look. *Language, Speech, and Hearing Services in Schools, 26*(1), 87–92.
Crais, E. R. (1990). World knowledge to word knowledge. *Topics in Language Disorders, 10,* 45–62.

Cromer, R. F. (1970). Children are nice to understand: Surface structure clues for the recovery of a deep structure. *British Journal of Psychology, 61*, 397–408.

Cromer, R. (1988). Differentiating language and cognition. In R. L. Schiefelbusch & L. L. Lloyd (Eds.), *Language perspectives* (2nd ed., pp. 91–124). Austin, TX: Pro-Ed.

Crystal, D., Fletcher, P., & Garman, M. (1976). *The grammatical analysis of language disability*. New York: American Elsevier.

Cummins, J. (1984). *Bilingualism and special education: Issues in assessment and pedagogy*. San Diego: College-Hill Press.

Cummins, J. (1988). Second language acquisition within bilingual education programs. In L. M. Beebe (Ed.), *Issues in second language acquisition: Multiple perspectives* (pp. 145–166). New York: Newbury House.

Cummins, J. (1989). A theoretical framework for bilingual special education. *Exceptional Children, 56*(2), 111–119.

Dale, P. S. (1972). *Language development: Structure and function*. Hinsdale, IL: Dryden Press.

deVilliers, J., & deVilliers, P. (1973). Development of the use of word order in comprehension. *Journal of Psycholinguistic Research, 2*, 331–341.

deVilliers, P. A., & deVilliers, J. G. (1979). *Early language*. Cambridge, MA: Harvard University Press.

Dicker, S. J. (1993). "Ethnic irrelevance" and the immigrant: Finding a place for minority languages. *The Educational Forum, 57*(2), 120–133.

Dillard, J. (1972). *Black English*. New York: Random House.

Dockrell, J., & Campbell, R. (1986). Lexical acquisition strategies in the preschool child. In S. Kuczaj & M. Barrett (Eds.), *The development of word meaning* (pp. 121–154). Berlin: Springer-Verlag.

Dollaghan, C. A., & Campbell, T. F. (1992). A procedure for classifying disruptions in spontaneous language samples. *Topics in Language Disorders, 12*(2), 56–68.

Donahue, M. (1984). Learning disabled children's conversational competence: An attempt to activate the inactive listener. *Applied Psycholinguistics, 5*, 21–35.

Donahue, M. (1997). Beliefs about listening in students with learning disabilities: "Is the speaker always right?" *Topics in Language Disorders, 17*(3), 41–61.

Donaldson, M., & Wales, R. J. (1970). On the acquisition of some relational terms. In J. R. Hayes (Ed.), *Cognition and the development of language* (pp. 235–268). New York: John Wiley.

Dore, J. (1974). A pragmatic description of early language development. *Journal of Psycholinguistic Research, 3*, 343–350.

Dowker, A. (1989). Rhyme and alliteration in poems elicited from young children. *Journal of Child Language, 16*, 181–202.

Dulay, H., & Burt, M. (1983). Goofing: An indicator of children's second language learning and strategies. In S. Gass & L. Selinker (Eds.), *Language transfer in language learning* (pp. 54–68). Rowley, MA: Newbury House.

Dunham, P., Dunham, E., & Curwin, A. (1993). Joint–attentional states and lexical acquisition at 18 months. *Developmental Psychology, 29*, 827–831.

Dunn, L., & Dunn, L. (1981). *Peabody Picture Vocabulary Test* (rev. ed.). Circle Pines, MN: American Guidance Service.

Echevarria, J. (1995). Interactive reading instruction: A comparison of proximal and distal effects of instructional conversations. *Exceptional Children, 61*(6), 536–552.

Echevarria, J., & McDonough, R. (1995). An alternative reading approach: Instructional conversations in a bilingual special education setting. *Learning Disabilities Research & Practice, 10*(2), 108–119.

Englert, C., & Mariage, T. (1996). A sociocultural perspective. Teaching ways-of-thinking and ways-of-talking in a literacy community. *Learning Disabilities Research and Practice, 11*, 157–167.

Ervin–Tripp, S. (1970). Discourse agreement: How children answer questions. In J. R. Hayes (Ed.), *Cognition and the development of language* (pp. 79–107). New York: John Wiley.

Fasold, R. W., & Wolfram, W. (1978). Some linguistic features of Negro dialect. In P. Stoller (Ed.), *Black American English* (pp. 49–83). New York: Delta.

Fazio, B. (1996). Serial memory in children with specific language impairment: Examining specific content areas for assessment and intervention. *Topics in Language Disorders, 17*(1), 58–71.

Feagans, L., & Short, E. (1986). Referential communication and reading performance in learning disabled children over a 3-year period. *Developmental Psychology, 22*, 177–183.

Felton, R. (1992). Early identification of children at risk for reading disabilities. *Topics in Early Childhood Special Education 12*, 212–229.

Fey, M., Catts, H., & Larrivee, L. (1995). Preparing preschoolers for the academic and social challenges of school. In M. Fey, J. Windsor, & S. Warren (Eds.), *Language intervention: Preschool through the elementary years*. Baltimore: Paul H. Brookes.

Fillmore, C. (1968). The case for case. In E. Bach & R. Harms (Eds.), *Universals in linguistic theory*. New York: Holt, Rinehart & Winston.

Fillmore, L. W. (1976). *The second time around: Cognitive and social strategies in second language acquisition*. Doctoral dissertation, Stanford University, Palo Alto, CA.

Fillmore, L. W. (1983). The language learner as an individual: Implications of research on individal differences for the ESL teacher. In J. Handscombe & M. Clarke (Eds.), *On TESOL 82: Pacific perspectives on language learning and teaching*. Washington, DC: Teachers of English to Speakers of Other Languages.

Flavell, J. H., Beach, D. R., & Chinsky, J. N. (1966). Spontaneous verbal rehearsal in a memory task as a function of age. *Child Development, 37*, 283–299.

Fokes, J. (1976). *Fokes Sentence Builder*. Boston: Teaching Resources.

Foster, S. (1986). Learning discourse topic management in the preschool years. *Journal of Child Language, 13*, 231–250.

Fraser, C., Bellugi, U., & Brown, R. (1970). Control of grammar in imitation, comprehension, and production. In R. Brown (Ed.), *Psycholinguistics: Selected papers*. New York: Free Press. (Original work published 1963)

Freeman, D. E., & Freeman, Y. S. (1994). *Between worlds: Access to second language acquisition*. Portsmouth, NH: Heinemann.

Fromkin, V., & Rodman, R. (1988). *An introduction to language* (4th ed.). New York: Holt, Rinehart & Winston.

Fujiki, M., & Brinton, B. (1994). Social competence and language impairment in children. In R. Watkins & M. Rice (Eds.), *Specific language impairments in children* (pp. 123–144). Baltimore, MD: Paul H. Brooks.

Gallagher, T. M., & Craig, H. K. Stuctural characteristics of monologues in the speech of normal children: Semantic and conversational aspects. *Journal of Speech and Hearing Research, 21*, 103–117.

Garcia, E. (1994). *Understanding and meeting the challenge of student cultural diversity*. Boston: Houghton Mifflin.

Garcia, G. E. (1992). Ethnography and classroom communication: Taking an "emic" perspective. *Topics in Language Disorders, 12*(3), 54–66.

Garcia, G. E., Pearson, P. D., & Jiminez, R. T. (1990). *The at-risk dilemma: A synthesis of reading research* (study 2.2.3.3b). Urbana-Champaign, IL: University of Illinois, Reading Research & Education Center.

Gardner, H., & Winner, E. (1979, May). The child is father to the metaphor. *Psychology Today*, 81–91.

Gardner, M. F. (1985). *Receptive One-word Picture Vocabulary Test* (rev. ed.). Novato, CA: Academic Therapy Publications.

Gardner, M. F. (1990). *Receptive One-word Picture Vocabulary Test* (rev. ed.). Novato, CA: Academic Therapy Publications.

Geller, E. (1991). The interplay between linguistic and social-cognitive knowledge in perspective–taking by autistic children. *Journal of Childhood Communication Disorders, 14*(1), 23–44.

Gentner, D. (1982). Why nouns are learned before verbs: Linguistic relativity versus natural partitioning. In S. A. Kuczaj II (Ed.), *Language development: Vol. 2. Language, thought and culture* (pp. 301–334). Hillsdale, NJ: Lawrence Erlbaum.

Gerber, S. (1991). Pragmatics in the 1990's: Perspective, retrospective, prospective. *Journal of Childhood Communication Disorders, 14*(1), 1–21.

German, D. (1992). Word-finding intervention for children and adolescents. *Topics in Language Disorders, 13*, 33–50.

Gerritz, K. E. (1974). *First graders' spelling of vowels: An exploratory study.* Unpublished doctoral dissertation, Harvard University, Cambridge, MA.

Gersten, R., Brengelman, S., & Jimenez, R. (1994). Effective instruction for culturally and linguistically diverse students: A reconceptualization. *Focus on Exceptional Children, 27*(1).

Gersten, R., & Woodward, J. (1995). A longitudinal study of transitional and immersion bilingual education programs in one district. *The Elementary School Journal, 95*, 223–239.

Gibbs, D. P., & Cooper, E. B. (1989). Prevalence of communication disorder in students with learning disabilities. *Journal of Learning Disabilities, 22*, 60–63.

Gillam, R. B., & van Kleeck, A. (1996). Phonological awareness training and short-term working memory: Clinical implications. *Topics in Language Disorders, 17*(1), 72–81.

Gitterman, D., & Johnston, J. (1983). Talking about comparisons: A study of young children's comparative adjective usage. *Journal of Child Language, 10*, 605–621.

Goldenberg, C. (1992–1993). Instructional conversations: Promoting comprehension through discussion. *Reading Teacher, 46*, 316–326.

Goldstein, A. P., Sprafkin, R. P., Gershaw, N. J., & Klein, P. (1980). *Skillstreaming the adolescent.* Champaign, IL: Research Press.

Goldstein, B. S. C. (1995). Critical pedagogy in a bilingual special education classroom. *Journal of Learning Disabilities, 28*, 463–475.

Goldstein P. A. (1994). *A comparison of language screening procedures in the identification of children with language delays in prekindergarten classes.* (Doctoral dissertation, Florida Atlantic University, Boca Raton, FL, 1994). *Dissertation Abstracts International, 55*(09), 2791.

Goodman, K. S. (1965). Dialect barriers to reading comprehension. *Elementary English, 42*, 853.

Goodman, K. S. & Buck, C. (1973). Dialect barriers to comprehension revisited. *The Reading Teacher, 25*, 6–12.

Graves, D. H. (1983). *Writing: Teachers and children at work.* Exeter, NH: Heinemann Books.

Graves, M., & Koziol, S. (1971). Noun plural development in primary grade children. *Child Development, 42*, 1165–1173.

Greene, J. F. (1996). Psycholinguistic assessment: The clinical base for identification of dyslexia. *Topics in Language Disorders, 16*(2), 45–72.

Grice, H. P. (1975). Logic and conversation. In P. Cole & J. L. Morgan (Eds.), *Syntax and semantics 3: Speech acts* (pp. 41–58). New York: Academic Press.

Guralnick, M., & Paul-Brown, D. (1980). Functional discourse analysis of nonhandicapped children's speech to handicapped children. *American Journal of Mental Deficiency, 84,*

Hakes, D. (1982). The development of metalinguistic abilities: What develops? In S. Kuczaj (Ed.), *Language development: Vol. 2. Language, thought and culture.* Hillsdale, NJ: Lawrence Erlbaum.

Hampson, J. (1989). *Elements of style: Maternal and child contributions to the referential and expressive styles of language acquisition.* Unpublished doctoral dissertation, City University of New York.

Hanna, P. R., Hanna, J. S., Hodges, R. E., & Rudorf, E. H. (1966). *Phoneme-grapheme correspondences as cues to spelling improvement.* Washington, DC: U.S. Department of Health, Education and Welfare.

Haring, K., Lovett, D., Haney, K., Algozzine, B., Smith, D., & Clarke, J. (1992). Labeling preschoolers as learning disabled: A cautionary position. *Topics in Early Childhood Special Education,12,* 151–173.

Hazel, J.S., Schumaker, J. B., Sherman, J. A., & Sheldon-Wildgen, J. (1981). *ASSET.* Champaign, IL: Research Press.

Heath, S. B. (1982). Questioning at school and at home: A comparative study. In G. Spindler (Ed.), *Doing the ethnography of schooling: Educational anthropology in action* (pp. 102–131). Orlando, FL: Holt, Rinehart & Winston.

Heimlich, J., & Pittelman, S. (1986). *Semantic mapping: Classroom applications.* Newark, DE: International Reading Association.

Hodson, B. (1994). Helping individuals become intelligible, literate and articulate: The role of phonology. *Topics in Language Disorders, 14,* 1–16.

Hodson, B. W., & Paden, E. P. (1981). Phonological processes which characterize unintelligible and intelligible speech in early childhood. *Journal of Speech and Hearing Disorders, 46,* 369–373.

Hodson, B., & Paden, E. (1991). *Targeting intelligible speech: A phonological approach to remediation* (2nd ed.). Austin, TX: Pro-Ed.

Hoffman, P. R. (1997). Phonological intervention within storybook reading. *Topics in Language Disorders, 17,* 69–88.

Hoffman, P. R., & Norris, J. A. (1989). On the nature of phonological development: Evidence from normal children's spelling errors. *Journal of Speech and Hearing Research, 32,* 787–794.

Hoggan, K. C., & Strong, C. J. (1994). The magic of "once upon a time": Narrative teaching strategies. *Language, Speech, and Hearing Services in Schools, 25,* 76–89.

Hopper, R., & Naremore, R. C. (1978). *Children's speech: A practical introduction to communication development* (2nd ed.). New York: Harper & Row.

Horgan, D. (1978). The development of the full passive. *Journal of Child Language, 5,* 65–80.

Horwitz, E. (1971). *The strange story of the frog who became a prince.* New York: Delacorte.

Hummel, L., & Prizant, M. (1993). A socioemotional perspective for understanding social difficulties of school-age children with language disorders. *Language, Speech, and Hearing Services in Schools, 24,* 216–224.

Hunt, P., Alwell, M., Goetz, L., & Sailor, W. (1990). Generalized effects of conversation skill training. *Journal of the Association for Persons with Severe Handicaps, 15,* 250–260.

Ingram, D. (1976). Current issues in child phonology. In D. M. Morehead & A. E. Morehead (Eds.), *Normal and deficient child language* (pp. 3–25). Baltimore: University Park Press.

Jakobson, R. (1971). Why "mama" and "papa"? In B. A. Bar-Adon & W. F. Leopold (Eds.), *Child language: A book of readings* (pp. 213–217). Englewood Cliffs, NJ: Prentice-Hall. (Original work published 1962)

Jenkins, R., & Bowen, L. (1994). Facilitating development of preliterate children's phonological abilities. *Topics in Language Disorders, 14*(2), 26–39.

Kamhi, A., & Catts, H. (1989). *Reading disabilities: A developmental language perspective.* Boston, MA: Little, Brown.

Keogh, B. K., Gallimore, R., & Weisner, T. (1997). A sociocultural perspective on learning and learning disabilities. *Learning Disabilities Research and Practice, 12*(2), 197–113.

Kessel, F. S. (1970). The role of syntax in children's comprehension from ages six to twelve. *Monographs of the Society for Research in Child Development, 35*, 6.

Kirchner, D. (1991). Using verbal scaffolding to facilitate conversational participation and language acquisition in children with pervasive developmental disorders. *Journal of Childhood Communication Disorders, 14*, 81–98.

Kit-Fong Au, T. (1990). Children's use of information in word learning. *Journal of Child Language, 17*, 393–419.

Klima, E. S., & Bellugi-Klima, U. (1971). Syntactic regularities in the speech of children. In B. A. Bar-Adon & W. F. Leopold (Eds.), *Child language: A book of readings* (pp. 412–424). Englewood Cliffs, NJ: Prentice-Hall. (Original work published 1966)

Knapp, L. (1972). *Nonverbal communication in human interaction.* New York: Holt, Rinehart & Winston.

Kotsonis, M., & Patterson, C. (1980). Comprehension-monitoring skills in learning disabled children. *Developmental Psychology, 16*, 541–542.

Krashen, S. D. (1992). *Fundamentals of language education.* Torrance, CA: Laredo.

Krashen, S. D., & Biber, D. (1988). *On course: Bilingual education's successes in California.* Sacramento: California Association for Bilingual Education.

Labov, W. (1969). *The logic of Nonstandard English.* Georgetown University 20th Annual Round Table. Monograph Series on Languages and Linguistics, No. 22.

Lahey, M. (Ed.). (1988). *Language disorders and language development.* New York: Merrill.

Lakoff, G. (1971). On generative semantics. In D. Steinberg & L. Jakobovits (Eds.), *Semantics: An interdisciplinary reader in philosophy, linguistics and psychology.* London: Cambridge University Press.

Langdon, H. W. (1996). English language learning by immigrant Spanish speakers: A United States perspective. *Topics in Language Disorders, 16*(4), 38–53.

Lapadat, J. C. (1991). Pragmatic language skills of students with language and/or learning disabilities: A quantitative synthesis. *Journal of Learning Disabilities, 24*(3), 147–158.

Layton, T., & Stick, S. (1979). Comprehension and production of comparatives and superlatives. *Journal of Child Language, 6*, 511–527.

Lazar, R., Warr-Leeper, G., Nicholson, C., & Johnson, S. (1989). Elementary school teacher's use of multiple meaning expressions. *Language, Speech, and Hearing Services in the Schools, 20*, 420–430.

Lederer, R. (1987). *Anguished English.* Charleston, SC: Wyrick.

Lederer, R. (1991). *Crazy English.* New York: Dell.

Lee, L. L. (1974). *Developmental sentence analysis: A grammatical assessment procedure for speech and language clinicians.* Evanston, IL: Northwestern University Press.

Leech, G. (1970). *Towards a semantic description of English.* Bloomington: Indiana University Press.

Lenz, B.K. (1983). Promoting active learning through effective instruction: Using advance organizers. *Pointer, 27*(2), 11–13.

Leonard, L. B., & McGregor, K. K. (1991). Unusual phonological patterns and their underlying representations: A case study. *Journal of Child Language, 18,* 261–271.

Limber, J. (1973). The genesis of complex sentences. In T. E. Moore (Ed.), *Cognitive development and the acquisition of language* (pp. 169–185). New York: Academic Press.

Linden, E. (1993, March 22). Can animals think? *Time,* 54–61.

Lindfors, J. W. (1980). *Children's language and learning.* Englewood Cliffs, NJ: Prentice-Hall.

Lindfors, J. W. (1987). *Children's language and learning* (2nd ed.). Englewood Cliffs, NJ: Prentice-Hall.

Lopez–Reyna, N. A. (1996). The importance of meaningful contexts in bilingual special education: Moving to whole language. *Learning Disabilities Research and Practice, 11*(2), 120–131.

Lovell, K., & Dixon, E. M. (1965). The growth of the control of grammar in imitation, comprehension, and production. *Journal of Child Psychology and Psychiatry, 5,* 1–9.

Lucas, E. V. (1980). *Semantic and pragmatic language disorders.* Rockville, MD: Aspen.

Lund, N. J., & Duchan, J. F. (1988). *Assessing children's language in naturalistic contexts* (2nd ed.). Englewood Cliffs, NJ: Prentice-Hall.

Lund, N. J., & Duchan, J. F. (1993). *Assessing children's language in naturalistic contexts* (3rd ed.). Englewood Cliffs, NJ: Prentice-Hall.

Lust, B., & Mervis, C. (1980). Development of coordination in the natural speech of young children. *Journal of Child Language, 7,* 279–304.

Maccarone, G., & Lewin, B. (1992). *Itchy, itchy, chicken pox.* New York: Scholastic.

MacDonald, G. W., & Cornwall, A. (1995). The relationship between phonological awareness and reading and spelling achievement eleven years later. *Journal of Learning Disabilities, 28,* 523–527.

Maratsos, M. P. (1974). Children who get worse at understanding the passive: A replication of Bever. *Journal of Psycholinguistic Research, 3,* 65–74.

Maratsos, M. (1976). *The use of definite and indefinite reference in young children: An experimental study of semantic acquisition.* Cambridge: Canbridge University Pres.

Maratsos, M. P., & Abramovitch, R. (1975). How children understand full, truncated, and anomalous passives. *Journal of Verbal Learning and Verbal Behavior, 14,* 145–157.

Maratsos, M. P., Kuczaj, S. A., Fox, D. E. C., & Chalkley, M. A. (1979). Some empirical studies in the acquisition of transformational relations: Passives, negatives, and the past tense. In W. A. Collins (Ed.), *Children's language and communication.* Hillsdale, NJ: Lawrence Erlbaum.

Martin, R. C. (1993). Short-term memory and sentence processing: Evidence from neuropsychology. *Memory and Cognition, 21,* 176–183.

Marvin, C., & Hunt-Berg, M. (1996). Let's Pretend! A semantic analysis of preschool children's play. *Journal of Children's Communication Development, 17,* 1–10.

McCord, J., & Haynes, W. (1988). Discourse errors in students with learning disabilities and their normally achieving peers: Molar versus molecular views. *Journal of Learning Disabilities, 21,* 237–243.

McGinnis, E., & Goldstein, A. P. (1984). *Skillstreaming the elementary school child.* Champaign, IL: Research Press.

McGregor, K., & Leonard, L. (1995). Intervention for word-finding deficits in children. In M. E. Fey, E. Windsor, & S. F. Warren (Eds.), *Language intervention: Preschool through the elementary years.* Baltimore, MD: Paul H. Brookes.

McLean, J., & Snyder-McLean, L. (1978). *A transactional approach to early language training.* Columbus, OH: Merrill.

Mclean, M., Bailey, D., & Wolery, M. (1996). *Assessing infants and preschoolers with special needs.* Englewood Cliffs, NJ: Prentice-Hall.

McNeill, J., & Fowler, S. (1996). Using story reading to encourage children's conversations. *Teaching Exceptional Children, 28,* 43–47.

Mellard, D. F., & Hazel, J. S. (1992). Social competencies as a pathway to successful life transitions. *Learning Disabilities Quarterly, 15,* 251–271.

Mentis, M. (1991). Topic management in the discourse of normal and language impaired children. *Journal of Childhood Communication Disorders, 14*(1), 45–66.

Mentis, M. (1994). Topic management in discourse: Assessment and intervention. *Topics in Language Disorders, 14,* 29–54.

Menyuk, P. (1977). *Language and maturation.* Cambridge: MIT Press.

Menyuk, P., & Menn, L. (1979). Early strategies for the perception and production of words and sounds. In P. Fletcher & M. Garman (Eds.), *Language acquisition: Studies in first language development.* New York: Cambridge University Press.

Merrill, E., & Bilsky, L. (1990). Individual differences in the representation of sentences in memory. *American Journal on Mental Retardation, 95,* 68–76.

Merrill, E., & Jackson, T. (1992). Sentence processing by adolescents with and without mental retardation. *American Journal on Mental Retardation, 97*(3), 342–50.

Merrill, E., & Jackson, T. (in press). Sentence processing by mentally retarded and nonretarded adolescents. *American Journal on Mental Retardation.*

Merritt, D. D., & Liles, B. Z. (1987). Story grammar ability in children with and without language disorder: A story generation, story retelling, and story comprehension. *Journal of Speech and Hearing Research, 30,* 539–552.

Milk, R., Mercado, C., & Sapiens, A. (1992). *Re-thinking the education of teachers of language minority children: Developing reflective teachers for changing schools* (FOCUS No. 6). Washington, DC: National Clearinghouse for Bilingual Education.

Miller, J. (1981). *Assessing language production in children.* Baltimore: University Park Press.

Miller, J., & Chapman, R. (1981). The relation between age and mean length of utterance in morphemes. *Journal of Speech and Hearing Research, 24,* 154–161.

Miller, W. R., & Ervin, S. M. (1971). The development of grammar in child language. In B. A. Bar-Adon & W. F. Leopold (Eds.), *Child language: A book of readings* (pp. 321–339). Englewood Cliffs, NJ: Prentice-Hall. (Original work published 1964)

Moats, L. C., & Lyon, G. R. (1996). Wanted: Teachers with knowledge of language. *Topics in Language Disorders, 16*(2), 73–86.

Montgomery, J. W. (1996). Sentence comprehension and working memory in children with specific language impairment. *Topics in Language Disorders, 17*(1), 19–32.

Morse, P. A. (1972). The discrimination of speech and nonspeech stimuli in early infancy. *Journal of Experimental Child Psychology, 14,* 477–492.

Moskowitz, A. (1970). The two-year-old stage in the acquisition of English phonology. *Language, 46,* 426–441.

Nabuzoka, D. & Smith, P., (1995). Identification of expressions of emotions by children with and without learning disabilities. *Learning Disabilities Research and Practice, 10,* 91–101.

Naigles, L., & Gelman, S. (1995). Overextensions in comprehension and production revisited: Preferential-looking in a study of "dog," "cat," and "cow." *Journal of Child Language, 22,* 19–46.

Naremore, R., & Dever, R. (1975). Language performance of educable mentally retarded and normal children at five age levels. *Journal of Speech and Hearing Research, 18,* 82–95.

Nelson, K. (1973). Structure and strategy in learning to talk. *Monographs of the Society for Research in Child Development, 38*(1/2), Serial No. 149.

Nelson, K. (1974). Concept, word, and sentence: Interrelations in acquisition and development. *Psychological Review, 8,* 267–285.

Nelson, K., Hampson, J., & Shaw, L. (1993). Nouns in early lexicons: Evidence, explanations and implications. *Child Language, 20,* 61–84.

Nelson, N. W. (1993). *Childhood language disorders in context: Infancy through adolescence.* New York: Macmillan.

Newman, B., Buffington, D., & Hemmes, N. (1996). Self-reinforcement used to increase the appropriate conversation of autistic teenagers. *Education and Training in Mental Retardation and Developmental Disabilities, 31,* 304–309.

Nicolosi, L., Harryman, E., & Kresheck, J. (1996). *Terminology of communication disorders: Speech-language-hearing* (4th ed.). Baltimore: Williams & Wilkins.

Nippold, M. A. (1985). Comprehension of figurative language in youth. *Topics in Language Disorders, 5,* 1–20.

Nippold, M. A. (1991). Evaluating and enhancing idiom comprehension in language-disordered students. *Language, Speech, and Hearing Services in Schools, 22,* 100–106

Nippold, M. A. (1992). The nature of normal and disordered word finding in children and adolescents. *Topics in Language Disorders, 13,* 1–14.

Norris, J. A. (1991). From frog to prince: Using written language as a context for language learning. *Topics in Language Disorders, 12*(1), 66–81.

Norris, J. A. (1997). Functional language intervention in the classroom: Avoiding the tutoring trap. *Topics in Language Disorders, 17*(2), 49–68.

Norris, J. A., & Damico, J. S. (1990). Whole language in theory and practice: Implications for language intervention. *Language, Speech, and Hearing in Schools, 21,* 212–220.

Nydell, M. K. (1987). *Understanding Arabs: A guide for westerners.* Yarmount, ME: Intercultural Press.

Obiakor, F. E. (1992). Embracing new special education strategies for African American students. *Exceptional Children, 59,* 104–106.

O'Connor, R. E., Notari-Syverson, A., & Vadasy, P. F. (1996). Ladders to literacy: The effects of teacher-led phonological activities for kindergarten children with and without disabilities. *Exceptional Children, 63*(1), 117–130.

Olswang, L., & Bain, B. (1991). Intervention issues for toddlers with specific language impairments. *Topics in Language Disorders, 11,* 69–86.

Ortiz, A. A. (1997). Learning disabilities occurring concomitantly with linguistic differences. *Journal of Learning Disabilities, 30*(3), 321–332.

Ortiz, A. A., & Garcia, S. B. (1990). Using language assessment data for language and instructional planning for exceptional bilingual students. In A. Carasquillo & R. Baecher (Eds.), *Teaching the bilingual special education student* (pp. 24–47). Norwood, NJ: Ablex.

Owens, R. E. (1988). *Language development: An introduction* (2nd ed.). New York: Merrill.

Owens, R. E. (1992). *Language development: An introduction* (3rd ed.). New York: Merrill.

Owens, R. E. (1995). *Language disorders: A functional approach to assessment and intervention* (2nd ed.). Boston: Allyn & Bacon.

Owens, R. E. (1996). *Language development: An introduction* (4th ed.). Boston: Allyn & Bacon.

Owens, R. E., & Robinson, L. A. (1997). Once upon a time: Use of children's literature in the preschool classrom. *Topics in Language Disorders, 17*(2), 19–48.

Palincsar, A. S., & Brown, A. L. (1984). Reciprocal teaching of comprehension-fostering and comprehension-monitoring activities. *Cognition and Instruction, 1*(2), 117–175.

Parenté, R., & Herrman, D. (1996). Retraining memory strategies. *Topics in Language Disorders, 17*, 43–57.

Parker, F., & Riley, K. (1994). *Linguistics for non-linguists: A primer with exercises* (2nd ed.). Boston: Allyn and Bacon.

Patterson, F. (1978). Conversations with a gorilla. *National Geographic, 154*(4), 438–465.

Pelligrini, A. D. (1984). The effect of dramatic play on children's generation of discourse text. *Discourse Processes, 7*, 57–67.

Perner, J., & Leekam, S. (1986). Belief and quantity: Three-year olds' adaptation to listener's knowledge. *Journal of Child Language, 13*, 305–315.

Peters, A., & Zaidel, E. (1980). The acquisition of homonymy. *Cognition, 8*, 187–207.

Piaget, J. (1959). *The language and thought of the child*. London: Routledge & Kegan Paul.

Plunkett, K. (1993). Lexical segmentation and vocabulary growth in early language acquisition. *Journal of Child Language, 20*, 43–60.

Prather, E. (1984). Developmental language disorder: Adolescents. In A. Holland (Ed.), *Language disorders in children* (pp. 159–172). San Diego, CA: College-Hill Press.

Prizant, B., & Wetherby, A. (1990). Toward an integrated view of early language and communication development and socioemotional development. *Topics in Language Disorders, 10*, 1–16.

Prutting, C. (1982). Pragmatics as social competence. *Journal of Speech and Hearing Disorders, 47*, 123–134.

Prutting, C., & Kirchner, D. (1987). A clinical appraisal of the pragmatic aspects of language. *Journal of Speech and Hearing Disorders, 52*, 105–119.

Quine, W. V. (1960). *Word and object*. Cambridge, MA: Harvard University Press.

Read, C. (1971). Preschool children's knowledge of English phonology. *Harvard Educational Review, 41*, 1–34.

Read, C. (1975). *Children's categorization of speech sounds in English*. Research Rep. No. 17. Urbana, IL: National Council of Teachers of English.

Reed, V. (1986). *An introduction to children with language disorders*. New York: Macmillan.

Reed, V. (1994). *An introduction to children with language disorders* (2nd ed.). New York: Merrill.

Rees, N. S., & Gerber, S. (1992). Ethnography and communication: Social-role relations. *Topics in Language Disorders, 12*(3), 15–27.

Reich, P. A. (1986). *Language development*. Englewood Cliffs, NJ: Prentice-Hall.

Reznick, J., & Goldfield, V. (1992). Rapid change in lexical development in comprehension and production. *Developmental Psychology, 28*, 406–413.

Rice, M. L., & Hadley, P. A. (1991). Conversational responsiveness of speech and language impaired preschoolers. *Journal of Speech and Hearing Research, 34*, 1308–1317.

Rice, M. L., Sell, M. A., & Hadley, P. A. (1991). Social interactions of speech and language impaired preschoolers. *Journal of Speech and Hearing Research, 34*, 1299–1307.

Roddie, S. (1991). *Hatch egg hatch.* Boston: Little, Brown.

Rosch, E. (1973). On the internal structure of perceptual and semantic categories. In T. E. Moore (Ed.), *Cognitive development and the acquisition of language* (pp. 111–144). New York: Academic Press.

Rosch, E., & Mervis, C. (1975). Family resemblances: Studies in the internal structure of categories. *Cognitive Psychology, 7*, 573–603.

Rosen, M. J. (1989). *We're going on a bear hunt.* New York: Simon & Schuster Children's Books.

Rosen, M. J. (1993). *Little rabbit foo foo.* New York: Little Simon.

Roser, N., & Frith, M. (Eds.). (1988). *Children's choices: Teaching with books children like.* New York: G. P. Putnam's Sons.

Ross, G., Nelson, K., Wetstone, H., & Tanouye, E. (1986). Acquisition and generalization of novel object concepts by young language learners. *Journal of Child Language, 13*, 67–83.

Roth, F., (1986). Oral narrative abilities of learning-disabled students. *Topics in Language Disorders, 7*, 21–30.

Roth, F., & Spekman, N. (1984). Assessing the pragmatic abilities of children: Part 1. Organizational framework and assessment parameters. *Journal of Speech and Hearing Disorders, 49*, 2–11.

Roth, F., & Spekman, N. J. (1986). Narrative discourse: Spontaneously generated stories of learning disabled and normally achieving students. *Journal of Speech and Hearing Disorders, 51*, 8–23.

Roth, F. P., Spekman, N. J., & Fye, E. C. (1995). Reference cohesion in the oral narratives of students with learning disabilities and mormally achieving students. *Learning Disability Quarterly, 18*(1), 25–39.

Sagan, C., & Druyan, A. (1992, June 7). How much are we like chimps? *Parade Magazine*, 10–12.

Sander, E. (1972). When are speech sounds learned? *Journal of Speech and Hearing Disorders, 37*, 55–63.

Schiefelbusch, K. (1993). Communication in adults with mental retardation. *Topics in Language Disorders, 13*, 1–8.

Schlesinger, I. (1971). Production of utterances and language acquisition. In D. Slobin (Ed.), *The ontogenesis of grammar.* New York: Academic Press.

Schober-Peterson, D., & Johnson, C. (1989). Conversational topics of 4-year-olds. *Journal of Speech and Hearing Research, 32*, 857–870.

Schwartz, R. G., Leonard, L. B., Folger, M. K., & Wilcox, M. J. (1980). Early phonological behavior in normal-speaking and language disordered children: Evidence for a synergistic view of linguistic disorders. *Journal of Speech and Hearing Disorders, 45*, 357–377.

Scott, C. (1988). Producing complex sentences. *Topics in Language Disorders, 8*(2), 44–62.

Searle, J. R. (1965). What is a speech act? In M. Back (Ed.), *Philosophy in America.* New York: Allen & Unwin.

Searle, J. R. (1976). The classification of illocutionary acts. *Language in Society, 5*, 1–24.

Seymour, H., & Ralabate, P. (1985). The acquisition of a phonological feature of Black English. *Journal of Communication Disorders, 18*, 139–148.

Seymour, H. N., & Seymour, C. M. (1981). Black English and Standard American English contrasts in consonantal development of four- and five-year-old children. *Journal of Speech and Hearing Disorders, 46*(3), 274–280.

Shachar, H., & Sharan, S. (1994). Talking, relating, and achieving: Effects of cooperative learning and whole–class instruction. *Cognition and Instruction, 12*(4), 313–353.

Shafir, U., & Siegel, L. (1994). Preference for visual scanning strategies versus phonological rehearsal in university students with reading disabilities. *Journal of Learning Disabilities, 27*, 583–588.

Shames, G., & Wiig, E., (1986). *Human communication disorders*, (2nd ed.). Columbus, OH: Merrill.

Shatz, M. (1994). *A toddler's life: Becoming a person.* New York: Oxford University Press.

Shatz, M., & Gelman, R. (1973). The development of communication skills: Modifications in the speech of young children as a function of listener. *Monographs of the Society for Research in Child Development, 38*(5, Serial No. 152).

Shekar, C., & Hegde, M. N. (1996). Cultural and linguistic diversity among Asian Indians: A case of Indian English. *Topics in Language Disorders, 16*(4), 54–64.

Shorr, D. N., & Dale, P. S. (1981). Prepositional marking of source-goal structure and children's comprehension of English passives. *Journal of Speech and Hearing Research, 24*(2), 179–184.

Shuy, R. W. (1967). *Discovering American dialects.* Urbana, IL: National Council of Teachers of English.

Skinner, B. F. (1957). *Verbal behavior.* New York: Appleton-Century-Crofts.

Slobin, D. (1971a). Developmental psycholinguistics. In W. Dingwall (Ed.), *A survey of linguistic science*, Linguistics Program, University of Maryland. Reprinted in C. A. Ferguson & D. I. Slobin (Eds.). 1973. *Studies of child language development.* New York: Holt, Rinehart and Winston.

Slobin, D. (1971b). Grammatical development in Russian-speaking children. In B. A. Bar-Adon, & W. F. Leopold (Eds.), *Child language: A book of readings* (pp. 343–348). Englewood Cliffs, NJ: Prentice-Hall. (Original work published 1965)

Slobin, D., & Welsh, C. (1973). Elicited imitation as a research tool in developmental psycholinguistics. In C. Ferguson & D. Slobin (Eds.), *Studies in child language development* (pp. 485–497). New York: Holt, Rinehart & Winston.

Smiley, L. R. (1977). Knowledge of phonological generalizations, orthographic patterns and eidontic deviance of American English in spelling disabled third and fourth graders (Doctoral dissertation, Georgia State University, 1977). *Dissertation Abstracts International, 38*(11), 6655.

Smiley, L. R. (1991a). Informal language assessment, Part I. *Learning Disability Forum, 16*(4), 23–26.

Smiley, L.R. (1991b). Language assessment, Part II. *Learning Disability Forum, 17*(1), 17–21.

Snow, M. A. (1990). Instructional methodology in immersion foreign language education. In A. M. Padilla, H. H. Fairchild, & C. M. Valadez (Eds.), *Foreign language education: Issues and strategies* (pp. 156–171). Newbury Park, CA: Sage Publications.

Spekman, N., & Roth, F. (1982). An intervention framework for learning disabled students with communication disorders. *Learning Disabilities Quarterly, 5*, 429–437.

Stampe, D. (1972). *A dissertation on natural phonology.* Unpublished doctoral dissertation, University of Chicago.

Stewart, W. A. (1969). On the use of Negro dialect in the teaching of reading. In J. C. Baratz & R. W. Shuy (Eds.), *Teaching black children to read.* Washington, DC: Center for Applied Linguistics.

Strickland, D., & Cullinan, B. (1991). Afterword. In M. J. Adams (Ed.), *Beginning to read: Thinking and learning about print* (pp. 425–434). Cambridge, MA: MIT Press.

Strohner, H., & Nelson, K. E. (1974). The young child's development of sentence comprehension: Influence of event probability, nonverbal context, syntactic form, and strategies. *Child Development, 45,* 567–576.

Supple, M. D. (19960). Prologue: Beyond bilingualism. *Topics in Language Disorders, 16*(4), 1–8.

Temple, C. A., Nathan, R. G., & Burris, N. A. (1982). *The beginnings of writing.* Boston: Allyn & Bacon.

Thal, D., & Bates, E. (1990). Continuity and variation in early language development. In J. Colombo & J. Fagen (Eds.), *Individual differences in infancy: Reliability, stability, prediction* (pp. 359–385). Hillsdale, NJ: Lawrence Erlbaum.

Tharpe, R. G., & Gallimore, R. (1988). *Rousing minds to life.* Cambridge, UK: Cambridge University Press.

Torgesen, J. K., Wagner, R. K., & Rashotte, C. A. (1994). Longitudingal studies of phonological processing and reading. *Journal of Learning Disabilities, 27*(5), 276–286.

Townsend, M., & Clarihew, A. (1989). Facilitating children's comprehension through the use of advance organizers. *Journal of Reading Behavior, 21,* 15–36.

Trantham, C., & Pedersen, J. (1976). *Normal language development.* Baltimore: Williams & Wilkins.

Treiman, R. (1992). The role of intrasyllabic units in learning to read and spell. In P. Gough, L. Ehri, & R. Treiman (Eds.), *Reading acquisition.* Hillsdale, NJ: Lawrence Erlbaum.

Trousdale, A. (1990). Interactive storytelling: Scaffolding children's early narratives. *Language Arts, 67,* 164–173.

Turner, E. A., & Rommetveit, R. (1967). The acquisition of sentence voice and reversibility. *Child Development, 38,* 649–660.

Tyack, D., & Gottsleben, R. (1977). *Language sampling, analysis, and training: A handbook for teachers and clinicians.* Palo Alto, CA: Consulting Psychologists Press.

Valletutti, P., McKnight-Taylor, M., & Hoffnung, A. (1989). *Facilitating communication in young children with handicapping conditions: A guide for special educators.* Boston: College-Hill Press.

van Kleeck, A. (1995). Emphasizing form and meaning separately in rereading and early reading instruction. *Topics in Language Disorders, 16*(1), 27–49.

Vellutino, F. R. (1991). Introduction to three studies on reading acquisition: Convergent findings on theoretical foundations of code-oriented versus whole-language approaches to reading instruction. *Journal of Educational Psychology, 83,* 437–443.

Vygotsky, L. S. (1934/1986). *Thought and language* (A. Kozulin Trans.). Cambridge, MA: MIT Press.

Wagner, R., & Torgesen, J. (1987). The nature of phonological processing and its causal role in the acquisition of reading skills. *Psychological Bulletin, 101,* 192–212.

Wales, R., & Campbell, R. (1970). On the development of comparison and the comparison of development. In G. B. Flores d'Arcais & W. J. J. Levelt (Eds.), *Advances in psycholinguistics.* Amsterdam: Elsevier North-Holland.

Wallach, G. P., & Butler, K. G. (1994). *Language learning disabilities in school-age children and adolescents: Some principles and applications.* New York: Merrill/Macmillan.

Walker, A. (1982). *The color purple.* Boston: G. K. Hall.

Walker, J. M., McConnell, S., Holmes, D., Todis, B., Walker, J., & Golden, N. (1983). *The Walker social skills curriculum: The ACCEPTS program.* Austin, TX: Pro-Ed.

Wanska, S., & Bedrosian, J. (1985). Conversational structure and topic performance in mother-child interaction. *Journal of Speech and Hearing Research, 28,* 579–584.

Warden, D. (1976). The influence of context on children's use of identifying expressions and references. *British Journal of Psychology, 67,* 101–112.

Wardhaugh, R. (1977). *Introduction to linguistics* (2nd ed.). New York: McGraw-Hill.

Wardhaugh, R. (1995). *Understanding English grammar: A linguistic approach.* Cambridge, UK: Blackwell.

Watson, M., Martineau, D., & Hughes, D. (1993). A case of phonological development in language delayed twins not enrolled in therapy. *Journal of Childhood Communication Disorders, 15,* 16–24.

Weaver, C. (1988). *Reading process and practice: From socio-psycholinguistics to whole language.* Portsmouth, NH: Heinemann.

Webster, P. E., & Plante, A. S. (1992). Effects of phonological impairment on word, syllable, and phoneme segementation and reading. *Language, Speech, and Hearing Services in Schools, 23,* 176–182.

Weir, R. H. (1962). *Language in the crib.* The Hague: Mouton.

Wells, G. (1985). *Language development in the preschool years.* New York: Cambridge University Press.

Westby, C. E. (1995). Culture and literacy: Frameworks for understanding. *Topics in Language Disorders, 16*(1), 50–66.

Westby, C., & Cutler, S. (1994). Language and ADHD: Understanding the bases and treatment of self-regulatory deficits. *Topics in Language Disorders, 14,* 58–76.

Wiig, E., Freedman, E., & Secord, W. (1992). Developing words and concepts in the classroom: A holistic–thematic approach. *Intervention in School and Clinic, 27,* 278–285.

Wiig, E., & Semel, E. (1984). *Language assessment and intervention for the learning disabled* (2nd ed.). Columbus, OH: Merrill.

Wilcox, M. J., Kouri, T. A., & Caswell, S. B. (1991). Early language intervention: A comparison of classroom and individual treatment. *American Journal of Speech-Language Pathology: A Journal of Clinical Practice, 1,* 49–62.

Williams, R. L. (1972). *The BITCH Test (Black Intelligence Test of Cultural Homogeneity).* St. Louis, MO: Robert Williams, Black Studies Program, Washington Universtiy.

Willig, A. C., Swedo, J. J., & Ortiz, A. A. (1987). *Characteristics of teaching strategies which result in high task engagement for exceptional limited English proficient Hispanic students.* Austin: The University of Texas, Handicapped Minority Research Institute on Language Proficiency.

Wilson, C. R., & Ferriss, W. (Eds.). (1989). *Encyclopedia of southern culture* (Vol. 1). New York: Anchor Books/Doubleday.

Wilson, K., Blackmon, R., Hall, R., & Elcholtz, G. (1991). Methods of language assessment: A survey of California public school clinicians. *Language, Speech, and Hearing Services in Schools, 22,* 236–241.

Wilson, M. (1996). Arabic speakers: Language and culture, here and abroad. *Topics in Language Disorders, 16*(4), 65–80).

Windsor, J. (1995). Language impairment and social competence. In M. Fey, J. Windsor, & S. Warren (Eds.). *Language intervention: Preschool through the elementary years.* Baltimore: Paul H. Brookes.

Wing, C., & Scholnick, E. (1981). Children's comprehension of pragmatic concepts expressed in "because," "although," "if," and "unless." *Journal of Child Language, 8,* 347–365.

Yonovitz, L., & Andrew, K. (1995). A play and story telling probe for assessing early language content. *Journal of Childhood Communication Disorders, 16,* 10–18.

Yopp, H. K. (1988). The validity and reliability of phonemic awareness tests. *Reading Research Quarterly, 23,* 159–177.

Yopp, H. K. (1992). Developing phonemic awareness in young children. *The Reading Teacher, 45,* 696–703.

Zoller, M. B. (1991). Use of music activities in speech–language therapy. *Language, Speech, and Hearing Services in Schools, 22,* 272–276.

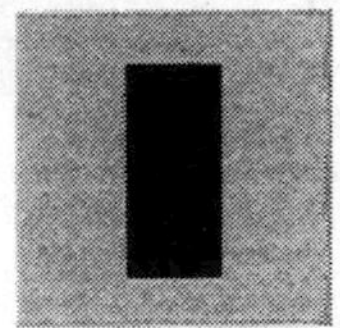

INDEX

C

D

E

F

G

H

I

J

K

L

R